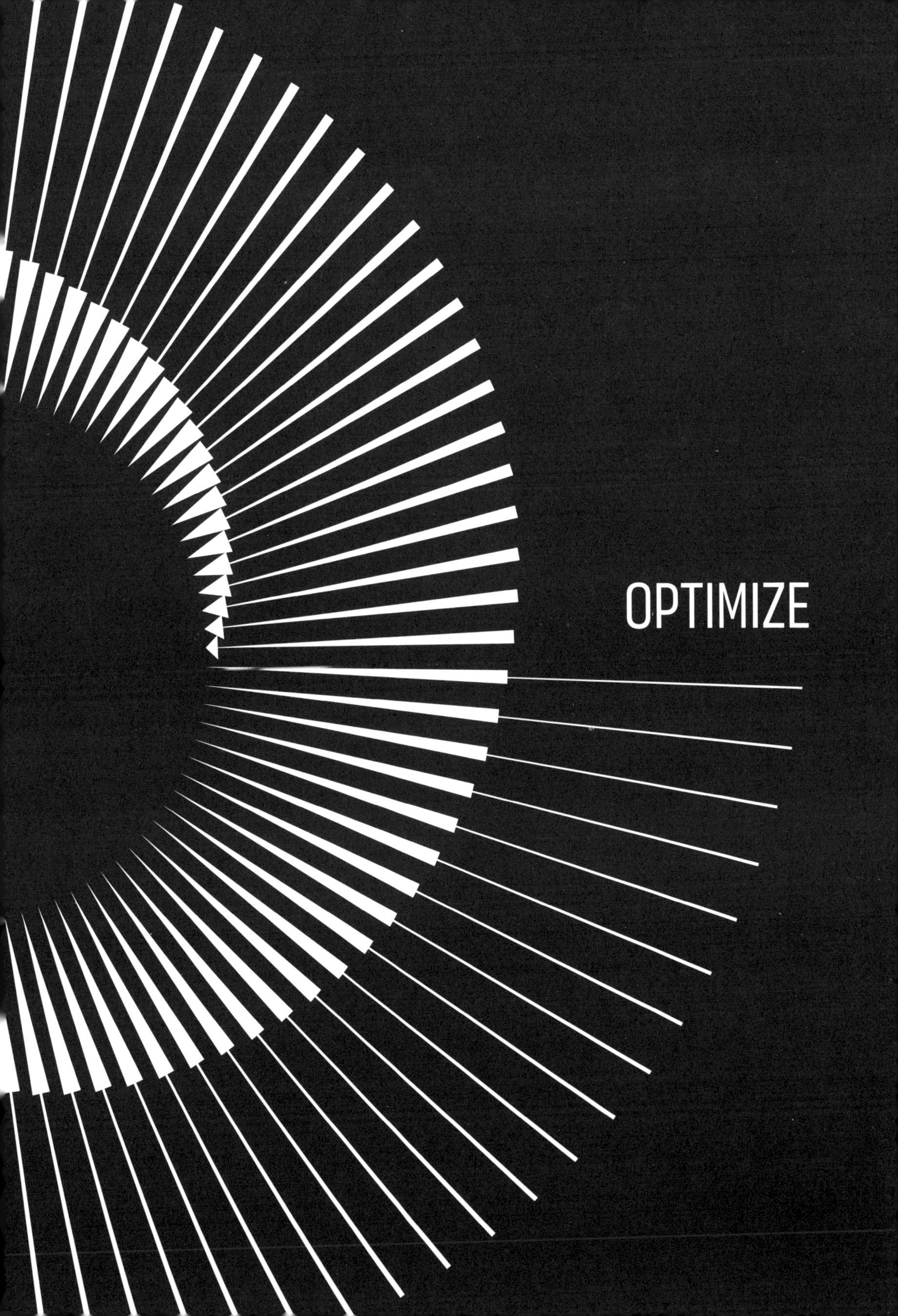
OPTIMIZE

Quarto.com

First Published in 2026 by Fair Winds Press,
an imprint of The Quarto Group,
100 Cummings Center, Suite 265-D, Beverly, MA 01915, USA.
T (978) 282-9590 F (978) 283-2742

EEA Representation, WTS Tax d.o.o.,
Žanova ulica 3, 4000 Kranj, Slovenia.
www.wts-tax.si

30 29 28 27 26 2 3 4 5

ISBN: 978-0-7603-9856-2

Digital edition published in 2026
eISBN: 978-0-7603-9857-9

Library of Congress Control Number: 2025943644

Design: Cindy Samargia Laun
Illustration: Justin Tran

Printed in Illinois, USA VP012026

The information in this book is for educational purposes only. It is not intended to replace the advice of a physician or medical practitioner. Please see your health-care provider before beginning any new health program.

OPTIMIZE

A Groundbreaking 7-Step Plan to Health and Longevity Through Quantum Biology

Dr. Catherine Clinton

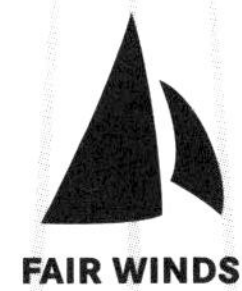

FAIR WINDS

*To my family:
my children, Kalea,
Kaemon, and Madison;
my husband, Drake;
and my mother and
father, all of whom
have spent countless
hours listening to me
talk about the contents
of this book for years.
Thank you for your
love and support.*

CONTENTS

INTRODUCTION

My name is Catherine Clinton. I'm a licensed naturopathic physician in Oregon. I teach people about and treat patients with the pillars of quantum biology for health: water, light, electricity, magnetism, coherence, resonance, and sound. Tending to these pillars changed my life and the lives of my patients. This book is a culmination of what I have learned, condensed into seven steps we can take to support health in a completely new way.

Until now, how the body works and how it stays healthy have been explained by a chemical-mechanical model. Action in the body and health comes from chemical activity, or direct physical contact, that causes mechanical change to the body's structure. Quantum biology speaks a language of *frequency* in the body. Each cell and every organ has its own unique vibration. These vibrations can orchestrate communication, energy transfer, and biological function in the body at a speed and efficiency unheard of in the current chemical-mechanical model. Applying the pillars of quantum biology to our daily lives can improve health and longevity in ways not currently addressed in conventional medicine.

When I was in my second year of naturopathic medical school—that initiation year when students are weeded out—I was diagnosed with two autoimmune diseases and Lyme disease. It was long hours of classes, boards exams in anatomy and physiology, cadaver lab, and stress after stress that kept piling on. My nervous system couldn't handle it.

The physician I was doing clinical rotations under, Dr. Satya Ambrose, was also my physician. She encouraged me to look at psychoneuroimmunology, or, in simpler terms, how our thoughts and emotions affect our health. At the same time, I was researching how mitochondria affect health and longevity, and I stumbled upon early research about quantum biology. My views of how the body works and what brings health began to shift. It was this very shift that brought me true healing and remission from my diagnoses.

Although I had spent years learning about how diet, lifestyle, vitamins, and supplements affected our health, this education provided a wealth of information about healing and disease, but it didn't provide a complete picture. When I began to learn how the thoughts and perceptions we hold create an environment all their own that directly affects our biology and health, a bigger picture of health started to emerge. Through a multitude of pathways, our thoughts exert a governing influence over our health. Our perceptions trigger the release of hormones, cytokines, neurotransmitters, pressure waves, and electromagnetic pulses that guide, educate, and inform our bodily processes. We are what we think we are.

The idea that our thoughts and emotions had predictable influences on our health blew me away. It opened a window into another level of healing, for my patients and myself. But this was only the beginning of an expanded understanding of health. I began researching how the body's cells are powered and how they communicate. I delved into the science behind how the microbiotic ecosystem in our microbiome fits into our greater ecosystem. This was very different from what I had learned in anatomy and physiology classes.

Our mitochondria, the little powerhouses of almost all our cells, can be fueled by the sun. Our body can repair when in contact with Earth. Our blood chemistry balances after a couple of days in the forest. And that's just the start. There is an invisible order that instructs, informs, and guides life as we know it. Health isn't just the product of a chemical reaction or a mechanical interaction. It is triggered by a sea of quantum biological action. The smallest pieces of our biology driven by electricity, sound, light, electromagnetic fields, water, vibration, and coherence can have the biggest impact on our ability to live a long and healthy life.

Our body communicates with the unseen forces of light, sound, electricity, magnetism, the biofield, electromagnetic fields, and more. These vibrations hold information that guides our immune system, hormonal balance, inflammatory pathways, metabolism, and more. We can do everything we know of to support our health, but if it's not in line with the unseen forces of life, we are missing a big piece of health. There is something deeper at play. The perfect diet, supplements, or exercise routines won't be as successful if you aren't being held by this world. At a quantum level, there are energies at play conducting life and, if ignored, our health suffers.

I wrote this book to share what I've learned about quantum biology and health, organized around seven steps that support health from a quantum biological perspective.

Step 1:
Tend to the water within us because it acts as the background for quantum biological action in the body.

Step 2:
As an extension of step 1, the second step is to support the liquid crystal structures in the body, such as DNA, microtubules, cell membranes, and fascia (connective tissue), that are sensitive to the forces of quantum biology. These liquid crystalline structures, along with the water that lines them, constitute a network that can communicate, transfer energy, and create biological action without depending on the chemical-mechanical model of life.

Step 3:
Tend to the electrical body.

Step 4:
Focus on aligning with the light in our environment and nourishing the light within us.

Step 5:
The next step supports the ability to sync with the natural forces around us, like the Earth, seasons, and the sights and sounds of nature.

Step 6:
Cultivate coherence within ourselves, our relationships, our communities, and with sound for better health and longevity.

Step 7:
This final step is about nourishing our immune system and the microbiotic community that lives intertwined with us.

Understanding and tending to these seven valuable aspects of our biology has the power to improve our health to a new level of vitality and longevity.

Quantum biology is a relatively new field. But the science continues to pour in and validate the idea that applying what is being discovered in quantum biology to health can be beneficial. There are Nobel Prize laureates who have been researching this field for decades, and the implications are becoming increasingly clear. Adhering to the old model excludes us from all the advantages that quantum biology can offer our immune system, metabolic balance, hormonal health, organ-specific function, mental and emotional health, and overall vitality.

The application of quantum biology in health holds an exciting future, but we don't have to wait to reap the benefits. There are ways to take advantage of what science is showing today. We can utilize light, sound, water, and the energy held in fields of frequency to optimize health and longevity. This book will teach and inform you about seven critical steps to do just that.

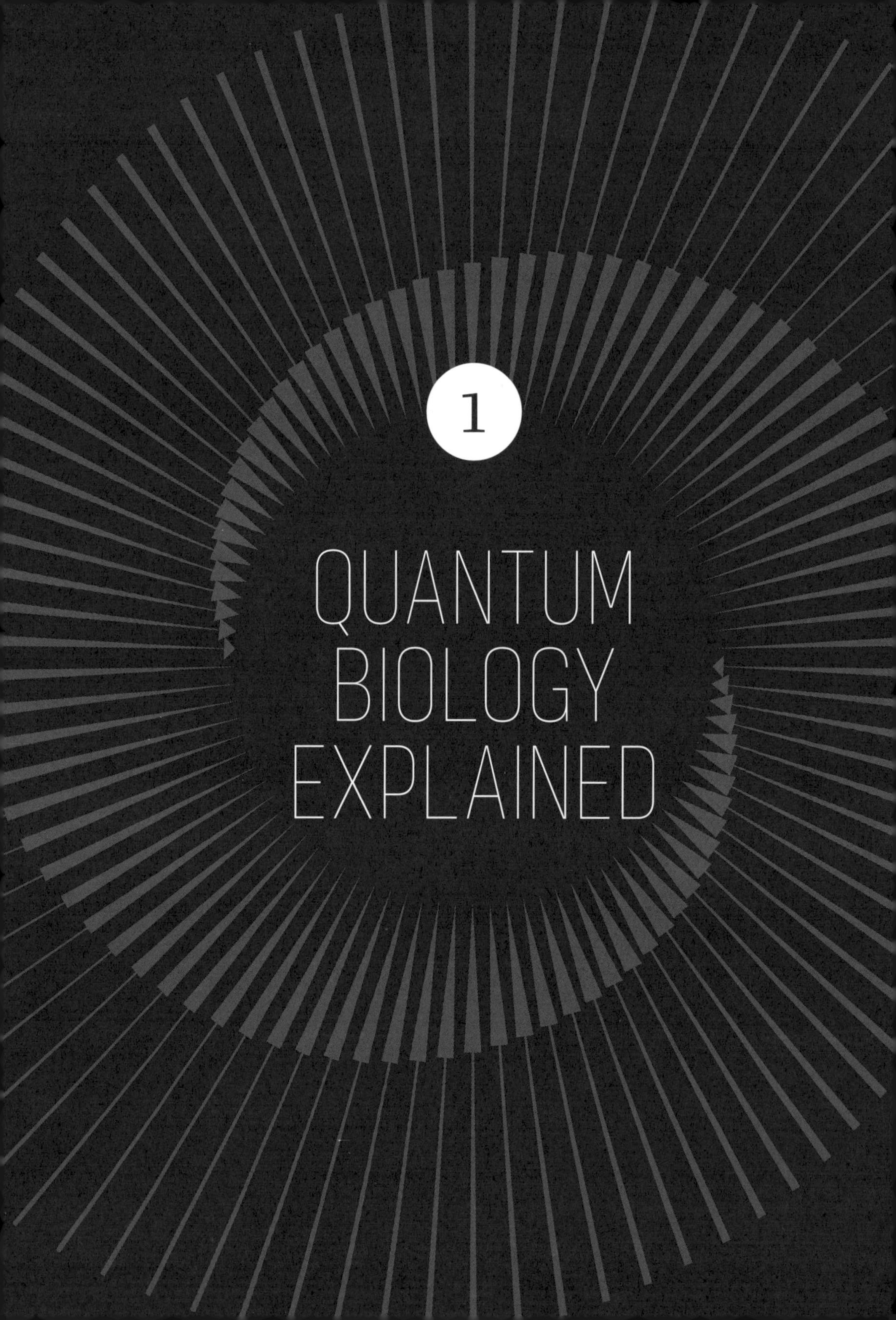
1
QUANTUM
BIOLOGY
EXPLAINED

Quantum biology offers a new perspective on health. It explores how the actions of quantum particles like electrons, protons, and photons influence the smallest parts of our biology. Our current health care model only explains so much. We must expand our knowledge and tool sets for healing. That is what quantum biology offers. By understanding a different perspective on the body, we increase not only our understanding of how the body works, but also our ability to heal and maintain health.

A quantum biological perspective of the body focuses on the body's energetic qualities, such as its electrical charge, its ability to entrain with the world around it, its propensity to build coherence, its electromagnetic field, and its more subtle biofield. Quantum biology opens a window to a whole new outlook on health, disease, and life in general. The impacts of light, sound, frequencies, and water offer a way to improve the immune system, metabolic pathways, hormonal health, mental emotional balance, and overall wellness.

It's time to redefine what it means to be healthy. Life expectancy is longer now. We are in the midst of an epidemic of chronic disease. Expanding our perceptions of health and disease has never been so important. Quantum biology is that expansion.

Life is beginning to shift. There is a momentum growing. Our understanding of biology, our expectations about health, our priorities in life are changing. We expect more now. The same old ways, the same old answers from science regarding health, no longer satisfy. We know there is more out there, and the rate at which we acquire new information is unprecedented. We're standing on the precipice of a new era, positioned between the current template and a catalyst into a new paradigm. The current template has brought us this far, but there's more to health and wellness. Applying quantum biology to health offers us that new paradigm.

A NEWTONIAN MODEL

Medicine across the globe has been focused on the Newtonian model of chemical and mechanical reactions. A Newtonian model of health sees the body as a machine, a compilation of gears. It reduces life down and separates the body into unconnected boxes, like breaking down a machine into its individual gears. Instead, quantum biology shows that it is the infinitesimally small pieces of our biology that can give rise to the interconnected picture of health. It shows how electrons, protons, photons of light, and vibrations from sound create a sea of action that creates what we observe with our eyes. There is an invisible order that guides life as we know it.

Our current understanding of biology relies on a model of the universe that is ruled by randomness, a model that puts random mutation and indiscriminate chance as the drivers of life. In the dominant paradigm, biology is ruled by arbitrary actions out of our control. In the current model, we have biological keys floating around the body looking for their biological receptor lock. These keys rely on random collision to bounce them around the body to find their receptor match in order to unlock the receptor and create biological action. That action can be an enzymatic function, a change in protein structure, or a biological cascade that creates activity in the body.

Each cell in the body completes more than 100,000 tasks each second, and we have trillions and trillions of cells in our body. This statistic is well accepted—it's not fringe science. Some scientists even estimate the tasks completed in a cell each second are in the millions. This is mathematically impossible within the current model. These reactions occur at nearly 100 percent efficiency. The speed and precision needed for this are impossible with randomness.

When we consider how densely crowded and tightly packed our cells are, the idea of random collision becomes even more problematic and unlikely. Quantum biology can help explain how these reactions can happen so quickly and so efficiently.

QUANTUM BIOLOGY: THE BASICS

Quantum biology is the study of quantum phenomena in living systems. It looks at the smallest pieces of the physical universe—the electron, the proton, and the photon—and how they affect our biology. Quantum phenomena, such as tunneling, entanglement, and coherence (which I cover later in the chapter), can account for this speed and efficiency in a purposeful way without writing it off as chance. Quantum biology offers an elegant understanding that takes us away from the randomness of biology and points to an invisible order that guides life. What a beautiful step for science to take.

Everything in our universe vibrates. Every living and nonliving thing has its own unique vibration, or frequency, that holds information and energy. What we talk about in this book—light, water, sound, electricity, magnetism, and energy in general—can be thought of as different energy fields vibrating at various frequencies, whether it's sound or an electromagnetic field. These unseen waves of light, sound, and energy have the power to guide life.

Quantum biology doesn't negate our current model of the universe. It adds another layer of explanation to how things function that extends the key and lock model. It's not that the key and lock receptor doesn't exist; it does. It just might not be driven solely by random collision.

There is an unseen order in the world that guides life on this planet. This order comes down to the flow of electrons, protons, photons, and even phonons of sound. It comes down to the effect that light, sound, magnetism, and electricity have on our biology. We are electric beings. We are sound beings. We are light beings. We are water beings tuned to the frequency of our environment. The frequency of our external terrain, the electromagnetic fields, the sound, the vibration, the light, as well as the frequency of our internal terrain, direct life. Quantum biology sets out to illuminate this invisible information and its role in biological function.

QUANTUM BIOLOGY: THE POSSIBILITIES

Understanding quantum biology ushers in a world of interconnection. When examining things at the scale of the photon, we see a universal flow of energy that enters our atmosphere and travels through every plant, animal, and human on this planet. Our health and vitality depend on our ability to participate in this flow of energy. And our body has a unique flow of energy of its own. There is a perspective of the body where pain, inflammation, and disease are associated with a decrease in electrical charge or electrons.

We don't end at the barriers of our skin. We are intimately and inseparably connected within ourselves, to each other, and to the world around us. Life is not just a series of random reactions. Life is guided by unseen information. This invisible order interconnects all life in a meaningful way. Ancient Indigenous cultures described our true place in this world as being part of a universal connection, bringing importance and necessity to all forms of life. This new science brings us back full circle to the ancestral idea of tending to the energetic flow in the body to increase vitality and treat disease.

Quantum Biology: Some Important Terms

Let's define some terms that are used frequently in the book to ensure you gain the most from the information here.

- **Quantum biology:** For purposes of this book, quantum biology refers to how the smallest building blocks of life—an electron, a proton, a photon, a vibration of sound, an exciton (an excited electron and its paired hole)—affect life. This includes circadian biology, light therapies, mitochondria science, electromagnetic influences on the body, sound therapies, psychoneuroimmunology, water research, the effects of nature, bioelectrics, and biofield therapies.
- **Frequency:** Frequency equals vibration. That vibration can be a wave of light or the vibration of an electromagnetic field. Vibrations can hold information and energy.
- **Frequency information** refers to information or energy held in vibratory wave form.
- **Coherence:** Coherence is when two or more things stay in sync with each other. Quantum particles can act like waves. When these waves are in harmony with each other, they can transfer energy and information between and among each other. Coherence brings shared information, harmony, intelligence, and efficiency. Consider a boat filled with rowers. If each rows at different times, the boat goes nowhere; it's incoherent. But if they all row in sync, the boat can smoothly navigate through the water—that's coherence.
- **Resonance:** Resonance occurs when something is exposed to its innate frequency and starts to vibrate at a stronger rate, like in a piano store. When you strike the middle C key on one piano, all the C keys in the other pianos throughout the store will also start to sing.
- **Resonant frequency:** Everything has a natural frequency, or resonance. In biology, when molecules and cells are exposed to light, sound, and electromagnetic fields at the right frequencies, they can begin to vibrate more, react faster, or even change shape. Some researchers propose this is how proteins find each other, how sound healing works, and how cellular communication happens at a distance.
- **Quantum phenomena:** When looking at how quantum particles influence action in the body, oftentimes, quantum phenomena such as tunneling, coherence, and entanglement are involved. This allows for a mode of communication and energy that is much faster than the current chemical-mechanical model.

I am not a quantum biologist. I am a naturopathic doctor searching for a new perspective on health because I've seen the limitations of our current approach. Some may vehemently disagree with my definition of quantum biology. Others may contend that living systems are too warm, wet, or chaotic for quantum phenomena. While others might say these phenomena are trivial and have no true impact on our biological function. Some want to keep quantum biology confined to the laboratory and to computer science, uncomfortable with any extrapolation to living systems. Others might argue that quantum biology is still in its infancy and no conclusions can be made.

Quantum biology is in its infancy; we're just beginning to unravel the mysteries it can explain. But there is also a wealth of information about how life works at the quantum scale, and we should be utilizing it in medicine. We understand the impact of light on the body, and that it touches every system in our biology. We understand the enormous effect sound has on our biology, and it's staggering. We know that the workings of our mitochondria and the flow of electrons, protons, and photons of light touch almost every modern disease as well as our capacity to navigate physical and emotional trauma. And there's more. That's what this book is about.

Although we are far from a scientific consensus, quantum biology, as defined for the purposes of this book, refers to quantum phenomena, such as quantum tunneling, entanglement, superposition, and coherence, at play in living systems. Quantum biology explores biology on the nanoscale—the workings of our mitochondria, our DNA, our proteins, and our fascia. It explores the impact of a photon of light or a frequency of sound or an electromagnetic field on the living systems of plants, animals, and our body. It endeavors to uncover the hidden order of life that structures biology. It goes beyond the chemical model of biology and unveils an expanded perspective of undeniable connection.

Quantum biology illuminates a world of interconnection that offers us better health and increased longevity: an interrelationship of all life on this Earth, with each organism possessing an individual contribution to the function of the whole; a world where the universal flow of electrons and protons travels from one living system to another, in a current that touches every living thing on our planet; and a worldwide tapestry of energy that links all beings in our ecosystem and begins to blur where one individual ends and another begins.

Quantum biology includes circadian medicine, light therapies, sound modalities, mitochondrial health, heart coherence, biofield medicine, and the role of maintaining our negative electrical charge. It does not negate the findings of classical physics or biology;

it simply adds another layer of understanding. When we learn to follow the clues that quantum biology offers—the influence of light, water, electricity, sound, and frequency—our understanding of health changes completely. With that new understanding comes an expanded toolbox with which we can improve our vitality and longevity.

QUANTUM PHYSICS EXPLORED

To understand quantum biology, we should have a familiarity with quantum physics. We don't need to be experts, but a basic appreciation will help with the application of quantum biology to health.

Classical physics explains how the matter we see with our eyes behaves, whereas quantum physics explores how the smallest pieces of nature, those we can't see with the naked eye, interact and affect their environment. At some level, we are all dancing in a sea of quantum music. Quantum physics is, arguably, the most successful scientific theory to date in its ability to explain the world around us. Quantum physics is an ever-expanding field, and this chapter aims at a basic understanding so we can more easily apply quantum biology to health. I'll keep it simple.

The study of quantum physics started in 1900 with Max Planck. Planck noticed that radiation emitting from a blackbody came in discrete packets of energy. Five years later, in 1905, Albert Einstein validated Planck's idea of quantized, or individual, packets of energy with his discussion of quantized light, or photons. This was revolutionary. Light was understood as a wave of energy, and this turned that idea on its head. These discoveries implied that light was not only a wave of energy, but it was also matter, something completely unheard of. Discovering that energy existed in packets as well as a continuous flow laid the foundation for quantum mechanics.

Einstein went on to test this idea with the photoelectric effect. He found that if the light was intense enough, it could knock an electron from the metal it was shining on. Almost like a strong wind knocking a leaf off a tree, these photons of light could dislodge matter in the form of electrons. Einstein's work with photons and the photoelectric effect earned him a Nobel Prize in Physics in 1921 and changed the way we understand subatomic reality.

The photoelectric effect becomes important to our understanding of how the body can create energy with exposure to the right spectrum of light. As you'll see, there is a way to look at health as an abundance of electrons, and disease, pain, or inflammation as a deficiency of electrons. Utilizing a similar photoelectric effect in the body, where

(continued on page 20)

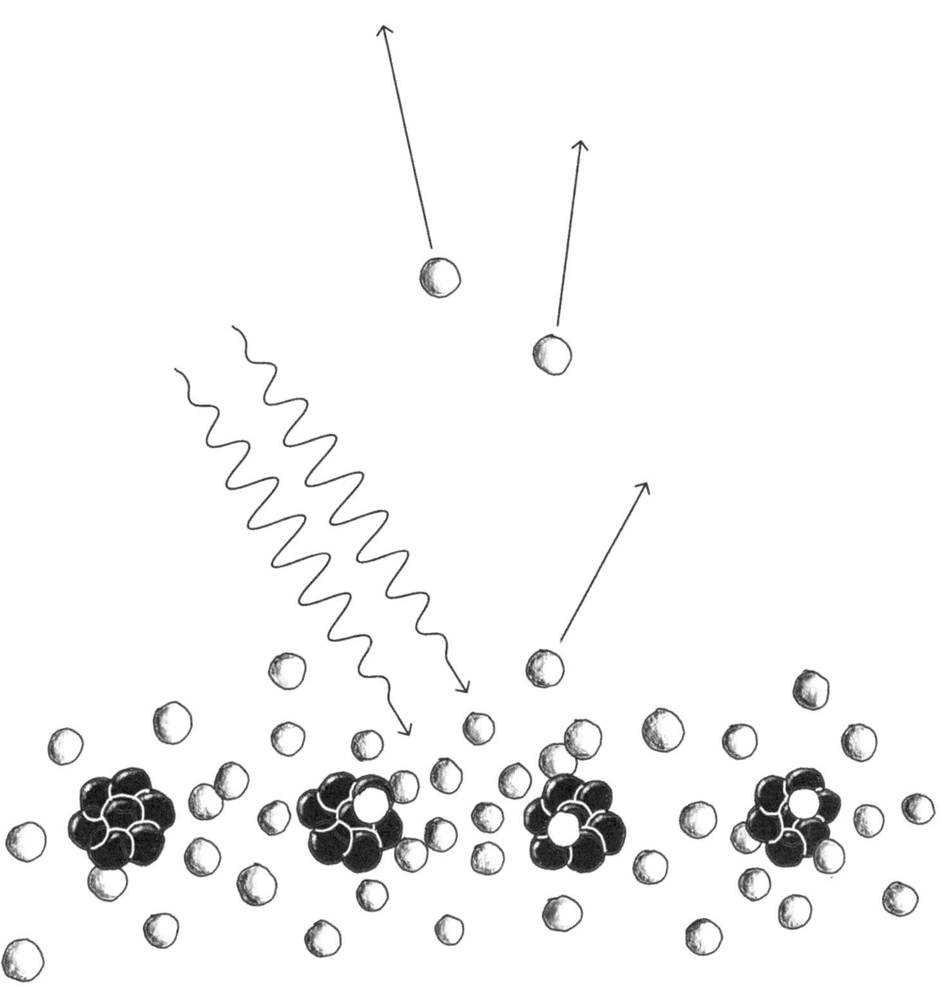

PHOTOEMISSION OF ELECTRONS FROM A METAL PLATE
ACCOMPANIED BY THE ABSORPTION OF LIGHT QUANTA-PHOTONS

The photoelectric effect describes how light of a certain intensity can knock electrons off the metal it hits, dislodging matter by certain light frequencies.

Double-Slit Experiment

Thomas Young's classic 1801 double-slit experiment had already shown that light behaved like a wave. The original experiment was set up with a beam of light directed at a solid metal sheet, which had two small parallel slits in it. Behind the double-slit metal sheet was a background wall to catch the light. The light traveled through the two slits like a wave, making an inference pattern of multiple bands as it hit the back wall. The pattern resembled the ripples that a pebble makes when tossed into a pond, demonstrating light's wave-like nature.

The double-slit experiment was repeated in 1927 by Clinton Davisson and Lester Germer after the acknowledgment that there was more to light than previously thought. This time, they used single photons rather than a whole beam of light. Unlike the previous double-slit experiment, which observed light as a wave of energy, Davisson and Germer found that photons acted like both waves and particles. The photons traveled through the two slits as a wave, yet when they hit the background wall, they collapsed into a particle. To discover that elements in our world could be both a wave of energy and a particle of matter was astonishing. This laid the foundation for the dual property of nature in quantum physics, where objects are both matter and energy, both a particle and a wave. This duality is what allows for the quantum phenomena that seem so strange in classical physics yet rule action on the quantum level.

Things got even stranger in future experiments when detectors, simple counting machines, were added to the slits to see which slit the photon traveled through it. Scientists found that the unobserved electron traveled as a wave, yet if observed by the detector, the electron would collapse into a particle. Not only were photons of light both particles of matter and waves of energy, but they also interacted with the world around them precisely enough to know when an observer was present. There was nothing in classical physics to account for this. This was more evidence that something beyond our everyday perception could be driving life.

WAVE PARTICLE WEIRDNESS

OBSERVING SCREEN OVER TIME

When quantum objects such as electrons are fired one by one through a pair of closely spaced slits, they behave like particles: Each one hits a screen paced on the far side at exactly on point. But they also behave like waves: Successive hits build up a banded interference pattern exactly like that generated by a wave passing through the slits (bottom). This wave-particle duality is described by a mathematical tool known as the wavefunction.

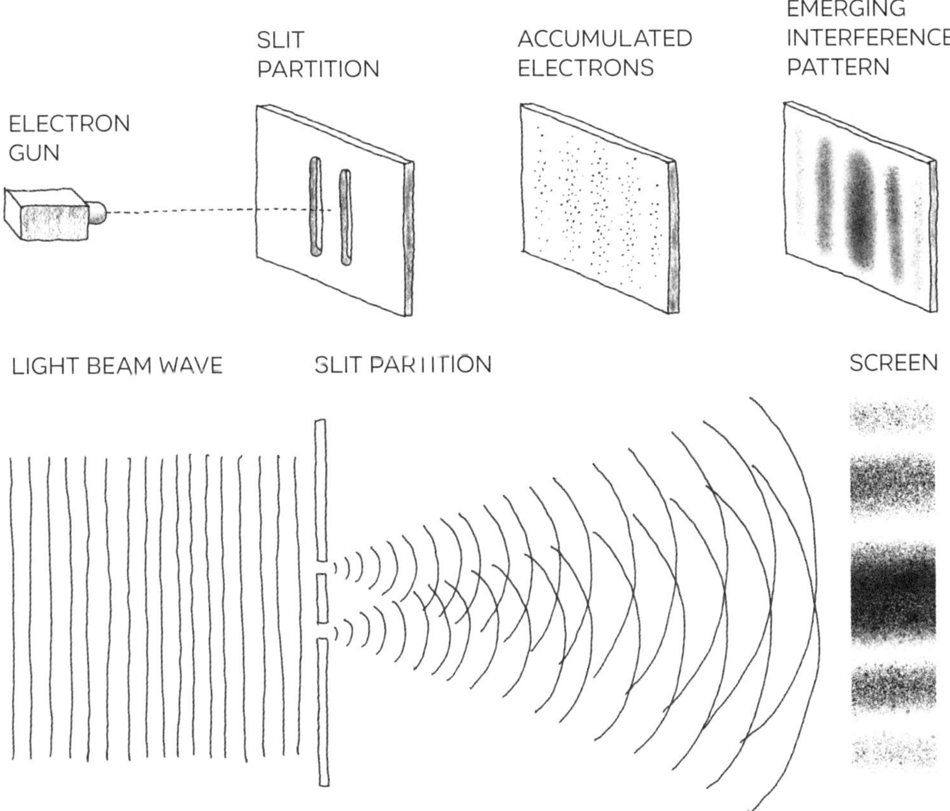

The double-slit experiment: When photons of light are directed through two narrow slits, they act like particles when they hit the background screen; they also act like waves of energy by creating interference waves exactly like a wave passing through two narrow slits would create.

light can excite electrons that can quench inflammation or stimulate action, can have numerous benefits—from our metabolism, mental emotional health, immune function, and hormonal balance to overall vitality.

WAVE-PARTICLE DUALITY

It was at that same time that Erwin Schrödinger introduced his wave function, known as the Schrödinger wave equation. Schrödinger's equation solidified the concept of the wave-particle duality of energy. The wave function proposes that a particle exists as a wave or cloud of possible locations as explained by probability percentages. Once observed or measured, the quantum particle's possibilities or wave function collapses into a particle, illuminating that wave-particle duality. Schrödinger's wave function is a mathematical attempt to describe the dichotomy that gives quantum physics its underpinning. This is pivotal because the dual nature of a wave of energy and a particle of matter in subatomic reality is the foundation of quantum phenomena. These phenomena help explain some of the quantum biological interactions we see with water, light, biofield therapies such as Reiki, and heart coherence exercises and how they benefit human health. They also hint at the notion that what we think of as discrete and separate objects, such as electrons, are really waves of energy possibly linked to a vast field of energy.

The wave-particle duality illuminates a world of unseen action. David Bohm referred to this hidden order as the "implicate order." Bohm talked about a veiled implicate order that gives birth to the explicate order we see in matter. He described an unseen implicate order of interconnectedness that gives rise to the explicate order we see as individual objects. This implicate order connects everything that was, that is, and that will be in the universe in a meaningful wholeness. The matter we see in everyday life springs from the deeper all-encompassing implicate order we cannot see.

This duality permits quantum effects like *quantum superposition*: the ability of quantum particles, such as an electron or group of protons, to be in multiple locations at one time. This concept of superposition extends to paths traveled as well. Because of the wave-particle duality, a particle doesn't have to travel only one path; it can travel multiple pathways at the same time.

The wave-particle duality also allows for *quantum tunneling*, which refers to the ability of a particle to cross unsurmountable barriers in energy, whether from repulsive forces or forces of a magnetic field or distance that cannot be crossed. In classical physics, a ball in a valley between hills needs to be kicked with enough energy to go up and over the hill, while quantum tunneling explains that the particle's wave function of possibility allows it a chance to appear on the other side of the hill without going over the hill. But we're not talking about hills and balls. We're talking about very small quantum particles and obstacles of temperature or distance. The particle can go straight through the obstacle because of its dual nature. The function of our essential enzymes and mitochondria depend on quantum tunneling. Quantum tunneling explains how electrons can travel through the electron transport chain within the mitochondria to generate the body' s vital energy currency, adenosine triphosphate (ATP). Without this, we wouldn't be alive, and if we can support tunneling in the mitochondria, we can improve our overall health and vitality.

The wave-particle duality also permits the strange phenomena of *quantum entanglement*, when two or more particles are inextricably linked, even at long distances apart. We can know exactly what is happening with one particle if we know what is happening to the other particle because of their inseparable nature. Quantum entanglement occurs when particles are generated together, have interacted together, or share space together. It usually refers to the relationship of the spin of the particle, like the example of a pair of shoes that you take on vacation: Upon arriving at your destination, you open your suitcase to find only the right shoe, knowing almost instantly that the left shoe remains at home where you left it. This becomes important in the nanosized signaling within living systems, including our body.

Schrödinger was one of the first to propose quantum mechanics could apply to our biology. His book *What Is Life?* posited quantum mechanics as a driving force in life. Schrödinger and Jordan Pascual both described the phenomenon of order from disorder. Small changes in oscillations or vibrations within the atom, electron, or photon can cause order on a larger sense. Pieces of the whole act independently yet work together as a cohesive collective. Like a wave in the ocean with individual water molecules participating in the collective action of the wave, coherence is an important piece of quantum biology. *Quantum coherence* explains how a quantum system creates an environment where quantum action can occur. Without quantum coherence there is no quantum action in a system.

WHAT IS QUANTUM BIOLOGY?

Long seen as a trivial piece in biology, critics argued that quantum biological effects are too small to have biological importance. Yet small units of organized action can have a much larger effect on the organism than their size warrants. Small, organized action in the form of DNA, microscopic enzymes, mitochondria, membrane-bound proteins, reactive oxygen species, and the like have an enormous effect on our overall health and function; they literally dictate life, death, and everything in between. These quantum particles drive the much bigger classical physics we see in the material world around us. The idea that actions at a quantum level cannot affect the larger system or organism holds less weight the closer we look. Sometimes, focusing on the smallest parts of our biology can have the biggest influence.

In the last fifty years, researchers have found mounting evidence of quantum mechanics at play in living systems. In 1966, Don DeVault and Britton Chance were studying electron transfer in the light-harvesting centers in photosynthetic purple bacteria and observed results that could not be explained by classical physics. In photosynthesis, a photon of light is captured by a chloroplast and transferred into the thylakoid stacks of chlorophyll as it works its way to the photosynthetic reaction center. If the photon does not get to the photosynthetic center, then photosynthesis does not take place.

DeVault and Chance were the first to show that electron transfer could successfully utilize quantum tunneling, constructing the framework for the concept of quantum electron tunnelling in biology. Of course, the idea of quantum effects in living systems was not readily adopted by the larger physics community. Historically, quantum physics experiments were set up to avoid heat and vibrations from noise that can destroy the delicate balance needed for quantum phenomena to occur in a laboratory setting. It was hard to believe that quantum phenomena could happen in a chaotic living system.

One main argument against quantum biology is that it cannot happen in the warm, wet, noisy world of living systems. When quantum mechanics are studied in a lab, scientists cool experiments to near absolute zero, where no life can exist. Scientists also shield the experiment from any external noise and vibration. Even the slightest disturbance or oscillation can destroy the complex balance of quantum coherence needed for quantum phenomena in the lab. From this viewpoint, the idea of quantum mechanics in the chaos of a living system seems impossible.

Each quantum phenomenon discussed, such as tunneling, entanglement, and superposition, depends on the delicate balance of quantum coherence. When particles are observed, they appear in one particular state, like the classical properties we see in the everyday world. For particles to exist in a quantum state in a laboratory setting, they need to be isolated from the environment for scientists to observe any quantum reactions. As soon as this system interacts with outside noise, it becomes "decoherent," collapsing the quantum phenomena into classical behavior. The more particles or objects involved, the faster the decoherence occurs, and the quantum state collapses because of the increased interference or noise from the external environment. There seemed to be no way to observe quantum phenomena in the chaotic world of living systems.

So how can quantum coherence exist in our noisy, hectic body? This question has puzzled scientists and fueled quantum biology critics for decades. While DeVault and Chance were exploring the quantum tunneling of quantum particles, Herbert Fröhlich was looking into the concept of quantum coherence in living systems. Fröhlich explained that living organisms are made up of dipolar molecules, molecules with a positive and a negative end, so closely packed together that they could epitomize a solid-state system that is constantly dancing in interacting forces—electromagnetic, electromechanical, and viscoelastic forces. Simply put, vibrations within a living system interact coherently with each other or act as a whole unit. This means they move in sync at a particular frequency, and structures such as proteins or enzymes can transfer energy and information through these vibrations. It theorizes that living systems can vibrate in unison, exchanging energy and information. For example, two proteins vibrating in unison could pass information and energy to each other. This provides a faster, much more efficient way to support health as compared to the chemical-mechanical model.

Molecules and membranes vibrate at characteristic frequencies that can build into collective vibrations or frequencies that could extend throughout the body. Fröhlich theorized that these long-range communications via collective oscillation were a guiding force within our biology. Although this contribution from Fröhlich was not enough to sway the larger scientific community, it mapped a path of possibility for quantum biological effects in living systems.

This idea of long-range communication through vibration or resonance is becoming more evident as research progresses. Excitation in subatomic particles leads to an electromagnetic field. This field can generate a flow of information, similar to what Frölich talked about. It doesn't have to be long-lived. That electromagnetic field can excite the electrons in some particles for a very short amount of time, and that excitement and communication can pass to another set of particles. As we'll explore later, the idea that structures in the body can communicate through vibrational resonance is an emerging field of science.

QUANTUM BIOLOGY EMERGES

In the early 2000s, evidence for quantum biological effects began to mount again. In April 2007, Greg Engel and Graham Fleming published a paper that claimed that certain photosynthetic bacteria used quantum mechanics to transfer excitons to the reaction center during photosynthesis. In the process of photosynthesis, a photon from the sun hits the chlorophyll held within the organism's chloroplasts. This creates an exciton that stores energy and information. This exciton needs to get to a reaction center within the chloroplast for photosynthesis to occur.

The problem is that chloroplasts are densely packed, making chlorophyll-to-chlorophyll transfer of the exciton too cumbersome to cover the distance in the time necessary. With a classical physics explanation, the exciton jumps from chlorophyll to chlorophyll ambling toward its goal. This explanation can't account for the time it would take to cover long distances nor the probability of the exciton getting lost on a meandering path. This is a big problem because of the high efficiency of photosynthesis. The transfer of excitons to a reaction center in photosynthesis has nearly 100 percent efficiency. Excitons can't afford a meandering path, nor can they get lost.

Engel and Fleming's research suggested that the exciton used quantum superposition and coherence to achieve the energy transfer of photosynthesis. They directed three successive pulses of laser light into the photosynthetic complex and measured the results. The research team from the University of California, Berkeley, found a quantum beat that correlated to the coherence of the excitons produced by the pulsed laser emissions. Further, they asserted it was this quantum coherence that kept the exciton on its path to the reaction center. The exciton was held on its path by the vibratory coherence, or what they called *the quantum beat*, from the proteins in the chlorophyll. It was like a ball headed toward its goal and kept on its path by the collective nudges from the crowd watching. This had never before been demonstrated.

These claims surprised most of the scientific community. As the story goes, researchers from the Massachusetts Institute of Technology (MIT) read the report of the research article in the *New York Times* and laughed at the preposterous conclusions. Among them was Seth Lloyd, a noted quantum physicist. Once Lloyd read the actual research, he understood the magnitude of the discoveries.

Engel and Fleming continued their research, confirming the initial quantum biological effects they found in green sulfur bacteria. Seth Lloyd and the team of researchers from MIT that initially mocked the idea also began to explore the quantum mechanical aspects of biology. They found that the random noise in living systems could account for the quantum coherence seen in photosynthesis. An exciton can sometimes get stuck at certain complexes in the photosynthetic chain, and Lloyd's research suggests that the environmental noise in a living system nudges the exciton forward without destroying its quantum properties. This quantum beat, or coherence, has been confirmed in biology many times, supporting the idea that quantum phenomenon can indeed occur in living systems. This is a huge discovery toward understanding the invisible order that seems to guide life as we know it, and, since then, several biological events have been attributed to quantum biology. A beautiful understanding that it is the chaos of a living system which allows for life to flourish.

QUANTUM BIOLOGY IN LIVING SYSTEMS

Enzymes are small proteins responsible for catalyzing, or speeding up, vital chemical reactions within our body. Without enzymes, no life could exist because they assist with digestion, metabolism, and a variety of biological actions. The traditional theory states that enzymes work through a lock and key, or the induced fit, model. Again, this Newtonian biological view of random collision is dubious at the scale of the cell. Judith Klinman was the first to postulate that enzymes used quantum tunneling in their ability to lower energy rates of reactions. This was later confirmed by several researchers across the globe. Tunneling in enzymes, DNA mutations, brain function, T cell function within the immune system, and mitochondrial formation of ATP have been proposed and experimentally confirmed. It seems it is not just enzymes, but also proteins within the body, that utilize quantum tunneling.

Groundbreaking research on microtubules could extend quantum biology to all life. Tryptophan is an amino acid found in the body. Tryptophan contains a benzene ring that allows tryptophan to absorb a photon of light and emit it again at a lower radiance. When tryptophan molecules are arranged symmetrically in protein structures like the microtubules in the neurons of the brain or in the microtubules in cytoskeletons of living organisms such as plants, animals, and microbes, this process is enhanced. The structures exhibit a quantum phenomenon known as *superradiance*. They can light up together in sync, like a choir hitting the high note together. This research suggests that neurons can communicate faster than we ever thought possible. The fact that superradiance takes place in microtubules hints at the possibility that quantum biology applies to all life, since microtubules exist in most living things.

Aromatic amino acids containing benzene rings, or six-sided rings, can be found in a variety of our biological structures, such as fascia, DNA, neurons, and collagen. And it's been postulated that the organized water that lines these structures contain six-sided ring formations as well. The benzene ring has three double bonds and each contains a pair of pi electrons. These six pi electrons can dislocate from the molecule, able to move freely around the molecule and even move to other molecules. Electrons are often thought of as billiard balls, or very small particles, but, really, they are more like waves of energy. These waves carry energy and information. So, rather than the idea of solid electron particles around a proton and neutron to form an atom, we are talking about waves of energy and information.

The pi electrons in benzene rings can become excited by light, magnetic, electric, and electromagnetic fields and carry that energy and frequency information to other molecules. It doesn't even have to be a local transfer. This transfer of energy and information can happen at a distance. The structure of the benzene ring allows us to utilize wave information and energy for health and longevity. Calculations with benzene rings show that even the zero-point field seems to be giving energy to benzene rings.

The total energy, structure, and reactivity of benzene rings cannot be explained without the addition of the zero-point energy, or energy that comes from the zero-point field or quantum field. This adds to the perspective that health comes from sufficient energy or electrons, and exposing ourselves to light, sound, and fields of energy such as electrical, magnetic, and electromagnetic fields can help quench the deficiency of energy or electrons we see in inflammation, pain, and disease. Benzene rings offer a mode of transfer for electrons in the body.

Researchers have suggested that our sense of smell also depends on quantum biology. Recent research has found that smell could depend on the oscillation of odor molecules being smelled and their ability to transfer electrons to receptors. Odorant vibrations seem to enhance the electron tunneling in the process of smell, meaning that the unique vibration of the odor excites the cell to provide the energy for electron tunneling and the resulting perceived scent.

We have olfactory receptors throughout the body, not just in the nose. Could this explanation of quantum smell allow for other areas in the body to receive these energetic messages? Smell receptors in the skin help with wound healing. Olfactory receptors in the kidneys help control metabolic function and blood pressure. Smell receptors in the prostate can inhibit the spread of cancerous prostate cells. Olfactory receptors in muscles help repair muscle tissue, and receptors in the lungs help constrict airways when we inhale a noxious odor. Olfactory receptors in the testes have even been found to act as a directional system guiding sperm to an unfertilized egg. This invisible sea of quantum effects commands our perception of the world.

Scientists have proposed that birds navigate in flight during their long annual migration with the help of quantum mechanics. Klaus Schulten, from the Max Planck Institute for Biophysical Chemistry in Göttingen, Germany, first proposed that the migratory bird relies on magnetically sensitive chemical transformations to make the long annual migration. Schulten was inspired by research that found radical pairs have unique properties that make their chemistry sensitive to weak magnetic interactions. Over the past forty years, researchers have conducted hundreds of lab studies validating that radical-pair reactions are affected by magnetic fields. Thought not to affect biology, magnetism seems to be one of the hidden orders that instructs life.

The light-sensitive cryptochrome protein in the bird's eye seems to sense Earth's magnetic field. As blue light hits the cryptochrome protein, two unpaired electrons in different parts of the protein are created and form a radical pair. A radical is an atom or molecule with at least one unpaired electron. When two unpaired electrons belonging to different molecules become entangled, they form a radical pair. This brief quantum entanglement lasts long enough to affect the reactions in the molecules they belong to and the bird's navigation. In the case of flight, the radical pairs react to the magnetic effect of Earth in the bird's biological compass, allowing it to fly great distances with precise accuracy.

The idea that fields of energy can guide life is an exciting turn for modern science to make. Recent research has found that people can detect Earth's magnetic field as measured through a change in brain waves. Recent research has also found that magnetic fields induce the radical pair mechanism, significantly affecting DNA synthesis. Scientists have observed what they proposed to be the production of entangled radical pairs from reactive oxygen species in human cells in reaction to magnetic fields.

Many biological processes are dictated by weak magnetic fields. Stem cell development and maturation, cell proliferation, and genetic repair are all influenced by magnetic fields. Weak magnetic fields influence a variety of actions in the body, including genetic expression and damage, cancer progression, immune system function, blood flow, pain, and metabolism. Even our circadian rhythms seem to be influenced by magnetic fields and the radical pair mechanism. Although not a common consideration in science and medicine, magnetism plays a pivotal role in the workings of our body. Interventions like pulsed electromagnetic field therapy and transcranial magnetic stimulation help support a multitude of conditions from inflammation, arthritis, bone fractures, pain, depression, and neurological disorders. This new understanding of how magnetism influences biology, once again, offers us an expanded perspective of the body and different ways to heal it.

In 2021, for the first time ever, scientists were able to visualize what they believe to be quantum mechanics at play in human cells. Researchers from the University of Tokyo exposed cells to blue light. Our body has flavins in it that are responsive to light. The light-responsive flavins in human cells began to fluoresce, or glow, in response to the light stimulus. Then, the researchers swept a magnet over the cells, creating radical pairs that dimmed the light emitted from the cells. Visualizing the changing light emission triggered by magnetic fields was something never witnessed before and implies a quantum biological action taking place in human cells. As you'll learn in future chapters, the benzene ring in our light-sensitive proteins, enzymes, hormones, pigments, and neurotransmitters is particularly suited for quantum phenomena. This is important because it gives us a fast and efficient option for healing a multitude of conditions.

The idea that fields of energy affect our biology is important. Understanding this language of frequency information can revolutionize medicine. We have relied on a model that involves slower chemical diffusion, random collision, or the necessity of direct physical contact. Utilizing fields of energy is a way for the body to communicate and transfer energy that is almost instantaneous. This enhances our ability to heal and stay healthy. Life is propelled by these unseen forces of electricity, magnetism, the flow of electrons, protons, and vibrations of sound. We can utilize these vibrational fields for better health and longer lives.

Quantum biology is a growing field exploding by leaps and bounds with new research. Universities such as the University of California, Los Angeles, the University of Chicago, University of Surrey, Howard University, the University of KwaZulu-Natal in South Africa, and the University of California, Berkeley, are adding dedicated quantum biology departments to their campuses. This is not to say there is unanimity in the scientific community regarding quantum biology. Although there is a lack of consensus, all the evidence starts to paint a convincing picture that certainly deserves a deeper look.

The light, the sound, the electrons, protons, and ions in our environment, the frequency of thoughts and emotions all affect our cell membranes, our mitochondria, our fascia, our DNA, and, from there, our biological function and health. They affect the smallest parts of our biology, seemingly starting the gears in motion in our larger biological actions. Health isn't just about chemical reactions; it seems intimately tied to the smallest pieces of life that connect us all. The things we seem to value the least in medicine—light, water, sound, energy—play an inseparable role in our health.

QUANTUM BIOLOGY AND OUR HEALTH

Quantum biology is more than just scientific discovery. It has powerful ramifications for our health and the future of medicine. The very essence of our health is dictated by the circadian rhythm of the sun, by the psychoneuroimmunology of our minds, by the vibrations of sound, and the forces that maintain or degrade our electrical charge. By understanding these forces, we have free access to incredible modalities for health and the prevention and treatment of disease.

As a review, for the sake of this book, I define and use the term *quantum biology* as the study of quantum particles, such as photons of light, electrons, protons, vibrations of proteins, frequencies of sound, and water molecules, and how they interact with our biology. This interaction often, but not always, seems to utilize quantum phenomena such as tunneling, superposition, and coherence.

We have a long history of thinking that we have finally arrived at the truth in science. As time passes and technology advances, we learn that the absolutism of that truth was held in the available understanding and technology of the time. Our understanding of the world around us, that elusive scientific truth, is always evolving. Quantum biology offers an opportunity to build our resilience and health so we can be the change we so desperately need.

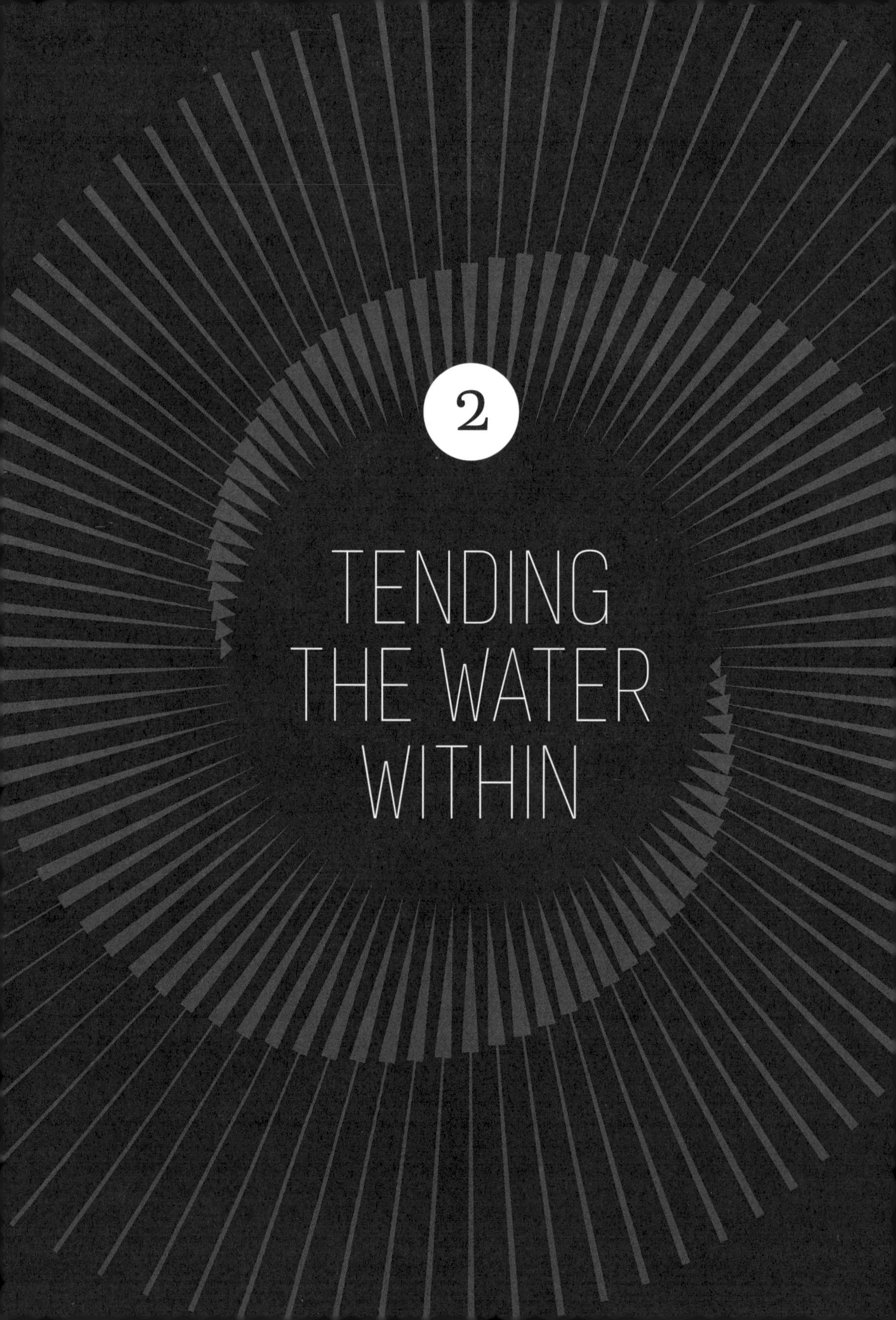

2

TENDING THE WATER WITHIN

When we talk about quantum biology within our body—the impact of light, sound, and vibrational frequency on biological action—we need to talk about water. Our body is around 70 percent water by weight. If we were to line up all the molecules in the body, because the water molecule is so small, we would find that 98 percent of the human body would be water molecules. We are water beings, and the water within us dances to the tune of the vibratory information in our environment. The vibration of light, sound, electricity, and the spin of an electron are all examples of frequency information that can act on water.

Water is foundational to our health and longevity, and it's vital to understand some of the roles it can play in the human body. Dehydration, or lack of water, can show up as fatigue, headache, chronic pain, accelerated aging, histamine intolerance, muscle tightness and weakness, cardiovascular dysfunction, blood pressure issues, and hormonal imbalance as well as immune dysregulations like autoimmunity and inflammatory conditions.

Hydration status influences almost every biological action in the body, from digestion to detoxification to immune balance to neurological function to cellular health. We live in a modern society that operates under constant stress, living mostly indoors with artificial heating and cooling, artificial lighting, and exposure to high amounts of nonnative electromagnetic frequencies, like Wi-Fi, all of which are dehydrating. Many people, as a result, experience a low to moderate level of dehydration. Most think that simply drinking more water will counteract this dehydration, but hydration is much more than that. When we start to explore the properties of water, we walk away with a completely new perspective on health and hydration.

One of the most underappreciated and overlooked substances *in* our body, water has a profound effect *on* our body. It helps translate those invisible vibrational instructions into numerous biological processes. While science still has more questions than answers when it comes to water, what we do know is starting to reveal a compelling picture of life and what it means to be healthy.

Within our body there exists a network formed by the interfacial liquid crystalline water that surrounds each and every cell, tissue, and organ. The communication that proteins engage in via frequency resonance seems to happen at the level of the liquid crystalline water that lines them. The spin of the entangled protons in the brain looks to take place in the water that surrounds the neurons. The microtubules that some point to as the receiver of consciousness are filled with this interfacial water. Water is part of every cell's ability to function. The ability of the proteins in our mitochondrial electron transport chain to capture, store, and emit light photons appears to happen in the water lining those proteins. The cell's action is dictated by the folding and unfolding of proteins. This, too, is enabled by the water that lines these proteins. The water within us is an essential part of our health.

TWO PHASES OF LIQUID WATER

Structured water, or exclusion zone (EZ) water, ordered water, bound water, biological water, interfacial water, and liquid crystalline water are all terms used to describe what researchers have found as a different organization of liquid water. We are all familiar with the three phases of water: gaseous vapor, solid ice, and liquid water. The theory that liquid water has two distinct phases has intrigued scientists for almost 150 years. These two phases of liquid water reflect two different states of energy and organization.

After Albert Szent-Györgyi received a Nobel Prize for his discovery of vitamin C, he turned his research to water. He saw water as a key component in living systems by contributing to the system's bioenergetics. Szent-Györgyi proposed that structured or organized water at the surfaces of living systems could induce long-lasting electronic excitation. The implication that water could provide a source of energy gives a whole new perspective on how biology works. This long-lasting excitation is the consequence of the two phases of water, which Szent-Györgyi called the "ground state" and the "excited state."

All atoms have two states: an excited, energized state and a ground, low-energy state. Szent-Györgi claimed that the same held true for water. He claimed that the transitions between these two states of water created long-lasting excitation that was enough to power biological processes. He also posited that there should be an electrical charge at the junction of these two phases of water.

His idea was that this long-lasting excitation formed a resonance vibration that could transfer energy to molecules from the excited water layer. All of this energy accumulation and transfer was to take place in the subatomic realm—the realm of quantum mechanics, which Szent-Györgi suggested was what powered chemical reactions in our body. It was not a random collision model that hoped for the chance meeting of biological keys and receptors. It was a language of frequency, of vibration, of oscillation that spoke to other molecules and proteins in the body, like the musician who holds two tuning forks set at the same frequency—when one vibrates, it entrains the other to play the same note even if the distance between them is large. Szent-Györgyi proposed that this was how biological reactions occurred.

Szent-Györgi claimed that the liquid crystalline water that lines a cell vibrates at a certain frequency. This frequency can attract other molecules and solutes to connect to the excited structured water. The long-lasting excitation of the structured water can also give the reaction between the cell and the biomolecule the energy it needs for the reaction to take place.

Gilbert Ling, cell physiologist, biochemist, and scientific investigator, also researched this different form of water and its ability to power life. Ling proposed that proteins, water, and potassium engage in multiple connections that form a biological protoplasm, or a source of biological energy. He theorized that this protoplasm came from switching the states of water from the resting state to the active state. This switch gives off energy and could provide the force needed to help power life. Ling proposed it was not the sodium potassium pump that gave the cell its negative electrical charge, but rather that the electrical charge came from the water lining the cell membrane.

The Fourth Phase of Water

In the 1990s, Gerald Pollack, professor from the University of Washington, made an incredible discovery. He was the first to identify a fourth phase of water, which is also the name of one of his books: *The Fourth Phase of Water*. Pollack was studying how water responds to hydrophilic, or water-loving, surfaces. He was looking at how water reacts with Nafion, a synthetic hydrophilic surface. These water-loving surfaces do not repel water. Instead, they allow water to come right up to the surface and, when it does, something incredible happens. Pollack found that when water comes to a water-loving surface, it takes on a distinctly different structure. It becomes more gel-like, more viscous in texture. Pollack explains that this water differs from regular bulk water, or H2O, and suggests it has a molecular structure of H3O2. The different molecular structure and textural change in this phase of water become very important to biological function and health as we'll see.

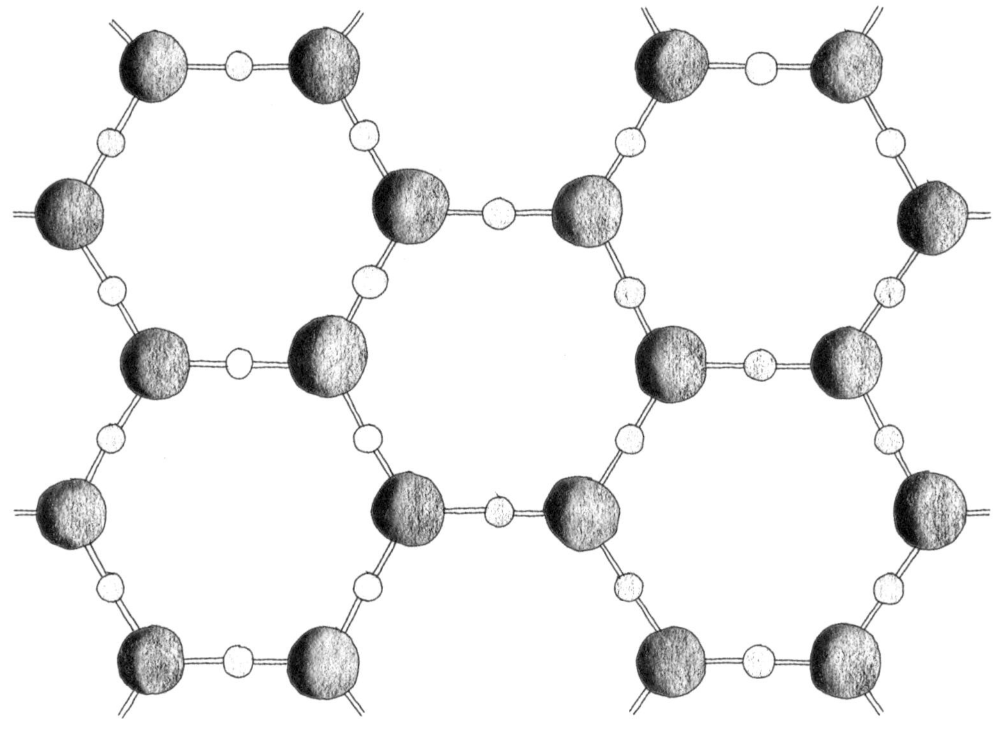

Pollack proposes that the structure of EZ water takes on a hexagonal lattice formation.

Pollack proposes that this interfacial water (the water at a surface) takes on a hexagonal lattice shape, much like a honeycomb. Although the structure is still in debate, the hexagonal shape aligns with the properties of the benzene ring that can capture, harness, and transmit energy. This liquid crystalline water is ordered and aligned. As one sheet of this latticed-structured water forms, it acts as a template for more sheets of liquid crystalline water to build. Pollack termed this fourth phase of water "exclusion zone" water, or EZ water, because as this lattice of organized water builds, it pushes out practically all particles or solutes.

It is infrared energy that causes this EZ structured water to build. By immersing Nafion in water and exposing it to an infrared lamp, Pollack and his team found the largest EZ water growth they had witnessed in the lab, and it steadily diminished after the light was extinguished. Pollack and other scientists have confirmed that EZ liquid crystalline water is, indeed, formed against hydrophilic surfaces and grows in size when supplied with a source of energy, light, or infrared heat. It's not just on synthetic hydrophilic surfaces that this happens. Pollack and others have done research with liquid crystalline water against hydrophilic surfaces in living systems such as plants, animals, and humans with similar results. Our cells, DNA, tissues, and fascia are all hydrophilic.

A WATER BATTERY WITHIN US

Pollack found that this EZ liquid crystalline water has a negative electrical charge. Our cells run on a negative electrical charge that's essential to a healthy cell and thus overall health. He also found that as this negatively charged liquid crystalline water builds, it pushes out a positively charged hydrogen or proton, creating what researchers are calling a proton-rich zone, or proton wire. As the negatively charged structured water forms against a water-loving surface, an oppositely charged positive zone of water forms right outside of it. This separation of charge, just like the separation in a nine-volt battery, creates potential energy.

Investigating further, Pollack and his team placed an electrode in the negatively charged liquid crystalline EZ water layer and another in the positively charged proton water that forms right outside the liquid crystalline EZ water layer. It created a biological battery between the two opposing charges that produced enough energy to power a small LED light bulb in the lab. This was an amazing discovery. To discover a potential source of energy in the body that does not come from chemicals or food intake requires a complete revision of our understanding of how the body works. It also provides us with a new set of tools for healing and longevity.

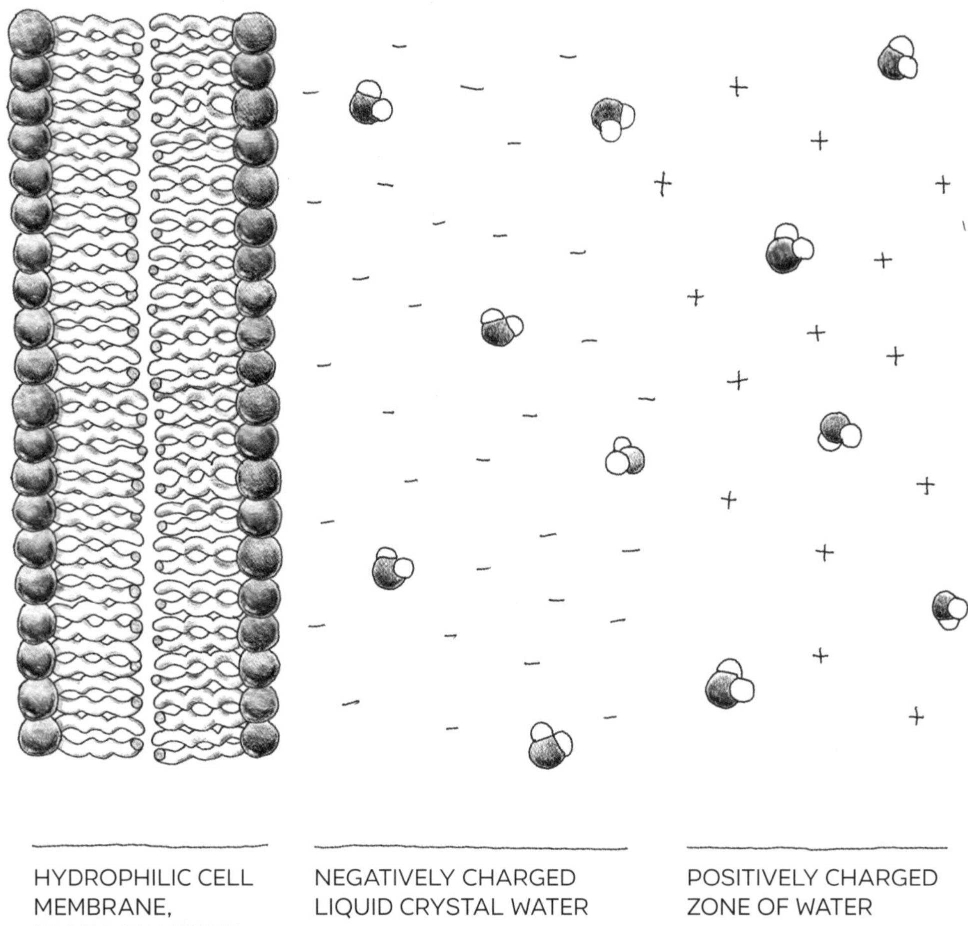

EZ liquid crystalline water forms against a water-loving surface and creates a gel-like negatively charged organization of water. As this liquid crystalline water forms, it creates a positively charged water zone directly outside the negatively charged EZ liquid crystalline water. This forms potential energy.

This is a dramatic shift from the chemical model of biology. It implies a source of energy from a water battery living within us, not solely from a chemical reaction or random collisions happening in the body. Organs, vessels, cells, and the microscopic organelles within cells are all lined with hydrophilic surfaces. The energetic input from our internal and external terrain has the potential to power this biological water battery within us. The implications of this are astonishing for health and longevity. We have worked under a chemical model for so long in biochemistry. It has been incredibly successful, and it has also led to dead ends. To view the body as an energetic being and to recognize the role that water plays in that gives us an opportunity to expand not only our understanding but our approach to health.

Professor Pollack then immersed a Nafion tube in water and applied infrared light. That liquid crystalline water battery started to form on the outside as well as the inside of the tube. Then, something astonishing happened: He witnessed the flow of water, particles, and protons being driven through the tube. This flow of fluid and protons continued as long as the infrared energy was present. There was no outside force pushing the water through the tube. This fits perfectly with the idea that the flow of water was propelled through the tube as a result of a water battery created by the negatively charged EZ water and the positively charged water outside of it. The energetic dance between the liquid crystalline water and the energetic input of the environment holds the power to direct the flow of information and energy.

It is not only infrared light that influences this liquid crystalline water. EZ water builds in the presence of electrical fields and visible light. Liquid crystalline EZ water is excited by ultraviolet light, creating an abundance of electrons. We have a collagen matrix lined with liquid crystalline water that spans from the most external layers of our skin to the most internal tissues of our body. This creates a bodywide network. This collagen grid, in conjunction with the water that lines it, could act as a reservoir of energy. We can look at biology as a dynamic flow of electrons in a living system. Symptoms of pain, inflammation, or illness can be seen as a deficiency of electrons. We have a network of collagen lined with EZ structured water that can act as repository of electrons that can be donated to quench inflammation and energy deficiency throughout the body.

CHARGED WATER

Research has found an association between the amount of cell-bound EZ water and a healthy cell. A diminished zone of EZ liquid crystalline water has been associated with cancerous cells whereas a robust zone of EZ water has been associated with healthy cells. Our cells run on a negative electrical charge, around –40 to –70 millivolts. We talk about this in depth in chapter 4, but I must mention it here. Professor Pollack proposes that it is the water's negative electrical charge that lines the outside and the inside of the cell that confers health. Once that negative electrical charge starts to erode so does the health of the cell. A diminished zone of liquid crystalline water has been correlated with pathology and an impaired immune function.

This water battery within us has also been proposed as a mechanism in the body's ability to circulate fluid through the body, such as blood, cerebrospinal fluid, and lymphatic fluid. Mathematically, it is difficult to explain how the heart's pumping is the sole force of blood circulating in the body because red blood cells need to be squeezed to fit through narrow capillaries. That requires considerable energy. Professor Pollack and his student Zheng Li have done several studies with blood circulation in chick embryos. After stopping the heart, the blood continues to flow as long as infrared energy is present. Incredibly, the circulatory system pump stopped completely yet the blood continued to flow for ten minutes or more in some cases. This implies that something over and above the heart pump must be at work. This fits perfectly with the idea that EZ liquid crystalline water builds against the inside of the vessel wall, creating a battery that powers the flow of fluid through the vessel with the help of infrared energy. It also suggests a mechanism for detoxification, where the EZ water pushes out any particles and pollutants, releasing them into the lymphatic system for removal.

THE QUANTUM ELECTRODYNAMICS OF WATER

Italian theoretical physicists Emilio Del Giudice, Guiliano Preparata, and Giuseppe Vitiello introduced the quantum electrodynamics theory of water. They also proposed that water has two liquid phases: a coherent excited state and a ground decoherent state. They described how water molecules can form clusters that synchronize their movements with electromagnetic fields via quantum coherence in formations called *coherent domains*. The vibrations of the coherent domain and the vibration of the electromagnetic field synchronize. This allows the water domain and the electromagnetic field to exchange information and energy, again, like two tuning forks. These coherent domains of water can trap and store electromagnetic energy. This could make water an active participant in health by organizing molecules, moving electrons, storing information, and acting as a liquid antenna that links frequency information to biological action.

Del Giudice, Preparata, and Vitiello claimed these water clusters of coherent domains allow for a fluid flow of energy that could help power life. Reminiscent of other work on the two energy states of liquid water, they describe a plasma of energy in the form of free electrons from a coherent domain of water even at room temperatures. They suggested that the EZ liquid crystalline water that Professor Gerald Pollack identified could be large coherent domains of water lining a cell. This explains how proteins, enzymes, and biological actions could use the energy from the coherent domain of water to both facilitate action and communicate within the body.

In simple terms, the quantum electrodynamics theory of water suggests that water can form clusters as coherent domains of water and can capture vibrational energy and information from electromagnetic fields. Rather than the key and lock model we learned about earlier that dominates science today, this theory talks of a language of frequency. The coherent domain of water acts as a communication beacon, sending information throughout the body almost instantaneously. Attracting reactants like a siren singing in the ocean to attract a passing ship, the water domains surrounding biomolecules sing throughout the body. This exchange of vibrational energy and information takes place at the subatomic level. It's the excitement of electrons and protons that seems to create energy and communication. Like an antenna picking up on the smallest frequencies, the water within biological systems have the potential to send and receive vibrations as well as emit energy that can potentially power reactions. This completely extends our understanding of biology.

Research over the last couple of decades has brought some validation to this theory. There's research showing that water has a regulatory function on cellular metabolism, the ability of coherent water to act as a semiconductor, a piezoelectric (able to produce an electrical current when pressure is applied) transducer, and as an antioxidant. There have been studies of models that find this liquid crystalline EZ water to have the ability to act on enzymes and proteins while acting as a source of energy and a system of communication, illustrating further the importance of water beyond the current understanding of hydration. Under this line of thought, it's not just about the amount of water one drinks. It is about how water can act as a source of energy, information, and communication in the body.

WATER HOLDS FREQUENCY

Ancient Indigenous cultures have always shown a deep respect and sacred rituals around water, including the worship of water gods and goddesses. Many of these cultures continue their reverence for water today.

The well-known Chinese text *Bencao gangmu* divides water into different types, such as rain, dew, and snow, according to the source. Each source confers a different healing mechanism.

Egyptian papyruses tell of how water created this world and can be used for purification and healing.

The Hindu Vedic texts also convey the importance of water in the creation of our universe and in purification and health. Water is said to be a healer, a purifier, acting as the container of life, strength, and eternity.

The Celtic tradition of Northern Europe revered the role of water in healing. Water was seen as a sacred portal to the Otherworld, with rituals to protect and respect it. Freshwater wells and springs were named after divinities and venerated for their magical and healing powers.

The Maya and Aztec cultures also had water as part of their creation lore. Water ceremonies and worship were commonplace in these cultures. The ancient Maya civilization of Tikal had sophisticated means of filtering and energizing water with zeolite and quartz crystals.

There has always been an acknowledgement of water's ability to hold energy. The more I study water, the more it seems to be a bridge for energy of all kinds: light, sound, electromagnetic frequency, the quantum field, and the frequency of thoughts. Water seems to be a bridge not only between the unseen blueprint of life and the concrete matter we see in the world around us, but also an amplifier of this invisible information.

The centuries-old practice of homeopathy also holds a relationship between water and energy. Homeopathic preparations are used to provide support in a variety of health conditions. To make homeopathic remedies, a small amount of an original substance is diluted in water through serial succussion and dilution. A small amount of a substance is placed in a vial of water and shaken vigorously. This process is called *succussion*, and the idea is that some energy and information transfer occurs between the substance and the water. Then, a small portion of the liquid is removed, placed into a new vial of water, and shaken vigorously again. This process is repeated until the desired level of dilution, or *potentization* as it is called in homeopathy, occurs. Often, the dilution continues until there is no detectable original substance left in the water—not even a molecule of the original substance is left in the diluted water. These different potencies are thought to hold different energetic imprints and information of the original substance and are used for different health benefits.

Different dilutions of homeopathic preparations have been found to hold and emit different frequencies of ultraviolet light. Even though they contain the same substance, the different amounts of dilution create a different spectrum of light. This research suggests that unique spectral patterns of light—specific to the original substance—can persist even after extreme dilutions, implying that energetic information may be transferred into water as light signatures. In other research, different substances were found to emit substance-specific ultraviolet transmission. Water has also been found to hold the electrical field of a homeopathic remedy. This also highlights how water can support health by more means than just hydration.

The work of Jacques Benveniste and Luc Montagnier are part of the controversial field of water memory. Jacques Benveniste was an immunologist studying the immune system and the cells that comprise it. He was studying how much of an allergen antibody it would take to produce an allergic reaction. Specifically, he was looking at basophils, the immune cells that degranulate the histamine that triggers the classic symptoms of allergies: runny nose, sneezing, itchy eyes, and scratchy throat.

As with many scientific discoveries, an error in Benveniste's lab unveiled an incredible insight into water's unique properties. A research student in the lab miscalculated the dilution calculations and ended up diluting the allergen antibody solution beyond the predetermined level. There was no detectable antibody in the solution. Yet, when the solution was applied to basophils, they reacted exactly as if there was an antibody present. Benveniste continued to reproduce this research with other substances. It appeared that the water was holding energetic information. Not only could the water hold immunological information, but that information could be received and used by cells to mount an allergic response.

Luc Montagnier was a French scientist whose work on human immunodeficiency virus, HIV, earned him a Nobel Prize. Soon afterward, he turned his research to water, believing these new ideas about water could change medicine. Montagnier found that highly diluted DNA from microbes could emit unique electromagnetic waves. Both Benveniste and Montagnier used a process of dilution similar to the process of potentization used in homeopathy. Montagnier took a sample of water in a glass container and placed a solenoid, a coil of wire, around the glass container to detect and amplify any electromagnetic signals emitted by the DNA. This container was placed by another container holding only ultrapure water. Though the two containers were close in proximity, they did not have direct contact to avoid any cross contamination. Next, Montagnier added building blocks of DNA to the second container of ultrapure water that had been exposed to the original electromagnetic field signal. The second container of water was able to construct DNA that was over 98 percent identical to the original. The electromagnetic field signal seemed to hold some information that allowed this to happen.

Montagnier then went on to record the unique DNA electromagnetic frequency, digitize it, and sent it to a different laboratory in Italy. Researchers in Italy played the electromagnetic field recording next to ultrapure water with nucleic acids for one hour. The Italian team produced DNA that was 98 percent identical to the initial DNA from Montagnier's lab under the influence of the electromagnetic field recording. Just the influence of the electromagnetic recording seemingly held the instructions for the DNA to build itself. The mind-blowing results of Benveniste's and Montagnier's research are incredible, yet they remain quite controversial in the scientific community.

The work of Hans Geesink and Dirk Meijer, two prolific researchers in the field of water biophysics and consciousness, has advanced our understanding of water even further. As we know, everything has unique vibrations or resonant frequencies. Geesink and Meijer have studied hundreds of resonant frequencies of living and nonliving substances. They have found that these frequencies occur in a natural harmonic ordering, like musical octaves. The frequencies of these substances, though different, take on a pattern of twelve distinct frequencies. Octaves are fractal in structure, the same pattern but at a different scale. Fractal octaves help maintain coherence. We see fractal octaves in the electromagnetic and vibrational modes of DNA, in brain wave rhythms (4 Hz, 8 Hz, 16 Hz, 32 Hz), and in the oscillations of the mitochondria, cell membrane, and ion channels. Some of the frequencies that Geesink and Meijer found can promote biological resonance and health whereas other frequencies degrade health. Their research could be used to diagnose illness through measuring these frequencies. It could also be used to bolster the health-producing frequencies, bringing health and balance back to the system. They have found all these frequencies present in the liquid crystalline structured water. Water can capture, store, amplify, and emit these frequencies so the system can work harmoniously—again, illustrating how important water is in creating health and coherence.

Masaru Emoto and Veda Austin, water crystallography researchers, have also done amazing research on the ability of water to hold information. Masaru Emoto began to explore the effects of human intention on water in the 1990s. He would take small samples of water and expose them to positive words, like love and hope, or to negative words, like evil and hate. Upon freezing, the water exposed to the positive words would form gorgeous, organized water crystals whereas the negative words would create disorganized, chaotic water crystals. His work is an exquisite collection of water crystals that suggests the power of human intention to organize water. Critics often dismiss Emoto's work as unscientific because he produced many different water crystal formations from the influence of words but only chose the most beautiful samples to demonstrate the positive influence and the most unorganized samples for the negatively influenced water. Emoto did later research that double blinded this research without the subjective practice of choosing the water samples, but it was not enough to silence his critics. Nonetheless, his work remains a beautiful example of water's ability to hold information.

Veda Austin has developed her own freezing technique to explore the relationship between human intention and water. She finds that when water is placed by an object or picture or exposed to human intentions it freezes with a reflection of the object or intention. Her book *The Living Language of Water* is filled with examples of water that is placed by objects and frozen to show a reflection of the image. Veda has found an incredible language of water crystals she calls "hydroglyphs."

After freezing hundreds of water-filled Petri dishes, Austin began to see repeated symbols in the water crystallizations that corresponded to a concept, as if water were trying to communicate. One example of a hydroglyph is the emanating seed, known as the creation glyph. This pattern resembles a seed emitting energy or growth and Austin found this glyph repeatedly in water samples from different kinds of water and different kinds of exposures. She explains it is water's way of conveying the concept of creation.

These researchers have all looked at water through different lenses and reached the same conclusion. Water can hold frequency and can impart energy and information to the body. Building on the idea that the water within us is crucial for health, these researchers propose that the water we drink can also transport energy and information from the world around us.

TRUE HYDRATION

Aging is a process of dehydration. Tissue stiffness and a diminished cell-bound structured water increases aging whereas an increase in hydration and the building of the cell-bound EZ water has been associated with a healthier, better functioning cell. The water that lines our proteins has a direct effect on their ability to change shape and thus function. Proteins within the cell membrane dictate the biological function of the cell. Decreases in our cellular hydration impairs this process, which has a detrimental effect on our overall health and longevity.

So, water is vital for our biology, but it begs the question, what is the best water to drink? From a quantum biological perspective, the water we drink is important for several reasons. It lays the potential foundation of hydration for the liquid crystalline cell-bound water within us that can act as a battery for biological action. In addition, the water we drink could serve as a potential reservoir of energy for the body to utilize. So, we need water that hydrates us and also has the potential to supply energy.

How to Hydrate

In 2020, Gerald Pollack and his team did research on the best ways to hydrate. He found that tap water was the least effective at hydration whereas mineral water was the most effective. This makes sense with what we know about osmosis. Water will follow the minerals, allowing the water to enter the body. Minerals not only help increase our level of hydration, but they also contribute to the energy or coherence of the water we drink.

There are several options for the type of water you drink to hydrate: alkaline, diluted sea water, sole water, electrolyzed, hydrogen, ionized, mineral, oxygen, spring, structured/coherent, and tap water. Tap water, however, has been found to contain a multitude of contaminants—from microbes to heavy metals to personal care products to medications to disinfectant by-products to herbicides, pesticides, and perfluorinated compounds.

Types of Drinking Water

Alkaline water refers to water that is less acidic. It can be found naturally in spring water or created by a process of electrolysis (see ionized water) or by adding electrolytes to water. Alkaline water only really refers to the pH, not the presence of ions, oxygen, or coherence.

Mineral water contains minerals. Mineral water can either be naturally formed or created by adding minerals to regular water. Both types are effective options for hydration. Remember, Pollack's recent research confirms that mineral water is optimal for hydration.

Spring water is naturally alkaline because of its mineral content. Spring water moves in a vortex motion that adds oxygen to the water. In the presence of minerals, the added oxygen creates more potential energy than regular water.

Diluted sea water mimics the electrolyte and mineral profile of our blood plasma and interstitial fluid. It can help replete the body's lost minerals while also ridding the body of toxins that accumulate in the interstitial fluid throughout. All hydration works on this level to some degree. Our interstitial fluid is constantly at work to help rid the body of toxic pollutants so options to foster this process can be helpful for our health.

Quinton marine plasma, discovered by Dr. René Quinton in 1894 while harvesting mineral-rich seawater from a plankton bloom on the coast of France, is another form of diluted seawater that has had decades of anecdotal benefits.

Sole water is created when sea salt is added to water until the water is so full of salt it can no longer be dissolved. Ancient Ayurvedic medicine has talked about the benefits of sole water for centuries. A teaspoon of this salt-rich sole water is added to a glass of drinking water for the added benefits of hydration, mineralization, and digestive health. This option, however, should be avoided for those on a salt-restricted diet or who have blood pressure issues.

Electrolyzed water is water that has been split into acidic and alkaline components. Electric current is applied to a saltwater solution in a membrane to create alkaline water at the cathode side and acidic water at the anode side. The alkaline water is used for drinking whereas the acidic water is used as a disinfectant.

Ionized water is another term for the alkaline part of electrolyzed water. It is also alkaline water because of the added ions but not because of added electrolytes.

Hydrogen water is water that has added molecular hydrogen. Hydrogen acts as an antioxidant in the body. Inflammation is associated with many chronic diseases, but it also serves a purpose. Steroids act as anti-inflammatories with a broad action: shutting down inflammation throughout the body without discrimination. This can cause many of the adverse side effects associated with steroid use. While inflammation can cause problems, it is also vital to many biological actions in our immune system, hormonal cascades, and metabolism. Interestingly, hydrogen water acts as a selective antioxidant, reducing inflammation judiciously, which makes it an effective option for helping improve many conditions. It also could benefit cell signaling and mitochondrial function. Research has shown that molecular hydrogen is beneficial for cardiovascular issues, cancer, nervous system dysregulation, mood, recovery in sports, and respiratory and neurological function.

Tabs of molecular hydrogen briefly supply extra hydrogen to the water. Hydrogen can also be added to water by adding hydrogen gas or through the process of electrolysis. Hydrogen content dissipates depending on exposure to air. If it is securely bottled, it can last days to months, whereas if it is exposed to air, it will quickly dissipate within ten minutes to a couple of hours.

Oxygen water has been infused with oxygen. Oxygen is dissolved in water by bubbling oxygen into water under pressure. There are claims of better oxygenation in the body, but oxygen is poorly absorbed by digestion and the gut.

Structured, or coherent, water has recently become a marketing trend with bottled water and devices being advertised as structured water or able to structure water. There is a common misconception that if we drink structured water, that structure and energy are preserved and completely transferred to the water battery within us. The liquid crystalline water within us is a different thing than coherent, energized drinking water. Water is dynamic, constantly changing structure. Drinking structured water seems to impart more energy and benefit to the body, but it's hard to maintain this higher energy state when it comes to bottling and storing. In line with the research on the quantum electrodynamics of water, domains of coherence could be created in the water that hold more energy.

We can create more coherent water by adding energy to it. Stirring or creating a vortex in the water, much like the natural vortex motion of spring water, can potentially add more energy. There are small metal devices on the market that create a vortex as water is poured through them. There are also specialized tools for stirring water to create more coherent water. Exposing the water to infrared energy in the form of sunlight, moonlight, and infrared saunas or devices can add energy to drinking water. Herbal teas, fruits, hydrated chia seeds, and vegetables are naturally abundant in liquid crystalline water. Many traditional medicinal remedies such as ghee, holy basil, probiotics found in fermented foods such as kimchee and sauerkraut, and turmeric have all been found to increase structured water.

Sound can also add structure to drinking water. The work of Veda Austin and Masaru Emoto suggest that our intentions and emotional state can affect the structure of water. The practice of approaching our food and drink with gratitude has always held a place of importance in health. The work of Austin and Emoto encourage a return to this practice.

What Is Structured Drinking Water?

Structured water, coherent water, magnetized water, and energized water refer to the organization and energy of drinking water.

Remember the two states of water that Albert Szent-Györgyi, Gilbert Ling, Gerald Pollack, and Emilio Del Giudice talked about? They refer to drinking water as well. Drinking water has the ability to capture, store, and transmit energy. The water in a glass can capture energy and potentially transfer that energy to us for biological action. The coherent domains or excited states of water that come from the addition of energy could provide health benefits. There is emerging research showing that structured, coherent, energized water has benefits for plants, animals, and humans. Some of this research comes from adding structure to water via magnets whereas other research comes from vortexing or using structured water devices like wands to add energy and structure to the water. While more research is needed, these results paint a promising picture of a noninvasive, inexpensive, accessible way to support health that has no known side effects.

Unfortunately, research on drinking energized water is limited and not well funded. The research that does exist seems to point to energized water's antioxidant capacity. There are several research studies on animals and plants showing that consumption of energized structured water improves immune health and organ health and improves the growth and health of crops. Research also showed that consumption of energized, structured water improved cardiovascular health, biochemical parameters, semen quality, and antioxidant status in animals.

- A research study out of India looked at thirty-eight human participants ages eighteen to sixty. Researchers found a 20 percent average increase in measured blood ATP as compared to the placebo group in those drinking energized structured water, indicating enhanced mitochondrial function. Improved ATP production is vital for our health and longevity.
- A pilot study found drinking structured water influenced the nervous system by improving heart rate variability, a sign that the nervous system is resilient to stress. This study also showed that consuming structured water increased fat loss. Visceral fat is the accumulation of fat around important organs such as the liver, stomach, and intestines and has been associated with an increased risk of heart disease, cancer, stroke, and Alzheimer's disease.
- A randomized, double-blind, placebo controlled study of sixteen healthy adults ages eighteen to seventy found that drinking 50 ounces (1.5 L) of coherent water for one hundred consecutive days improved the gut dysbiosis score by 16 percent over placebo, indicating improved balance of the gut microbiome.
- A case study followed one person for three years and measured cellular parameters before and after drinking energized water. Results showed that drinking energized structured water decreased resting energy expenditure (REE) by 18.3 percent and resting oxygen consumption rate decreased. The subject showed enhanced cellular energy expenditure and resilience to cellular stress.
- A small study of nineteen people found improved inflammatory markers in seventeen of the participants who drank energized structured water, leading to an average biological age reduction of 3.79 years as measured by the GlycanAge test. The GlycanAge test analyzes the presence of pro-inflammatory glycans that increase with age and anti-inflammatory glycans that are associated with youth. More coherent, energized water also improved protein folding, which is important to biological function overall and especially in conditions like Alzheimer's disease.
- A study with human cancer cells in vitro found cancer growth suppression after exposure to energized, structured water.

Though the research is still emerging, the implications are remarkable and deserve further investigation. Drinking energized water is an easy, inexpensive, and accessible way to support health that has no known adverse effects.

Filtering Your Drinking Water

The water available to most of us is filled with contaminants—from heavy metals to herbicides to nanoplastics to pesticides to pharmaceutical medications and birth control. Our drinking water contains substances we don't want to drink. Although clean water is something everyone deserves, many of us have access only to tap water. I believe that even tap water can serve its purpose when approached with gratitude.

In light of all these contaminants, there are a variety of water filters available that fit most budgets and needs. Although filters can do a wonderful job at filtering out most contaminants, they can also strip the minerals and salts out of the water. There are filter options that put the minerals back into the water before completing the filtration process, or this can be done manually. Also, FindASpring is an app that can help you find a clean, natural spring in your area.

Which Water Filters Are Best?

There are so many different types of water and water devices on the market, it can get confusing to know which is best for us. Exploring the various options will offer a better idea of what we should be drinking.

Filtered Water

When it comes to filtered water, there are nine common ways to filter:

1. Reverse osmosis
2. Distillation
3. Activated carbon filters
4. Ion exchange filters
5. Ultraviolet disinfection filters
6. Ultrafiltration
7. Activated alumina filters
8. Nanofiltration
9. Graphene-based filters

Reverse osmosis utilizes pressure to reverse the natural flow of liquids through semipermeable membranes, which can remove up to 99 percent of contaminants, microbes, chemicals, and particles. This is a great way to filter, but it does waste a fair amount of water in a time when water conservation is important.

Distillation uses heat to boil the water and remove most contaminants, microbes, minerals, and solutes. This is one of the best ways to remove toxins because most do not evaporate in the process and are left behind to be discarded. Both distillation and reverse osmosis are the most effective ways to filter water.

Activated carbon filters come in either activated carbon blocks or granulated activated carbon filters. They remove organic contaminants, some but not all heavy metals, pesticides, chlorine, fluoride, lead, copper, and disinfectant by-products such as trihalomethanes. Some activated carbon filters have been found to remove 70 to 90 percent of perfluorinated compounds, or forever chemicals as they are popularly referred to, while reverse osmosis filters remove 99 percent.

Ion exchange filters use ion exchange resins that contain positively charged hydrogen ions (H+). They remove contaminants by attracting them with the same charge and can remove contaminants such as pesticides, microbes, heavy metals, and perfluorinated compounds.

Ultraviolet filters remove only microbial presence in water, leaving other contaminants in the water.

Ultrafiltration units remove less than reverse osmosis filters due to their bigger pore size on their filter membrane although nanofilters can match reverse osmosis filters' efficiency.

Activated alumina filters remove only arsenic and fluoride.

Nanofiltration uses nanomaterials like carbon nanotubes to remove even the smallest contaminants, including heavy metals and pathogens, with greater efficiency than traditional reverse osmosis.

Graphene-based filters use graphene membranes to filter. Graphene membranes are ultrathin and highly effective at filtering out contaminants, including microplastics and viruses, while maintaining high water flow rates.

BUILDING THE WATER BATTERY WITHIN

How do we build that water battery within us? Although structuring our drinking water and structuring the water within us is different, the process is similar in many ways. Basically, we must add energy into the system to build energized water. Our sun is the most abundant source of infrared energy. Safe sun exposure has the potential to build the water battery within us and the potential energy it creates. It doesn't need to be a gorgeous sunny day to get infrared energy. Any time the sun is up, even on a rainy or cloudy day, there is an abundance of infrared energy present. Sitting in the shade on a sunny day also provides infrared exposure. The tree canopy absorbs the sun's ultraviolet rays and the leaves allow the infrared rays to pass right through, providing plenty of infrared energy. Indoors, modern LED lighting has moved away from the infrared spectrum of light, but halogen, incandescent, and specialty infrared bulbs provide infrared exposure. Infrared energy in the form of movement, moonlight, sitting fireside, snuggling, time in saunas and warm baths, sound immersion, and infrared devices all have the potential to build the liquid crystalline water within us.

Other easy ways to build that water battery within include:

- Adding a blanket or an extra layer of clothes to increase internal infrared energy
- Breathwork, nasal breathing
- Drinking warm beverages or eating warm food can also increase the infrared energy internally
- Movement: dancing, exercise, Qigong, walking, yoga
- Snuggling with a loved one or pet
- Tending to mitochondrial health (which also has the potential to create metabolic water and act as a source of hydration; see chapter 5 for more on this)

TENDING TO YOUR WATER BEING

Staying hydrated is the foundation of tending to the water within. Being hydrated allows our proteins and cellular action to function with ease. Dehydration is a major obstacle for health and has major negative impacts on longevity and the aging population. Choosing water with mineral content or adding minerals and electrolytes can help the hydration process. Remember, true hydration has to do with the water inside our body so things like mitochondrial function, earthing (coming in contact with Earth's surface and the free electrons that line it), movement, breath, and safe sun exposure can be extremely hydrating.

Choose clean water sources or filter water. There are a variety of water filters that fit most budgets and needs. From distillation to reverse osmosis to activated charcoal to ultra-filtration, filtering your water is an important step toward tending to your water being.

Add energy to your water. There are several ways to add energy to your water. Exposure to sunlight, moonlight, and infrared saunas or devices all have the capacity to increase energy in water. There are several devices on the market today that claim to structure water, but not all of them do. If you choose this route, make sure the device has some research behind its claims. You can also add energy to your water by stirring or creating a vortex in the water for thirty seconds to a few minutes, which exposes it to more oxygen and increases its energy. Drinking water out of a glass container allows the water to meet the surface of the glass and build that liquid crystalline structure. Even approaching the water with a sense of reverence, gratitude, and awe seems to create more structure in the water.

Build EZ cell-bound water within. Exposure to healthy infrared energy has the potential to build that interfacial liquid crystalline water.

Avoid activities that are dehydrating or act as an obstacle to building that water battery within:

- Artificial lighting can dehydrate via its potential to inhibit mitochondrial function and thus the water the mitochondria produce.
- Living indoors with constant heat and air-conditioning can both dehydrate and act as an obstacle to building liquid crystalline water. Take breaks outside and open the windows as much as feasible.

- Menstruation, pregnancy, breastfeeding, diabetes, advanced age, certain medications, and supplements all require more hydration.

- Mouth breathing is dehydrating as it bypasses the natural route of hydrating air that happens during nasal breathing.

- Nonnative electromagnetic fields, like Wi-Fi, can be both dehydrating and act as an obstacle to building cell-bound water. Unplug your Wi-Fi router when not in use and during sleep and consider using the Internet through wired means. Put your phone on airplane mode when not in use and do not sleep with your phone in the room. Wireless headphones also expose you to nonnative electromagnetic fields and can be switched to wired alternatives.

- Stress can be extremely dehydrating. Stress management tools are essential to most living in this modern world (see chapter 7 for more resources).

Finally, support your collagen fascial network that has the potential to build liquid crystalline water (see chapter 3 for more on this) and support your mitochondria, which produce metabolic water (see chapter 4 for more on this).

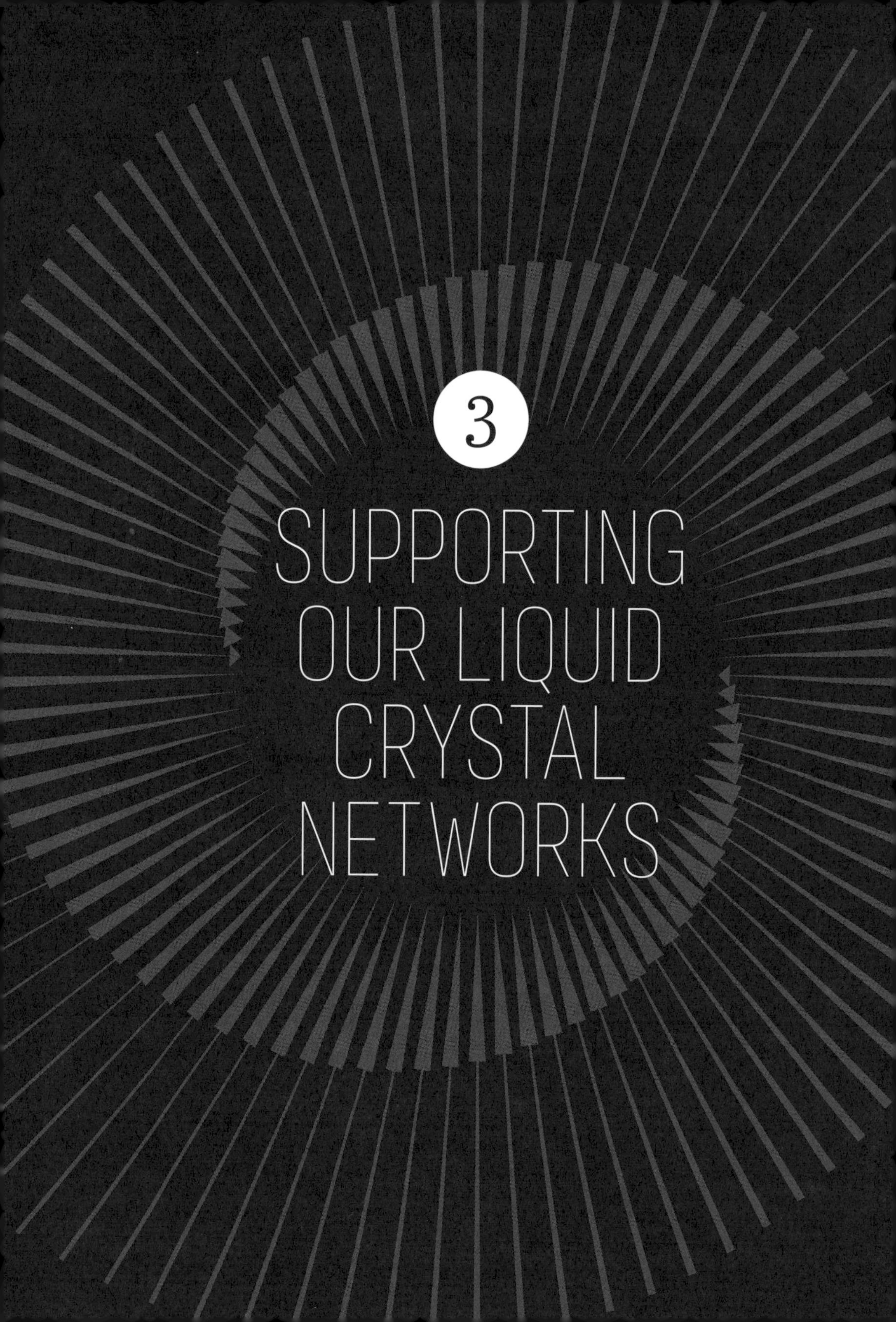

3

SUPPORTING OUR LIQUID CRYSTAL NETWORKS

Certain structures in our body, such as DNA, cell membranes, and fascia, along with the water that lines those structures, have a liquid crystal structure. We are much more than the chemical-mechanical machines we were taught about in school. We are liquid crystal beings. We have the ability to react to the invisible information of light, sound, and the frequency of vibrations around us. Tending to our liquid crystal nature reinforces a mode of communication and function in the body that is not reliant on the chemical model of biology. While working in tandem with the chemical model, it is faster and more efficient at communicating and transmitting energy. Our liquid crystal nature has a powerful influence on our health and longevity. It gives the body a mode of interaction and energy transfer that is more proficient at supporting health than the chemical model alone.

LIQUID CRYSTALS

Liquid crystals are in a mesophase between a liquid and a solid. Liquid crystals are aligned and ordered with the ability to respond to electrical currents or fields of energy. All of the molecules in a liquid crystal are organized and when exposed to light, electrical currents, or magnetic fields, change direction as a cohesive group, much like a wave in the ocean made up of individual water molecules yet acting in one coherent wave motion.

You might not be familiar with the term *liquid crystal*, but liquid crystal technology is something most of us use daily. The screens on our computers, smartphones, and televisions all utilize liquid crystal technology. Each of these screens has a thin liquid crystal component that covers the screen. As the liquid crystal component is exposed to an electrical stimulus, the organized molecules all react as a collective. Like synchronized swimmers moving to the same music, the molecules rearrange as a unified collective group. This lets in a different arrangement of light and creates the beautiful imagery we see on the screen.

Liquid crystals can engage precisely with a variety of frequencies, including light, heat, pressure, sound, electricity, biophotons, magnetism, and electromagnetic field waves. This is what makes them the perfect technology for our TV, computer, and smartphone screen.

That same mechanism allows our liquid crystalline DNA, cell membranes, and fascia within us to act as a network, communicating and responding as a collective. The liquid crystalline water lining our organelles, cells, and vessels can act as a conduit for quantum information. It allows for the capture, storage, and movement of vibration, electrons, protons, vibrations of sound, and photons of light. This mode of efficient communication and rapid source of energy is foundational to our health and longevity. Without it, biology would be stuck in the slower time scale of chemical diffusion or random collision.

Marcel Vogel was an IBM scientist who worked on the liquid crystal displays in use in today's technology. Vogel hypothesized that crystals, particularly quartz crystal, could store and direct subtle energy, promoting healing and energetic coherence. His experiments explored how focused intent amplified through crystals could improve plant health, change water structure, and foster a connection with humans for better health.

Within the world, there are a variety of forces that comprise the field of physics. The interaction between electricity and magnetism is at play in all these forces except for gravity (as far as we know). Electromechanical forces arise due to the interaction between electromagnetic fields and solid, elastic structures or rigid bodies. Solid objects, like the proteins within our body, can experience these forces and change shape, activating biological switches in the immune system or inflammatory pathway, for example. Forces like the electrostatic and the magnetostatic forces that exist between electrical charges at rest or the underlying magnetic field are constantly at play. The piezoelectric and piezoresistive forces describe how certain materials, like our fascia, can be deformed with pressure and accumulate electrical charge as a result.

BIOLOGICAL LIQUID CRYSTALS

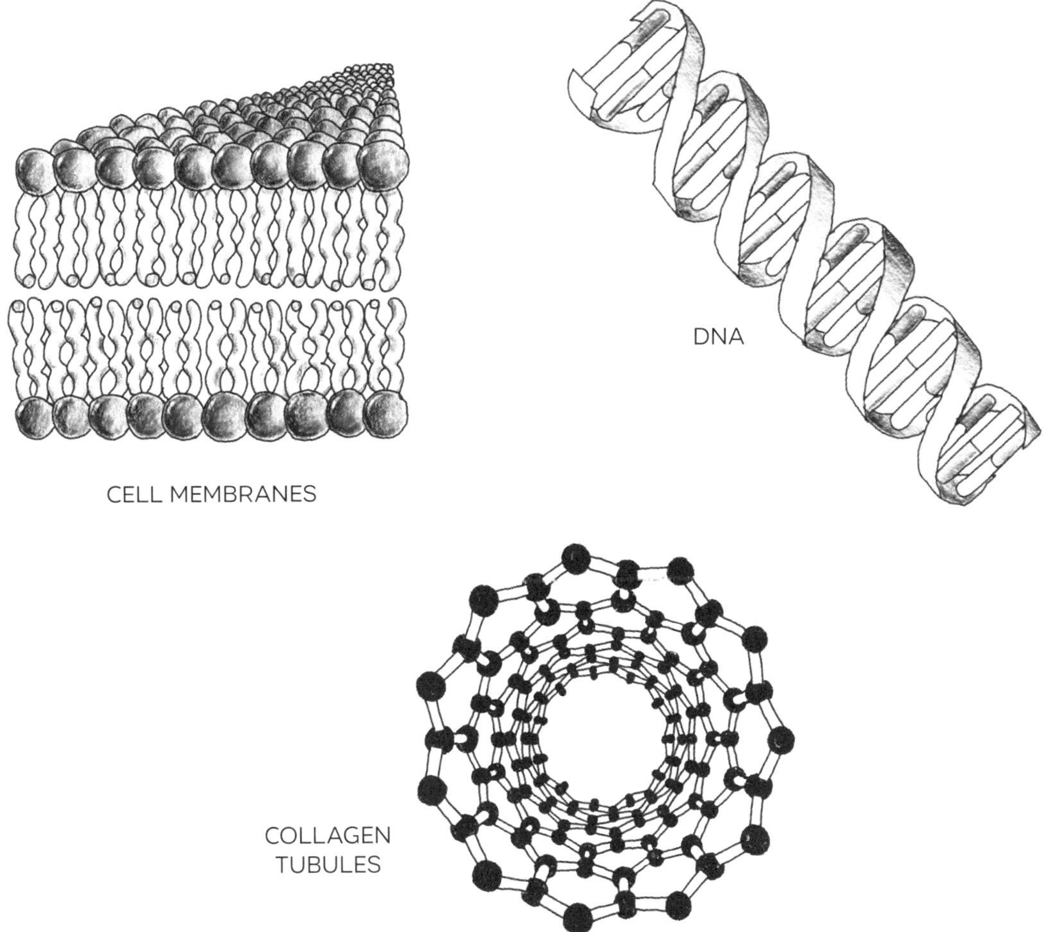

DNA, cell membranes, and the collagen tubules of fascia are all liquid crystal in nature. The molecules within them are organized and aligned, in a mesophase between a solid and a liquid.

The physical structures within us are constantly exposed to a sea of varying forces and changing charges while at the same time emitting their own forces. When we talk about forces, we often use individual examples and forget that we live in an ocean of charge, a sea of forces, a tide of frequencies. These invisible forces guide life as we know it. They lay the foundation for a quantum biological approach to wellness and longevity. Tending to the structures that conduct these forces allows for a much faster form of communication in the body than from chemical signals. This can allow for rapid cell signaling, healing, the maintenance of health, and thus longevity.

When looking at structures in the body, we find that DNA, cell membranes, fascia, and the water that lines them all have liquid crystal properties. This is important because liquid crystal formations are sensitive to vibrations. They are sensitive to the frequency information we have been talking about. This is where quantum biological action takes place. These liquid crystal structures have a crucial role in electrical and resonant cellular communication. They assist the flow of energy and information while supporting stability in DNA, cell membranes, and fascia.

Fascia, cell membranes, DNA, and microtubules all contain benzene rings that can capture frequency information. When excited by a vibration, the pi electrons in the benzene ring are free to move around the molecule and even relocate to other molecules. They are not tightly bound to the molecule as would normally occur with electrons. This represents a mode of energy and information transfer that does not depend on direct physical contact or chemical action. It is a language of frequency that has the potential to initiate biological activity such as enzymatic reactions, immune cascades, hormone signaling, and cellular function. Even quartz crystals have six-sided rings in their silicon lattice, pointing back to Marcel Vogel's ideas on crystal formation and the transfer of healing energy.

Aging and disease are associated with damaged DNA and a decrease in the liquid crystal capacity of cell membranes. Damaged DNA is correlated with disease of all kinds. A disruption in the bioelectrical conductivity and increase in the stiffness of fascial collagen has also been associated with aging. From a quantum biology perspective, a decrease in the ability to vibrate, to resonate, will impair the ability to transfer information and energy. This disrupts the physical, chemical, and electrical environment needed for proper cellular signaling, which impairs the immune, hormonal, and nervous systems. A youthful cell, in contrast, can maintain cell communication, fostering a robust immune system and a balanced nervous system. This makes nourishing the liquid crystal structures in the body a top priority for good health.

RAINBOW LIQUID CRYSTALS

Biophysicist Mae-Wan Ho made an astonishing discovery about biology. She was studying a fruit fly larva with a polarized light microscope, which is used to look at nonliving liquid crystals. But this was a living larva, and it was displaying the same brilliant rainbow interference colors of a liquid crystal. The only way that was possible was if the molecules in the living worm were aligned like a liquid crystal and moved together coherently. That was something completely unheard of in biology.

Ho soon discovered that living cells and life forms display this liquid crystal organization under a polarized light microscope, as did the water lining them. This was an incredible discovery that highlights how the body can respond to signals of light, electromagnetic fields, and the biofield, not just chemical and mechanical inputs. It explains how we can utilize the energy and data of vibration.

Mae-Wan Ho contributed an important understanding of biology. She proposed that energy flows coherently through the body by way of liquid crystal structures and the liquid crystalline water that lines them. This exemplifies the quantum coherence needed to have fast, efficient, and long-range vibrational communication in the body. This well-organized system is what allows quantum biology to occur, resulting in an effectual system in the body able to respond rapidly to healing interventions to support overall health and vitality.

From her research, Ho suggested that the liquid crystalline state of biological structures is highly organized yet flexible. This allows for coherent electrical and vibrational energy transfer, meaning that energy can travel in an organized and efficient way. This provides a faster mode of energy transfer than chemical diffusion, making interventions that utilize liquid crystalline structures more efficient at supporting health, vitality, and longevity. She also proposed that communication within living cells and the water that lines them can be stored and transmitted because of their liquid crystal nature, like electrical capacitators. Capacitators can store electrical charge for use when needed. Cell membranes and their liquid crystalline structure act as electrical capacitators, storing charge until needed.

When studying biology in a Petri dish, we miss out on the vital aspects of life. What a paradox that we remove anything living to study life. Ho's use of the polarized light microscope on living organisms brings a completely new understanding of what it means to be alive. Liquid crystals work with frequencies, not chemicals. This means there is a *language of frequency* in living systems that is separate from the chemical model of life.

It's a revolutionary perspective that changes our understanding of life and well-being, extending it beyond only chemical-mechanical controls and into the influences of vibration, energy, and resonance. It gives us an expanded perspective of the body with new tools for healing that shouldn't be ignored.

A LANGUAGE OF FREQUENCY

Irena Cosic and colleagues have put forward the Resonant Recognition Model (RRM), which proposes that proteins, biomolecules, and specifically the water that lines them can vibrate at frequencies that can travel long distances in the body. These proteins can communicate and interact through electromagnetic fields. These vibrations serve as nonlocal resonant communication signals that travel much faster and more efficiently than chemical signaling.

Traditional biochemistry explains that proteins interact through direct physical contact. The Resonant Recognition Model proposes that proteins can recognize each other and communicate at a distance via electromagnetic resonance. Like two tuning forks tuned to the same frequency—when one plays a note the other also sings that same note, even if separated by distance. This allows for a transfer of energy, information, and function. Separate research demonstrates how light in the spectrums of ultraviolet, visible, and infrared can be used as a form of communication in the body (I talk all about this in chapter 5). The Resonant Recognition Model expands this idea into a wide range of electromagnetic frequencies that are also used for communication.

The Resonant Recognition Model uses mathematical modeling to demonstrate the feasibility of a language and communication of resonance in the body. It has been explored for peptide-based drugs and identifying cancer biomarkers. Recent experimental measurements found that biomolecular recognition can occur over distances through resonant electrodynamic intermolecular forces. Simply put, biomolecules can recognize and communicate via electromagnetic energy transfer. Each observed protein interaction and function can be associated with a specific frequency, forming a language of resonance and frequency in the body.

In a study of the Resonant Recognition Model, peptides were synthesized based on their resonant frequencies. Antibodies are proteins produced by the immune system that recognize and bind to other proteins called *antigens*. These are recognized and predictable reactions that happen throughout the body at all times. Researchers began with a known antigen protein that had a well-defined biological function and that triggered a predictable immune response. Then, the dominant vibrational frequency peaks were detected and a resonant frequency of the antigen was identified. Researchers then designed a new, short peptide with the purpose of emitting the same resonant frequency as the antigen protein. The new peptide with the original antigen's resonant frequency was exposed to antibodies. The peptide bonded to the antibody, just like the antigen protein would have.

This was a huge discovery. The peptide was made with the purpose of emitting a specific resonant vibration. The peptide stimulated action with the antibody as if the peptide was the antigen, even though it did not have the same shape or composition. But it wasn't dependent on direct contact or molecular shape. It was a recognition and interaction of resonant frequency, bringing more validation to the Resonant Recognition Model.

The Resonant Recognition Model explains a new view of the body where direct chemical or physical contact is not the only way for action to happen in the body. In a body with trillions and trillions of cells that are completing hundreds of thousands of tasks each second, we need a better explanation of how biology works than the random collision or chemical diffusion models. The Resonant Recognition Model gives that explanation: The body also uses frequency to recognize, communicate, and trigger action. And by supporting the structures that allow for this type of communication and energy transfer, we have powerful tools for health and longevity that are currently not being addressed in conventional medicine.

LIQUID CRYSTAL DNA

DNA and the water bound to it are liquid crystalline, making DNA sensitive to information in vibration of light, sound, and fields of energy. DNA's double helix is formed by two coiling, negatively charged backbones. These backbones hold between them positively charged base pairs that make up the internal ladder of the helix. The ladder rungs comprise two nucleotide pairs that fit together like puzzle pieces. Protons are able to quantum tunnel between rungs of the base pair ladder. Proton tunneling has been proposed to play a role in DNA mutation and replication.

DNA emits light in the form of biophotons. It also emits longitudinal waves in the form of magnetic scalar waves from the vibration of DNA. Longitudinal waves are produced by vibrations in a medium. They hold information and can pass through all four phases of matter: liquid, solid, plasma, and gas. Some research suggests DNA displays characteristics of a molecular quantum wire, allowing for coherent charge transfer. This long-range charge transfer is vital for biological processes such as gene expression, repair mechanisms, and replication, which are foundational for overall health and well-being in aging. This long-range energy transfer and the liquid crystalline state of DNA are essential to these crucial biological functions.

DNA contains benzene rings that have pi electrons, or free electrons, that can delocalize, meaning the electrons are not tightly bound to the molecule and can move around and even be donated to other molecules. This can be a source of energy in the body as well as a source of biological communication that coordinates action in the body. DNA and proteins can resonate at specific frequencies, permitting long-range coherent energy signaling that is much faster than the Newtonian model provides for. Rather than casting dye into water and waiting for it to spread or randomly knocking on doors to find the right address, resonant communication is more like two tuning forks—where when one is struck, the second begins to ring out in that same tune, or frequency, transferring energy and instructional information.

The entire DNA structure is completely surrounded by a layer of crystalline water. This layer of water allows for quantum coherence, proton tunneling, energy storage, and a communication network of vibrational resonance. Water surrounding DNA has been proposed as the facilitator for energy waves of phonons to travel across DNA with little resistance, akin to a semiconductor. Because both DNA and the water that lines it are organized like liquid crystals, rapid signaling can occur, which offers both a new understanding of biology and new ways to support it. Supporting the liquid crystalline nature of DNA and the water that envelops it provides a powerful way to aid overall health and vitality.

Supporting DNA's health is paramount to its liquid crystal and quantum biological properties. Maintaining cell-bound water and proper lipid composition helps support the liquid crystalline state of DNA. Polyphenols found in richly colored fruits and vegetables or compounds like resveratrol and quercetin activate the protein SIRT1, which promotes stability and integrity in DNA. Telomeres are the protective ends of the chromosomes in DNA. The shortening of telomeres is associated with accelerated aging. Omega-3 fatty acids from seafood, such as fish, fish roe, and algae, lower inflammation, which reduces the rapid aging associated with telomere shortening.

Making sure mitochondria are working efficiently promotes healthy autophagy, the natural process of breaking down and removing damaged cells, which supports DNA integrity. We explore this in depth in the next chapter. Optimizing circadian rhythm encourages circadian DNA repair cycles. Grounding, coming in direct contact with the electrical charge of Earth, can help reduce inflammation, thereby stabilizing the liquid crystalline structure of DNA. Tending to the liquid crystalline water battery within us also has the potential to enhance DNA stability and conduction.

Minimizing nonnative electromagnetic frequencies, like Wi-Fi, that have been proposed to increase DNA mutations via increased proton tunneling, can also support DNA health.

Our DNA's liquid crystal structure can pick up on the invisible frequencies of the electromagnetic field. Steer clear as best as possible of insecticides, herbicides, pesticides, plasticizers, heavy metals, processed food, excessive alcohol, smoking, and endocrine-disrupting chemicals that can lead to mutations and accelerated aging. Even social and psychological stress can damage the liquid crystal properties of DNA. Stress management and meditation help protect telomere length and the liquid crystal structure of DNA.

LIQUID CRYSTALLINE MEMBRANES

The cell membrane is made of two layers of fats in its bilipid membrane. This membrane is 10,000 times thinner than the width of a human hair and consists of two layers of phospholipids, which have a hydrophilic (water-loving) phosphate group head and two hydrophobic (water-fearing) fatty tails. These phospholipids arrange themselves with the phosphate heads on the outside of either side of the cell membrane and the water-fearing fatty tails meeting in the middle of the membrane.

In the cell membrane, the phospholipid heads create a structural barrier while the tails create a fluid yet organized structure that gives the membrane a liquid crystal quality. They align in a certain order and can be influenced by fields of energy—magnetic and electric—to align in a different order. They can also help regulate electron and proton tunneling, maintaining critical electrochemical gradients. This liquid crystalline arrangement also allows structured water to form on the outside and inside of the membrane. Both the cell's liquid crystal structure and the liquid crystalline water that lines it are major players in the ability of the body to communicate with resonance. Again, the ability of resonance to stimulate biological action brings us a new understanding of the body as well as offering new tools for health and longevity. It's a revolutionary new way to support the body that has effects on immune system health, nervous system balance, and hormonal homeostasis.

Cell membranes have an important role in our health. They must be fluid, able to flex and bend while at the same time maintaining integrity and strength. Although phospholipids account for half of the mass of the cell membrane, cholesterol, sphingomyelin, and proteins also make up the cell membrane. Lipids influence the fluid qualities of the membrane, cell signaling, and cell recognition. Cholesterol helps regulate the rigidity of membranes, maintaining the organization of proteins within the membrane, which dramatically affects cellular and mitochondrial function. If membranes are missing these lipids or they are oxidized or replaced with processed trans-fat, the liquid crystal capacity falters, and communication and energy transfer collapses.

Adequate levels of phospholipids are associated with liver, brain, cardiovascular, mitochondrial, and gastrointestinal health. As phospholipids decline with age, there is a correlation with decreased liver and mitochondrial function, memory issues, Alzheimer's disease, and metabolic syndromes such as obesity and insulin resistance. The cell membrane's liquid crystal function depends on phospholipid content in the architecture of the membrane.

Phosphatidylcholine is the major phospholipid that makes up about half of the cell membrane. Phosphatidylcholine's headgroup is made from choline, which is not synthesized by the body. Choline is found in organ meat like liver and kidney, egg yolks, fish, fish roe, beef, chicken, turkey, cottage cheese, shiitake mushrooms, wheat germ, and cruciferous vegetables like broccoli and brussels sprouts. Phosphatidylcholine can integrate into the cell and repair damage while helping preserve membrane fluidity and integrity. Antioxidant-rich food and polyphenols can protect the cell membrane from damage.

Cardiolipin is found almost exclusively in the mitochondrion's inner membrane where the electron transport chain is located. Mitochondria are the cell's powerhouses, creating the energy currency of the body, ATP. A decrease in mitochondrial function has been associated with aging, disease, and almost every modern disease out there. Having a fluid, yet strong, inner mitochondrial membrane allows the electrons to quantum tunnel through the electron transport chain and create heat, water, and ATP.

Omega-6 fatty acids, such as those found in unprocessed sunflower, safflower, hemp, chia, pumpkin, walnuts, and sesame seeds as well as soy and avocados, help protect the cell membrane and the inner mitochondrial membrane. Cold exposure has also been found to reinforce the amount of cardiolipin in the inner mitochondrial membrane. C15 fatty acids, found in full-fat dairy and fish, embed into the membrane phospholipids and support resilience.

Earthing, or grounding, has shown promise in supporting the cell membrane. Research has found that grounding could help maintain membrane integrity, which is vital for cell membrane health and function. Other research has found that earthing can bolster the membrane electrical potential, possibly affecting membrane fluidity and function. Earthing has also been shown to decrease inflammation, which is another avenue of possible protection against damage to the cell membrane.

QUANTUM FASCIA

Fascia is another liquid crystal structure in our body. Fascia is the thin white layer we removed during cadaver lab in naturopathic medical school to study an organ, or the thin white layer that many peel away from a chicken breast when cooking. It has been considered the scaffolding of the body but nothing more than that.

Are Omega-6 Fatty Acids Bad for Us?

There is a lot of discussion on whether omega-6 fatty acids are bad for us. There is little doubt that industrialized seed oils or the heavily processed seed oils we see in ultra-processed foods are not good for us. They contain trace amounts of the solvents, like hexane, that are used to extract the oil from the seed or grain. Seed oils are usually processed using high heat and pressure, leaving them oxidized, which can lead to inflammation when consumed. Unfortunately, omega-6 fatty acids have become synonymous with processed foods, and this is where most people get omega-6 fatty acids in their diet.

But omega-6 fatty acids are essential. Our mitochondria rely on natural forms of omega-6 fatty acids to function properly, and we know how important mitochondria are. Research has shown that higher linoleic acid intake, the most common omega-6 fatty acid, is associated with reduced rates of heart attacks and cardiovascular diseases. Omega-6 fatty acids help maintain healthy cell membranes, which are foundational to overall health. Linoleic acid is converted into gamma-linoleic acid that seems to help with inflammation.

Healthy omega-6 fatty acids are found in almonds, avocado, eggs, soybeans, sunflower seeds, and walnuts. Nutrients such as magnesium, vitamins B3, B6, and C, and zinc help convert omega-6 fatty acids in the body into their anti-inflammatory forms. What we really want is a diet rich in whole, real foods and low in toxin-laden processed foods. A diet with quality fats of all kinds—polyunsaturated fats like omega-3, -6, and -9 as well as monosaturated fats like avocado and olive oil and saturated fat from quality sources of organic, grass-fed/pasture-raised meat, butter, ghee, and quality dairy if tolerated—promotes healthy DNA, cell membranes, and fascia.

There is a new understanding of fascia starting to emerge. Fascia is essential for living a healthy long life. It helps facilitate movement throughout the body, which becomes increasingly important as we age. Fascia creates a bodywide network, connecting to every structure in our body. It is as if our bones are a loom and the fascia is the fabric, fashioning an all-encompassing, intertwined tapestry of the body. This interconnected web of fascia builds a quantum communication network of energy and information in the body.

Fascia is an important energy source and information highway in the body. It's intimately connected with the immune system, the lymphatic detoxification system, and in powering the muscular system. Dysfunctional fascia is associated with aging, nervous system dysregulation, and pathologies such as cancer and immune system imbalance. Supporting our fascial network is imperative to our health and longevity.

Fascia is made up of mostly connective tissue, which is mainly collagen. This collagen network starts at the most external layers of our skin and extends to the most internal parts of our anatomy. Our bones are covered in fascia. Collagen is a semiconductor of energy, meaning this collagen fascial network has the capacity to receive, store, and transmit electrical energy. Fascia can even transfer information into the cell's cytoskeleton via transmembrane receptors called *integrins*. Integrins take the vibratory information that the fascia holds and brings it into the environment of the cell. This creates a quantum communication network and energy reserve made of fascia that spans the entire body—from the bigger structures to the individual cell.

Fascia is produced by fibroblast cells, which are densely packed with mitochondria. The integrins that connect fascia to the intercellular environment have been found to affect mitochondrial function. Both the mitochondrial membrane potential that powers the assembly of ATP and the production of reactive oxygen species from the mitochondria that serve as messengers are influenced by the action of the integrins. This creates a continuum from the extracellular matrix and fascia into the cell and mitochondria. What an incredible interconnected web of communication fascia produces, allowing for a seamless transfer of information throughout the body. Research has found that myofascial trigger points, areas in the fascia that are irritated and painful, might be linked to mitochondrial dysfunction. Tending to mitochondrial function like we talk about in the next chapter is an important piece of caring for the fascia.

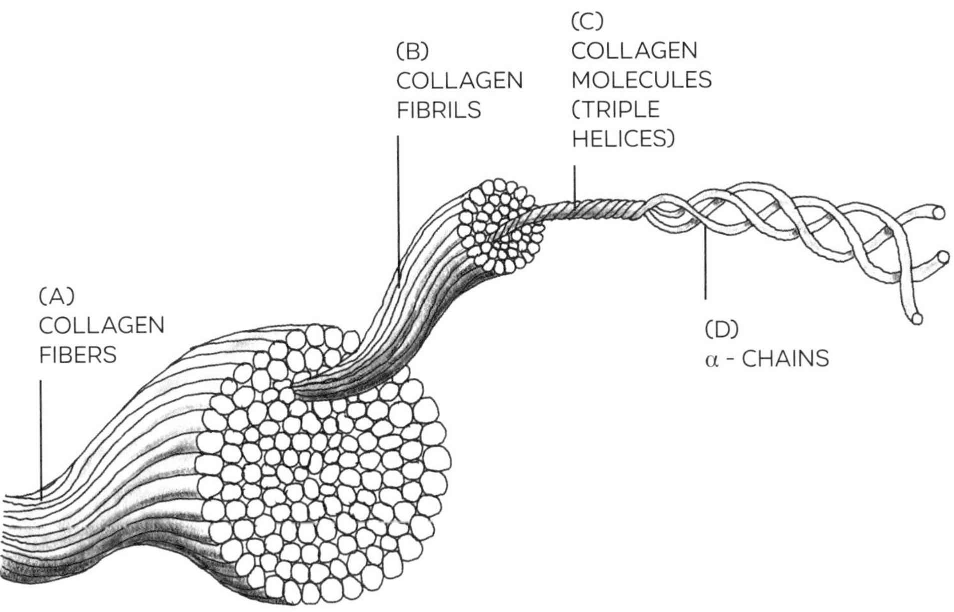

The collagen in fascia forms tropocollagen nanotubules, which come together to form fibrils, which then form the fibers of fascia.

Fibroblasts also have a close relationship with the immune system, nervous system, and mitochondria. Recent research has found that the fascia system directly recruits and directs lymphatic cells, acting as a conductor of the immune system. Macrophages, cardinal players of the immune system, together with fibroblasts direct the deposition of new collagen. Our immune system directly affects our state of wellness and vitality by keeping inflammation at bay while maintaining a healthy interaction with the microbes and toxins we encounter.

Fascia, Pain, and Emotions

We know how important emotional and mental health are to our overall wellness. Fascia has been posited as the receiver and container of emotion and trauma—it's all connected. With the potential to absorb and store emotional trauma, our fascia can act both as an obstacle in healing trauma and as a gateway to releasing trauma. Bodyworkers have long reported a link between the fascia and emotions. Science now seems to be adding some validation to this idea.

Fascia can be thought of as our largest sensory organ. Fascia is abundantly innervated with more than 250 million nerve endings. It has significantly more sensory nerves than motor neurons. There are 25 percent more nerve endings in fascia than skin, and 1,000 percent more than muscle. Fascia contains sensory nerve endings, including nociceptors, or pain receptors. These pain receptors can release substance P in response to mechanical stress, injury, or chronic tension. Substance P is a neuropeptide that plays a central role in pain perception, inflammation, and emotional processing. Substance P increases inflammation and pain sensitivity, which has been shown to lead to fascial stiffness or discomfort.

Substance P mediates the intersection of emotional stress, pain, and fascial tension. Emotional stress triggers the release of substance P, which can interact with brain regions involved in emotional processing, such as the amygdala and hypothalamus. Prolonged stress and anxiety increase the levels of substance P, which can potentially cause chronic muscle pain and tightness and stiffness of the fascia. Higher levels of substance P are found in individuals with depression, post-traumatic stress disorder (PTSD), and anxiety, suggesting a direct link between emotional distress and bodily pain. Reducing its activity through relaxation techniques, movement, fascial release, and therapy can help alleviate physical, mental, and emotional upset.

Research continues to make a connection between emotions and fascia. Adhered dysfunctional fascia that is stuck together and cannot move effectively has been associated with pain and depression. In a study analyzing patients who had major depressive disorder and examining fascia health, individuals exhibited adhered, stiff, and reduced elasticity in the fascia of the neck and trapezius muscle compared to nondepressed participants, suggesting a link between adhered, stuck fascia and depression. In other research, fascial maneuvers that release adhered fascia have been found to decrease feelings of anxiety and depression.

Different research found that fascial release could activate Ruffini mechanoreceptors, which communicate directly with the nervous system. This can improve heart rate variability, soothe the nervous system, and promote a parasympathetic response, the response needed for cellular healing. Again, there appears to be a connection with fascia, our emotions, and the state of the nervous system. What an extraordinary understanding of how the body connects with emotions. By simply tending to the fascia with hydration and fascial maneuvers or release, we open a powerful window into releasing trauma and negative emotions.

In a fascinating study with fascial maneuvers, researchers looked at a group of overworked and stressed-out workers in the fashion industry. They divided the group into two. They asked one group to simply rest and relax. The other group received a fascial release to the occipital area, at the base of the skull. The people in the group who received the fascial release had a marked improvement in heart rate variability. Higher heart rate variability has been associated with better health, a longer life, and a more resilient nervous system. This is another incredible example of the connection between our fascia and our nervous system.

Fascia as an Antenna

Fascia also has remarkable properties that illustrate why it is an important piece of our quantum terrain. Fascia is piezoelectric, like a quartz crystal. When a quartz crystal is exposed to pressure, it creates an electrical current. Fascia does the same thing. When deformed by the pressure of movement, such as exercise and stretching, or by manual bodywork such as massage and fascial release, fascia generates an electrical current. This electrical current also produces infrared energy, the same energy needed to build liquid crystalline water.

Fascia is circadian in nature. The laying down of new fascia, the hydration of fascia, and the scavenging and repair of damaged fascia are all connected to the rhythm of the sun. Fascia has been found to produce biophotons, the light that our cells emit. Fibroblasts in fascia have been shown to emit and respond to biophotons. Emerging research shows that fascia can reflect, transmit, and even guide near infrared light, like fiber optic cables. Biophotons from fascia follow not only a circadian rhythm but also a seasonal rhythm. Researchers postulate that biophotons are a form of communication, and this extends to fascia. Both melatonin and circadian cycles influence biophoton emissions in fascia, which may affect how the fascia stores and releases energy throughout a twenty-four-hour cycle.

Fascia creates and communicates with light and electricity as well as sound. Recently discovered fasciacytes (cells within the fascia) are involved in shearing actions and sounds. The sound from the shearing and gliding provides valuable information about the environment and health of the fascia.

Fascia not only makes sounds, but also responds to sounds. A review by Dr. Bruno Bordoni, a researcher, physiotherapist, and osteopathic physician, and his colleagues suggests that the shearing sounds of fascia along with the biphotonic light that fascia emits form a communication network that extends past a chemical model. Different research proposes that sound can increase flow pressure through the fascia. The vibratory oscillations of sound can trigger the release of hyaluronic acid, increasing water in the area and increasing the flow of fascia.

Fascia participates in an intimate dance with water. Recent research found that dehydrated fascia dramatically increases the tensile stress within it, inhibiting its ability to glide. Adhered and dehydrated fascia does not make the same sound as hydrated fascia. Dehydrated fascia is not an effective conduit of energy and sound. It's much less conductive of electrons, electricity, and these regenerative bioelectric signals. Hydrating the fascial network is paramount to health and biological communication—and it's not just drinking water that hydrates fascia. The hyaluronic acid found in fascia helps with hydration as well.

Hyaluronic acid is secreted by the fibroblast cells in fascia. Hyaluronic acid has a full hydration shell of water, meaning that a molecule of hyaluronic acid is completely surrounded by a shell of liquid crystalline water. Recent research found that the structured liquid crystalline water layers on one molecule of hyaluronic acid can extend up to 1,600 water molecules. When the fascia is exposed to pressure from movement, massage, stretching, or manual therapy, it releases hyaluronic acid. This release of hyaluronic acid brings fresh liquid crystalline water and hydration to the collagen within fascia. It is strange to think of movement as hydration, but it's true!

Helene Langevin, famed fascia researcher and director of the National Center for Complementary and Integrative Health (NCCIH) at the National Institutes of Health (NIH), has found that adhered fascia creates chronic inflammatory conditions. Her research shows that gentle stretching of fascia can hydrate it and decrease the growth of breast cancer tumors. Langevin took mice that had tumors and put them through a process of daily stretching. The arms of the mice held on to a bar as they were gently stretched, creating a line of extension through the arms and chest. The group that received daily stretching reduced tumor growth by 52 percent compared to the control group.

Previous research found that stretching just ten minutes a day twice a day decreases connective tissue inflammation and fibrosis. Gentle stretching is a potent way to support our fascial health and hydration. This influences the ability of our fascial network to generate energy and serve as a communication network in the body.

We also have a large fascial pad on the bottom of our feet. James Oschman has done amazing research on earthing. Oschman posits that when we place our bare feet on the Earth, the fascial pad on the bottom of the foot and the water that lines it can capture electrons that line the Earth and conduct them where needed in the body. This would make both maintaining the liquid crystalline water in fascia and earthing powerful ways to support our fascial network.

Fascia as a Quantum Highway

Now we have a better understanding of fascia, that liquid crystal network that connects to every structure in the body. This network is semiconductive and piezoelectric, able to create and transmit electricity. It is intimately connected with the function of the nervous system, immune system, and mitochondria. But there's more.

The collagen within fascia forms specialized small tubules. We are accustomed to visualizing the double helix of DNA, but collagen creates a triple helix tubule. These tubules are called *tropocollagen nanotubules*, meaning they are so small they register on the nanoscale. We have a bodywide network of collagen tubules that are so small they can facilitate quantum phenomena.

Those nanoscale-size tubules of collagen that make up our fascial network have different properties than larger tubules that researchers call *confined space thermodynamics*. Nobel Laureate Albert Szent-Györgi proposed that electrons in confined spaces were free to flow; they are not readily bound to their molecules as they normally are. The tubes of collagen in fascia create confined spaces. Szent-Györgi found that electrons within crystalline networks like connective tissue are free to migrate. Electrons are not bound to the orbit of one single atom as we would assume but can move throughout the fascial network. So, movement in the fascial network creates electrons that can flow, bringing energy and information throughout the body.

Mae-Wan Ho put forth the idea that the thermodynamics of collagen tubules epitomize quantum coherence in living systems. She illustrated how our collagen network possesses the quantum property of semiconduction, allowing for the transfer of protons throughout the body. Current research on the proton wires that form adjacent to liquid crystalline water and proton conduction show precisely this. These wires can conduct protons at incredibly fast speeds for incredibly long distances. Nassim Haramein, physicist and head researcher at the International Space Federation, has shown that a proton can hold a vast amount of information, making these tubes of fascia an ideal mode of information transfer.

Remember Gerald Pollack's research on water and water-loving Nafion tubules (see page 33). Pollack and his team furthered this research by looking at collagen tubes, similar to the collagen tubes we have connecting every structure in the body. He placed a molded collagen tube in a container of water, mimicking the aqueous environment of the human body. Then, Pollack exposed the collagen immersed in water to infrared light. What he saw was truly astonishing.

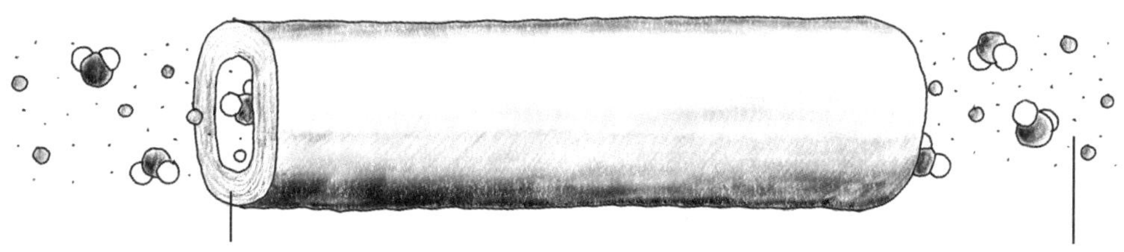

Example of a tube of fascial collagen creating a potential water battery that propels water, particles, and protons through the collagen tube.

Pollack observed EZ structured water form on the inside of the collagen tubule. Then, he saw that liquid crystalline water formed on the inside of the collagen tubule. This interior liquid crystalline water created the water battery we discussed in the previous chapter. Not only did the negatively charged EZ water and the positively charged water form, but it also powered a propulsion of water through the collagen tubule, driving the flow of water, of particles and of protons. There was no outside force driving the flow; seemingly it was just the liquid crystalline water battery and infrared energy that provided the force.

We are accustomed to thinking about the flow of electrons as energy. We plug our appliances and devices into the electrical outlet and the movement of electrons creates the electricity that powers our devices. It also produces fields of energy that can transmit energy to whatever is within that vicinity. Protons also create energy. Protons are quantum particles that create energy when in flow. They also can hold a surprising amount of information. Our fascia is a conduit of flowing protons that hold energy and information that travels via quantum mechanics throughout the body.

When we move, we create a piezoelectric charge in our tropocollagen tubules. This electrical charge produces infrared energy, which could further build the water conduction through the nanospaces of collagen that extend throughout our fascial network. This water battery within the semiconductive collagen tubes can produce a reservoir of electrical energy—a flow of energy and information from the movement of protons as well as a reservoir of electrons, both of which can potentially be directed to where there is an energy deficiency in the body. Remember, there is a way to look at the body where pain, inflammation, and disease are an energy deficiency, a deficiency in electrons. Fascia and the water that lines it can create a reservoir of free electrons that can help reduce this energy deficiency and improve symptoms.

Fascinating connections have also been made between our fascia, the meridian system, or energy flow throughout the body, and the biofield. The meridian system is the body-wide network of energy that acupuncture and acupressure utilize. From a quantum biological perspective, our fascia is more than scaffolding; it creates a vast system that communicates via light, sound, and electricity. Fascia connects into cells within our body. It covers every organ, every nerve, every structure. It not only covers these structures, but it also runs throughout these structures. Fascia runs through our nervous system and neurological network. It is inserted into the cytoskeleton of our cells, making fascia the largest, most extensive connective network in the human body.

Interesting research has made an association between the fascia and the meridians used in Chinese medicine. In the 1960s, Dr. Bong Han Kim discovered the primo vascular system. This vessel system is distinct from the blood and lymphatic vessels, and it flows throughout the fascial network. Convincing evidence suggests that the meridian system corresponds to the fascial network, or the primo vascular system, or both. While more research is needed, it's fascinating to think that fascia, with its liquid crystal structure, could act as an antenna for frequency information and energy described by meridians and acupuncture.

Recent research discovered that the electrical impedance on the skin was lower at acupuncture spots, meaning that the mechanical act of deforming the tissue at acupuncture points could transfer energy more readily at these points. Other research points to the association between meridians and biophoton transmission routes. Remember that when fascia is deformed by manual pressure, like that of an acupuncture needle being inserted or an acupressure point being pressed, it could create a piezoelectric charge. And the collagen tubules of fascia could transmit this electrical current. More and more, fascia appears to be the antenna and conduit for frequency energy of all kinds in the body.

TENDING TO YOUR LIQUID CRYSTAL BEING

We now have an astonishing view of the human body—one where liquid crystal structures within the body can act coherently as a collective when exposed to vibration information and energy. Our DNA, cell membranes, fascia, and the liquid crystalline water that lines them can act as an antenna for this frequency information. This creates a network that spans the body, potentially sending energy and information where it is needed in a much faster way than chemical diffusion or random collision. Tending to this liquid crystal matrix is foundational to our health and longevity.

Tend to your water body. The water within is foundational for your ability to capture, store, utilize, and transmit the vibrational information of light, sound, electricity, magnetism, electromagnetism, and fields of energy. Tending to the liquid crystalline water within is vital for the function and health of the liquid crystal structures in the body (see chapter 2 for more on this).

Tend to your liquid crystal DNA. Polyphenols found in richly colored fruits and vegetables or compounds such as resveratrol and quercetin, as well as omega-3 fatty acids, reduce inflammation, which reduces rapid aging associated with telomere shortening. Stress management and meditation also help protect telomere length and the liquid crystal structure of DNA.

Supporting mitochondrial health for optimal DNA function (see chapter 4 for more on this) and tending to mitochondrial function is an important part of maintaining fascial health.

Optimize circadian rhythm and cultivate a routine of grounding to help reduce inflammation and protect DNA.

Avoid electromagnetic frequencies like Wi-Fi when possible, as well as insecticides, herbicides, pesticides, plasticizers, heavy metals, processed food, excessive alcohol, smoking, and endocrine-disrupting chemicals that can lead to DNA mutations and accelerated aging.

Tend to your liquid crystal membranes throughout the body. Eat a diet rich in quality fats, C15 fatty acids, phospholipids and omega-3 fatty acids, to support membrane health. Incorporating choline into the diet helps provide building blocks of phosphatidylcholine, the major constituent of the cell membrane. Consuming omega-6 fatty acids helps protect the cell membrane as well as the inner mitochondrial membrane. Antioxidant-rich foods and polyphenols are excellent ways to protect the membranes. Appropriate cold exposure and grounding daily are wonderful ways to support the electrical capacity and integrity of the liquid crystal cell membrane.

Tend to your fascia. Fascia's liquid crystal properties make it an antenna to frequency information and cultivating an environment of healthy frequencies is a wonderful way to support the health of your fascia. Good nutrition is also a great way to support the fascia. Collagen is the building block of fascia and has been shown to be beneficial to its health and function. Vitamin C is also very important in its ability to support healthy fascia. Aligning your circadian rhythm and getting adequate natural light throughout the day can also support healthy fascia.

Daily movement to hydrate and remove adhesions in the fascia is critical: Walking, gentle exercise, yoga, Qigong, gentle stretching, dance, and movements of all kinds induce a piezoelectrical current and infrared energy in the fascia that potentially builds the liquid crystalline water while signaling the fibroblasts to release hyaluronic acid and, with it, more water. Consider fascial maneuvers, bodywork, and myofascial release to address any areas of fascial adhesion you can't address on your own.

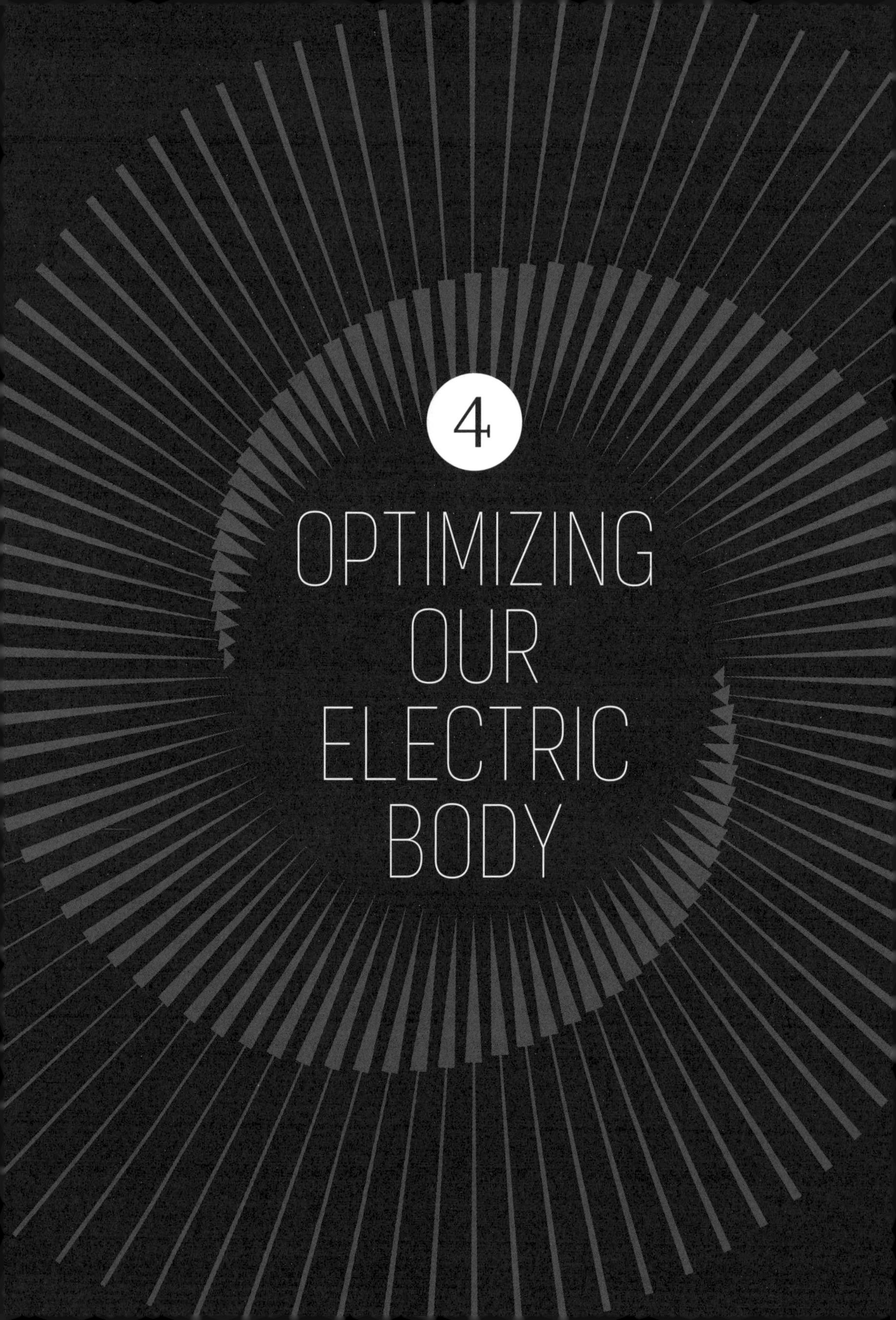

4

OPTIMIZING OUR ELECTRIC BODY

One of the fundamental forces guiding our biology is electricity. We are more than gears in a machine. We are more than the chemical reactions within our body. We are electric beings. We are part of a universal flow of energy that flows in from the universe and through every plant, animal, and human on this planet. These fields of energy excite the smallest pieces of us, giving rise to biological action. This imperceivable current of energy guides everything, including our biology. The flow of electrons, protons, ions, and electromagnetic fields throughout the body can be harnessed for better health. This flow of energy powers a balanced nervous system, healthy cells, a stable hormonal network, and a healthy immune system. Tending to this flow of energy is foundational for health.

Our cells communicate via electricity. When an electrical current moves, it creates an electromagnetic field—a combination of an electric field and a magnetic field. The electromagnetic field of cells can drive biological processes, guiding our immune system, inflammatory state, and hormonal state as well as the function of our vital organs such as the heart, lungs, digestion system, and elimination. Emerging research shows us that our cells are regulated by electromagnetic communication. The cell has its own unique electromagnetic field, and that field regulates the essential physics of cell biology.

Our body runs on electrical charge. Our cells run on a net negative charge. As you read previously, the cell membrane maintains a negative electrical charge of between −40 and −70 millivolts. Our cells use electromagnetic signals to direct migration, behavior, and cell differentiation, whether a cell becomes an ear or an elbow. Our body depends on the electrical flow of electrons through the mitochondria. The same goes for our heart, respiratory, digestive, immune, and nervous systems. The bioelectric view of the body has been established as a guiding force in biology. Although it's rarely talked about, the movement of electrons and protons is vital for our health. Maintaining our electric nature is crucial for our overall wellness and longevity.

There's a way to look at health as a matter of electrical charge. Pain, inflammation, disease, and aging are all conditions that represent a decrease in negative electrical voltage. From a quantum biological perspective, maintaining or reestablishing negative electrical charge has the potential to decrease these ailments and slow aging. The body has an innate electrical grid that can shuttle electrical charge where needed. This grid of electricity consists of proteins, collagen, DNA, fascia, cell membranes, nerves, mitochondria, and the water that surrounds them. The body's electrical grid and the water that lines it can be charged by the unseen vibrations of light, electricity, magnetism, the quantum field, thoughts, and emotions. We truly are electric beings, guided by invisible forces of fields of energy that shape our biology and health.

WHAT IS ELECTRICITY?

There may be some misconceptions about electricity that should be cleared up before advancing. Electricity is often thought of as moving in a physical line, like water in a hose. The electrons travel down a wire until they get to the device being powered, again, like water in a hose bringing hydration to a garden. That's only partly correct.

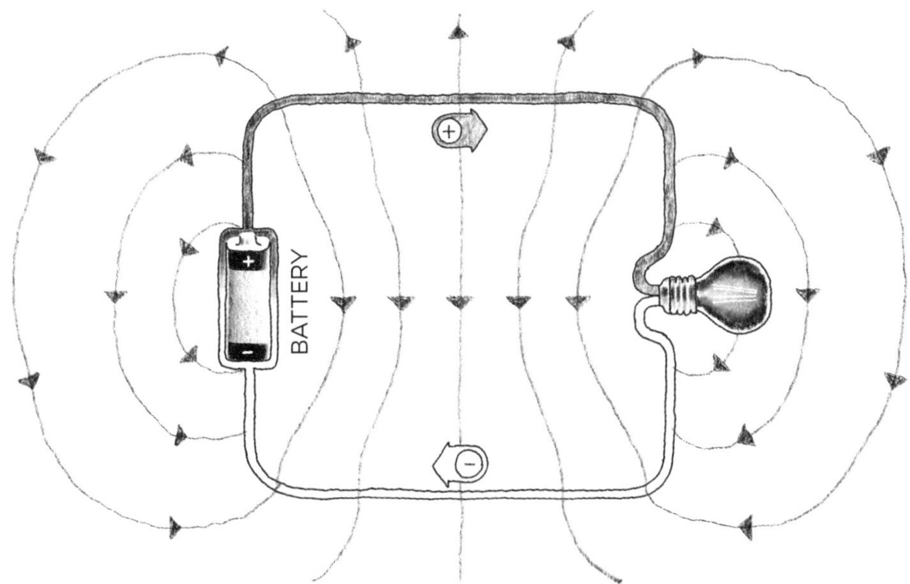

Electrons starting to flow from the battery create excitement in the electrons in the wires that lead to the light bulb. Almost instantaneously, this creates an electromagnetic field that holds the energy that excites the electrons in the light bulb and produces light.

It's not just the electrons that carry energy. It's also the electromagnetic field formed by the movement of electrons that carries energy. The Poynting vector principle describes the concept that the directional flow of electrons in a direct current creates an energy field in the space between the conductors at the speed of light. Using the example of a battery lighting a light bulb through a wire, there is an electromagnetic field created by the battery as well as the wire. The battery begins a flow of electrons that creates an electromagnetic field in the wire. This produces energy that is transferred almost instantaneously to the light bulb. The energy is held in the field, not in the wire.

Biology often describes bioelectricity in the form of ion flow through nerves and tissues. If energy transfer in the body follows the Poynting vector principle, then electrical signals in the body aren't governed solely by the direct flow of ions. Electrical signals also propagate through electromagnetic fields surrounding cells and tissues. This fits with what research has found on nonlocal electromagnetic field communication in cells and proteins.

It could also fit with the idea of liquid crystal cell-bound water, which may allow electromagnetic fields to propagate along the water lining cells and tissues. This water acting as a capacitor, storing electromagnetic energy and releasing it when needed, also aligns with the Poynting vector principle. This explains how liquid crystalline water could transfer rapid, long-range biological signaling. Remember Irena Cosic's Resonant Recognition Model (see page 60). Applying the Poynting vector principle to EZ liquid crystalline water could explain how energy and information transfer happen so quickly and efficiently in this model, which facilitates rapid communication and healing.

THE ELECTRIC BODY

While there is more recognition now, this idea of bioelectricity is not new. Albert Szent-Györgyi pioneered the idea that the body maintained an electrical charge and communication. Szent-Györgi proposed that life is, fundamentally, an electronic process, during which electron flow and electrical charge transfer are vital to biological reactions. He theorized that proteins, like the collagen in fascia, DNA, enzymes, cell membranes, mitochondria, molecules like flavin, and quinones like coenzyme Q10, are all semiconductors. Semiconductors can capture, harness, store, and transmit energy. Szent-Györgi was the first to propose that cancer started with a decrease in electrical charge, a concept that is now gaining evidence. I will focus on how to support the body's electrical charge as a way to influence the decrease in electrical charge being associated with cancer and other illnesses later in this chapter.

Szent-Györgi theorized that the protein chains in collagen and actin conduct electrons, creating an energy source for biological action in the body. That sounds exactly like fascia! These electron donor bridges in the body are essential to the flow of energy. At the time, the world was enamored with a chemical view of biology and Szent-Györgyi's ideas about bioelectricity did not gain traction. We now know that collagen, cell membranes, flavins, proteins, and enzymes can act as semiconductors. Electrons in peptide bonds found in proteins, enzymes, and collagen can delocalize and be conducted through this semiconductive material. Pi electrons in aromatic rings found in many amino acids and proteins in the body have even more freedom to move and be conducted. This allows electrons to travel throughout the body and potentially quench the symptoms of electron deficiency, such as pain, inflammation, and disease.

Robert Becker, an orthopedic surgeon and researcher looking at the effects of electrical fields on healing, regeneration, and cellular communication, also contributed to the field of bioelectricity. Becker found that living systems produce an intrinsic direct current of electricity. A direct current of electricity moves in one direction from the negative charge to the area of positive charge. He discovered that bone fractures and wounds generated specific electrical currents that were essential for healing. Becker confirmed that bones are piezoelectric—they can create an electrical charge when exposed to pressure. By applying electrodes with these specific weak direct electrical currents to the bones and wounds, Becker found they would heal much faster. He found that electrical stimulation could cause cells to revert to a regenerative state.

Becker investigated the process of regeneration in salamanders. When salamanders lose a limb, they can grow a new one in its place. Becker found that this process of regeneration was directed by distinct electrical currents. Becker could apply the specific currents with electrodes to the tissue and stimulate limb regeneration. Unlike the fast, alternating electric current of the nervous system, the body has an underlying direct electrical current, Becker's research suggested. Becker was also the first to warn of the dangers of human-made electromagnetic fields, like electric power lines.

Michael Levin, a prominent researcher in the field of bioelectricity and morphogenesis at Tufts University, continues this research on bioelectricity today. His work focuses on the electrical potential across cell membranes and how the cell uses these bioelectric signals to communicate, direct development, and even regenerate tissues. His research suggests that bioelectric signals play a major role in guiding embryonic development, tissue regeneration, and tumor suppression. His research could be applied to diagnosing illness and disease through electrical charge or creating electrical devices that can bolster the electrical charge of a cell and thus its health and function.

Moving beyond the idea that genes are the sole guiding force of growth and development, Levin proposes the driving force of bioelectricity as another primary influence. Taking genetics out of the driver's seat and replacing it with a language of bioelectricity completely changes our current understanding of biology. Levin works with worms because of their ability to regenerate. If you cut a planarian worm in half, the bottom half will regrow a head and the top half will grow back a tail, creating two whole worms. No matter how many times you cut the worm, it will regenerate the pieces into whole worms. In astonishing research, Levin created a two-headed worm, something not seen in nature. He did this not by changing genetics but by applying the appropriate bioelectrical signal for regenerating a head where a tail should have been—an incredible illustration of the power that bioelectricity has to guide life.

Levin has made important contributions to the field of cancer research as well. He found that depolarized cells, cells with less negative charge, were more likely to display cancerous properties. He found that depolarization can cause tumor-like growth or rapid cellular division like what we see in cancer. This loss of negative charge seemed to travel beyond individual cells, influencing nearby cells to become cancerous as well. By repolarizing the cell, Levin's team was able to reduce tumor growth. Although a loss of negative charge can be associated with cancerous changes, when the negative charge is reestablished, the cancerous changes slow or disappear. What a profound understanding about a devastating disease that our chemical approach to life has yet to remedy.

Levin has also suggested that aging is a decline in essential bioelectrical signaling and proposes bioelectrical interventions as a solution. Levin describes how the use of electroceuticals (devices that use electricity to support health) has evolved and will continue to evolve. The first generation of electroceuticals, of pacemakers, cardiac defibrillators, cochlear and retinal implants, transcutaneous electrical nerve stimulation, spinal cord stimulation, and deep brain stimulation, has been successful using simple electrical waveforms for broad action. Second-generation electroceuticals have developed into more precise vagus nerve stimulation, and Levin predicts even more specific targeting in the future.

Recent research found that the electrical charge of cells was responsible for the movement of cells, especially important when studying cancer. Tatsat Banerjee, a graduate student researching cell biology and electrical charge at Johns Hopkins University, saw something previously unknown. Negatively charged lipid or fat molecules on the inner layer of cell membranes didn't all act the same, as everyone previously thought.

Banerjee and team found that the outcropping produced on the cell membrane to prepare the cell for movement was associated with a corresponding reduction in negative electrical charge. John Hopkins researchers found that the negative electrical charge of the cell's inner membrane was necessary to produce the cascade of biological action found in cell movement. This research shows that cell movement is guided by electrical patterns, not just chemical patterns. This points us away from the idea that biology is driven solely by chemical action.

Different research discovered that the cell produces its own electromagnetic field. These self-generated electromagnetic fields guide cell behavior and migration and were also found to govern the process of cell differentiation—whether a cell becomes a nose or a knee. This is a truly astonishing perspective on the body—one driven by electricity rather than chemicals.

ELECTRIC WATER

The role of cell-bound EZ water shouldn't be ignored when talking about the electric nature of the body. The water that lines our cells takes on a unique organization. This liquid crystalline water carries a negative electrical charge. This electrical charge is conveyed to the structure it envelops, whether that be collagen, cell membranes, fascia, enzymes, or proteins.

As discussed in chapter 2, some researchers have proposed that the negative electrical charge of the cell membrane comes from the negatively charged water that is bound to it. As we walk through the electric structures in the body, we must remember the negative electrical charge that cell-bound liquid crystalline water has. This liquid crystalline water can act as a reservoir of electrical charge. It grows with exposure to infrared light and, to some degree, visible light. Ultraviolet light excites it, creating a plasma of free electrons. Liquid crystalline water holds free electrons that can disassociate and flow, creating an electrical current. Mae-Wan Ho called this a "redox pile," meaning a reservoir of energy in the form of free electrons that can go where needed in the body to be donated where there is an energy deficiency, such as in areas of pain, inflammation, and illness. What a paradigm shift!

Just like the research suggesting that negative electrical charge of the cell membrane comes, in part, from the charged water that lines it, there is a similar connection in DNA. Although several research studies have found DNA to be conductive, it was recently discovered that it was in the water of hydrated DNA that could hold and transfer an electrical charge. This highlights the valuable role that negatively charged water has in imparting charge to biological structures.

We'll continue to return to the electrical charge of the liquid crystalline water that lines our cells in this chapter. It's hard to distinguish between the physical structure and the water that encircles it. In the body, it is all interconnected.

ELECTRIC FASCIA

As you read in chapter 3, fascia is a fundamental component of our electric being. From a quantum biological perspective, our fascia is more than scaffolding; it creates a vast system that communicates via light, sound, and electricity. It is easy to imagine fascia as an electrical grid of the body. This collagen network of fascia starts at the most external layers of our skin and extends into the most internal parts of the body. It is comprised of mainly connective tissue, which is mostly collagen. This collagen is semiconductive, meaning it can receive, store, harness, and transmit electrical energy. This is important when looking at the body from an electrical perspective because the body needs a way to transmit energy to areas that are deficient in charge.

The entire fascia network is lined with semiconductive liquid crystalline water. The free electrons in the collagen within fascia as well as the free electrons in the liquid crystalline water that lines it can potentially travel throughout the fascial web, donating electrons and charge where needed. This could help quench inflammation, improving pain and symptoms throughout the body.

The tropocollagen fascial tubules can utilize mechanical energy from the movement of the fascia. The collagen in fascia has a triple helix shape that is piezoelectric, meaning it creates electricity when you apply pressure or movement to it. Research has found that electrical fields, like those created by the piezoelectrical currents in fascia, play a role in cell movement, growth, activation of secondary cellular cascades, and differentiation to different lineages in a variety of tissues. This is one reason tending to the electrical capacity of our fascia is so important for our health.

It is not only movement and deformation that create an electrical charge in fascia. Fascia's piezoelectric nature also creates infrared energy as the electrical current flows. This infrared energy is perfectly suited to build the water battery within the body. The liquid crystalline water that lines fascia has the capacity to create a negative electrical charge. This highly organized EZ water also produces free electrons that could travel the body's water system. On top of that, the positively charged water that forms just outside the negatively charged liquid crystalline water creates a water battery of potential energy that powers the flow of protons. Incredible! All three of these—the negatively charged liquid crystalline water, the water battery, and the flow of protons—offer potential sources of energy for the body independent of the chemical-mechanical model.

The water lining this collagen network can excite when exposed to light. When exposed to ultraviolet light, infrared energy, and electrical charge, the water that lines collagen could create a repository of electrons to be shuttled where needed in the body. The combination of the piezoelectric fascia and the water that lines it could form a fount of electrons and electrical energy that not only produces an abundance of electrons when healthy, but also constructs a network for this energy to flow within.

ELECTRIC CELL

Research suggests that cell depolarization, or loss of the negative electrical charge, also has an adverse effect on the immune system's cells. When an immune cell maintains its negative electrical charge, it functions properly. T cells and macrophages are white blood cells and are vital pieces of the immune system that recognize, communicate, and rid the body of infected or damaged cells. When they are depolarized, they become more positive as they lose their negative electrical charge and cannot perform these crucial actions properly.

Depolarized T cells dampen immune signaling and decrease immune activation and the turning on of cytokine genes. Cytokines are the messengers of the immune system and have a systemic effect throughout the body by influencing the immune, inflammatory, hormonal, and metabolic pathways. The electrical membrane potential sets thresholds for immune system activation. Without it, immune cells can become activated when they shouldn't be. Maintaining negative electrical charge is needed for differentiation, proliferation, and cytokine expression. It is essential to a healthy functioning immune system, which helps control inflammation, supports robust interactions with microbes, and promotes healing and recovery.

A depolarized T cell, which includes many immune system cells, can induce a state of inflammation. A depolarized T cell can trigger NLRP3 inflammasome activation and initiate cell death. T regulatory cells function as an anti-inflammatory branch of the immune system. They travel throughout the body putting out inflammatory fires. When a T regulatory cell becomes depolarized, it can no longer reduce inflammation properly. On both accounts, the loss of the negative electrical charge causes an increase in inflammation, which contributes to heart disease, diabetes, depression, and autoimmune conditions. So when an immune cell loses its negative electrical charge, it doesn't perform its normal functions properly. Therefore, it can send out inappropriate signals for cytokine production, which can derange health throughout the body and T regulatory cells, the anti-inflammatory arm of the immune system, no longer put the brakes on inflammation.

There is a similar association in autoimmune reactions. In autoimmune conditions such as multiple sclerosis, lupus, rheumatoid arthritis, and type 1 diabetes, there is an association with a hyperpolarized cell. Hyperpolarized means that the negative electrical charge is increased beyond the normal charge. The autoreactive immune cells in these conditions become hyperpolarized, which causes them to become overreactive. Depolarized T cells can dysregulate immune activation thresholds, which can lead to the hyperreactive immune responses seen in autoimmunity.

In other words, the loss of the immune cells' negative electrical charge causes T cells and macrophages to not function properly. When they are depolarized, the immune system activation thresholds are dysfunctional and the immune system can be activated when it shouldn't be. This is what we see in autoimmune reactions. The autoreactive immune cells are hyperpolarized because they receive dysfunctional signals from the immune cells that have lost their negative charge. Add to this the inability of depolarized T regulatory cells to decrease inflammation, and the immune system enters a state of chaos.

Researcher Gerald Pollack suggests that the cell's electrical charge comes from the EZ liquid crystalline water that surrounds it and exists within it. All of the research on electrical charge and the immune system looks at ion channels in the cell. A research study with rats found that dehydration increased the calcium current associated with depolarization. The study didn't provide evidence of cell depolarization, but it is certainly a possibility with an increased calcium current. EZ liquid crystalline water is ignored, but if it imparts a negative electrical charge to the cell, then it would be a key player in immune regulation. A decrease in EZ liquid crystalline water would lead to the loss of proper function in the adaptive immune cells and the loss of appropriate thresholds for immune activation, which creates the hyperreactive cells in autoimmune reactions. A loss of liquid crystalline water in T regulatory cells could further this immune dysfunction by impairing their ability to inhibit inflammation, leaving one vulnerable to inflammatory conditions like cardiovascular disease, diabetes, and autoimmune diseases.

This would make interventions like building liquid crystalline water within the body (like we talked about in chapter 2), earthing, and supporting mitochondrial health important considerations for supporting the immune system. Getting morning sunlight and safe daytime sun, lowering the lights at night, cold and heat exposure, and movement are effective ways to support the water within and mitochondria, which could help maintain the immune system's negative charge.

ELECTRIC MITOCHONDRIA

Within the cell live all the microscopic organelles. Mitochondria are among the most fascinating organelles within our cells. Mitochondria have a wide range of actions in the body. The most commonly known role mitochondria play is that of the powerhouses of the cell, making ATP, the energy currency in our body. Our mitochondria produce our body weight in ATP each and every day. Even small decreases in mitochondrial function make enormous changes in the way our body functions. Electric mitochondria are essential to our electric charge.

Researcher Douglas Wallace has spent years researching mitochondrial function. Our mitochondria have their own unique electromagnetic frequency. Wallace found, and others have confirmed, that most modern diseases start when there is a decrease in mitochondrial voltage. This makes tending to our mitochondria vital to our overall health.

Mitochondria have an outer membrane and an inner membrane. The folds in the inner membrane, called *cristae*, house the electron transport chain. This transport chain ushers electrons along the chain to produce energy in the form of ATP, water, biophotons, and infrared energy. There are four protein complexes that make up the electron transport chain, with a fifth protein, ATP synthase, at the end. Electrons are tunneled from protein complex to protein complex until they reach the fifth complex, ATP synthase, and ATP is formed. Mobile electron transfer carriers, ubiquinone and cytochrome c, complete the chain. Different research shows that the spacing between the electron transport chain's protein complexes has a tremendous effect on the voltage and function of the mitochondria. If the complexes are spread too far apart, the electrons cannot quantum tunnel and water, heat, and ATP cannot be made.

Mitochondria create what are called *super complexes* in the inner membrane, more like circles than linear chains. These protein complexes of the electron transport chain must be assembled into precisely configured super complexes to function properly. If the protein complexes in the chain are too far apart, the electrons cannot quantum tunnel along it and mitochondrial function suffers. Research shows us that the quantum tunneling of electrons can only happen when the protein complexes in the electron transport chain are properly spaced. This makes tending to the liquid crystal nature of the inner membrane important to mitochondrial health and our overall wellness. We talked about this in chapter 3: A diet rich in omega-3 fatty acids and quality fats and cold exposure can help maintain integrity in the mitochondrial membranes.

As complex I, III, and IV accept electrons along the chain, they become electrically charged, which allows them to transfer a proton from the inside matrix of the mitochondria to the inner membrane space between the inner and outer mitochondrial membrane. Recent research shows the electron transport chain complexes act like

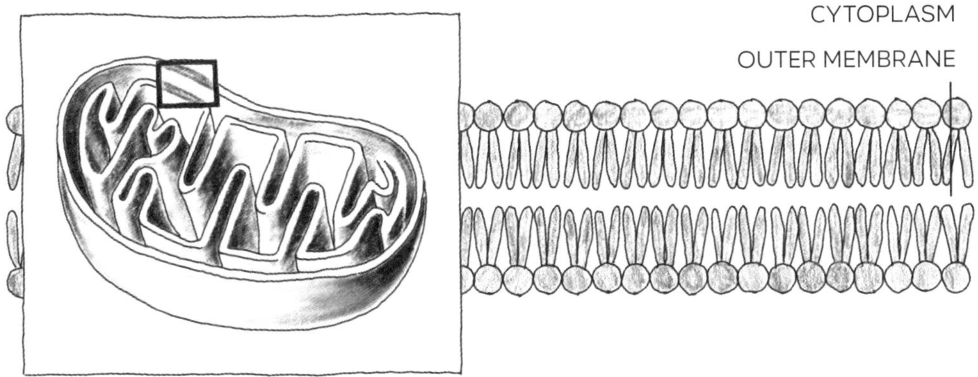

INTERMEMBRANE SPACE

INNER MEMBRANE

4H⁺ 4H⁺ 2H⁺ nH⁺

Q

Cyt C

2e⁻ 2e⁻

I II III IV

NADH NAD⁺ + 2H⁺ FADH FAD + 2H⁺

$[2H^+ + \frac{1}{2} O_2 + 2e^- \rightarrow H_2O] \times 2$

ADP ATP

ELECTRIC TRANSPORT CHAIN

MITOCHONDRIAL MATRIX

The mitochondrion has an outer membrane that faces the cytoplasm of the cell and an inner membrane that faces the inside matrix of the mitochondrion. Within the inner membrane, the electron transport chain consists of four protein complexes with a fifth and final complex ATP synthase. As electrons are tunneled down the chain and protons are tunneled through complexes, metabolic water, ATP, and infrared energy are created.

individual batteries, charging and discharging electricity, highlighting the importance of maintaining the electrical charge in our mitochondria. The proton gradient between the inner membrane space and the mitochondrial matrix drives the turning of the final protein complex, ATP synthase. This creates a magnetic pull that attracts the proton through the complex, resulting in infrared heat and ATP.

QUANTUM MITOCHONDRIA: LIGHT, WATER, AND ENERGY

We should not think of mitochondria as working in isolation. Rather than just the solitary batteries of the body, mitochondria also form vast social networks. Our mitochondria act as a collective, passing genetic information and electrons between each other. They can change shape, place, and function in response to the signals from the world around us. Mitochondria can stretch out to form networks that can shuttle electrons to other organelles within the cell that need electrical charge. They can form interconnected networks outside the cell to transfer electrons to other cells experiencing an electrical deficit, like a conveyer belt delivering goods to the areas that need it the most.

When looking at biochemistry in the body, we see it is a dance of redox—the state of having energy or electrons to donate. Oxidants are molecules or substances that need extra energy or electrons. We have heard a lot about the oxidative damage that too many oxidants can cause. Reductants give electrons; oxidants take electrons. Within the body, we are in constant energy flux, with electrons flowing where needed. Having an adequate redox potential means having enough electrons to donate, giving the body the capacity to donate electrons where there is an energy deficiency. As mentioned earlier, pain, inflammation, and disease can be viewed as a deficiency in energy. A deficiency in electrons translates into a deficiency in energy and the beginning of dysfunction in the body. Mitochondria are crucial to the body's redox capacity. We must have healthy functioning mitochondria to shuttle energy where needed in the body.

It's not just the quantum flow of electrons in the mitochondria that drives ATP. It's also the flow of protons from the inner membrane space that regulates ATP production. The liquid crystalline water that lines the inside pore of the proteins in the electron transport chain is what the protons travel through. This liquid crystalline water allows for the quantum jump conduction of protons. This is similar to what we saw in the fascia. One study estimated 275 structured water molecules help conduct protons from the inner membrane space to the inner mitochondrial matrix so ATP can be made.

The final electron acceptor in the electron transport chain is oxygen, forming water. Electrons from food enter the chain and ATP, infrared heat, and deuterium-free water are produced along the way. Mitochondria produce metabolic water in complex 4 of the electron transport chain and the next protein complex, ATP synthase, produces infrared heat and ATP. Metabolic water and infrared heat are created right next to each other. It couldn't be more perfect for building liquid crystalline water in the cell. A healthy functioning mitochondrion can support that water battery within us.

Research has also found that infrared energy and red light improve the function of mitochondria and that near infrared (NIR) and red light stimulate cytochrome c oxidase, improving cellular respiration and ATP production while reducing reactive oxygen species generation. Red light and NIR have been found to improve aging eyesight and blood sugar regulation via their effects on the mitochondria. Infrared energy and red light are also the perfect ingredients for building a liquid crystalline water repository of electrons. Being outside exposes us to abundant amounts of infrared energy. Red light is also abundant at sunrise and sunset. Getting safe sun exposure is a wonderful way to support mitochondria. Utilizing red and infrared light devices can also support healthy mitochondrial function.

Mitochondria also have a circadian rhythm and are tuned to the light in the environment. The circadian rhythm of mitochondria is associated with immune and metabolic health. Aligning with the rhythm of the sun by getting natural light exposure in the morning and throughout the day and lowering the lights when the sun goes down support mitochondrial health. Artificial light at night is damaging to mitochondria. It blocks the release of melatonin that helps mitigate oxidative damage in the mitochondria as well as initiating the cleanup crew of autophagy and apoptosis. Autophagy is the natural process of breaking down and recycling damaged cells; apoptosis is the normal process of cell death to eliminate damaged or unwanted cells from the body. Both are vital ways to rid the body of damaged and dysfunctional cells that we don't want to inhibit with artificial light. Limiting artificial light at night is a great way to support mitochondrial and cellular function.

Mitochondria also serve as a communication hub of the cell and throughout the body. Mitochondria convert cholesterol into pregnenolone, the backbone of sex hormones. They also produce heme, which is essential to hemoglobin, myoglobin, and various enzymes, with downstream effects on oxygen delivery to the body. They also produce melatonin, a master antioxidant involved in more than 250 biological pathways such as metabolism, inflammation, and the immune system. Mitochondria are involved in the synthesis of serotonin and dopamine through tyrosine conversion. They help synthesize acetylcholine for neurotransmission and muscle activation. Mitochondria produce glutamate, the major excitatory neurotransmitter, and help synthesize GABA, the primary inhibitory neurotransmitter. They help convert thyroid hormones, insulin, norepinephrine, and epinephrine. Simply put, mitochondria are critical for metabolism, hormonal balance, cell signaling, immune response, and cell death. Their biochemical products affect everything from aging to cancer, neurodegeneration, metabolism, mood, and immune function.

Each time a mitochondrion produces ATP, it produces biophotons. We'll talk about biophotons more in the next chapter. For now, it's important to know that biophotons are very weak light emissions made from metabolic processes in the mitochondria. Research suggests that biophotons serve as light communication in the body—even in mitochondria. We've been so focused on the input of food into the electron transport chain for energy production without acknowledging the impact of electrical charge, light, and infrared energy in the equation.

Mitochondria drive a powerful and sophisticated communication web in the body. In the mitochondria, electrons can leak out of the electron transport chain as they tunnel down the chain. These electrons turn into reactive oxygen species. These reactive species are messengers, responding to our environment, to our thoughts and perceptions. Low reactive oxygen species are necessary for cell signaling and adaptation in cell growth, differentiation, and immune responses. High reactive oxygen species levels lead to oxidative stress, which can damage lipids, DNA, and proteins, contributing to aging and disease. Luckily, mitochondria produce melatonin, a master antioxidant. With exposure to infrared energy, the mitochondria produce melatonin in the exact location where prooxidant reactive oxygen species are produced.

Putting the Brakes on Mitochondria

Mitochondria are usually associated with energy production, like a race car is associated with speed. But the mitochondria have built-in mechanisms to slow energy production and even initiate cell death. Just like a race car must be able to quickly and efficiently accelerate, it also requires the ability to shift gears and apply the brakes. Mitochondria are similar. They must generate light, messengers, and energy while, at the same time, being able to conserve energy production and start the recycling, repair, and death of cells with autophagy and apoptosis.

There are proteins in the electron transport chain interspersed among the five major protein complexes that are called *uncoupling proteins*. These proteins uncouple the membrane potential of the inner membrane of the mitochondria. This dissipates the proton gradient across the inner membrane, allowing protons to flow out of the inner membrane space back into the inside matrix of the mitochondria. Rather than energy going into ATP, it is released as heat in a process called *thermogenesis*. Thermogenesis has the power to burn body fat and help with weight loss. With mitochondrial uncoupling, ATP, reactive oxygen species, and biophoton production slows, conserving the life span of the mitochondrion. Slowing ATP production signals mitobiogenesis, the creation of new mitochondria. Uncoupling in the mitochondria decreases reactive oxygen species production, increases the ability to burn fat, and prolongs the life span of the mitochondrion while creating more new mitochondria.

Polyphenols in colorful foods and spices help induce mitochondrial uncoupling. Berries, pomegranate, olives, dark chocolate, black tea, coffee, turmeric, cinnamon, ginger, and cumin are all high in the polyphenols that stimulate mitochondrial uncoupling. Cold exposure, such as cold plunging, cold face plunging (putting your face in a basin of cold water), ending a shower with cooler water, and facilitating safe cold exposure while exercising in winter, all provoke mitochondrial uncoupling. Long chain fatty acids, like in olive oil and avocados, and omega-3 fatty acids found in seafood also stimulate uncoupling in the mitochondria. Ketosis and ketogenic diets can also uncouple mitochondria. While not directly stimulating, eating resistant starches and probiotic foods support the gut microbiome, which can indirectly affect mitochondrial uncoupling.

Infrared exposure from saunas, movement, and warm baths are all soothing ways to induce mitochondrial uncoupling. Movement also affects mitochondrial health. Exercise helps boost ATP production and stimulate new mitochondria growth. Earthing has been found to decrease signs of oxidative stress and inflammation. Researchers suggest that earthing can promote a state of homeostasis in mitochondria, supporting their life span.

Molecular hydrogen, which can be added to water via tablets or electrolysis, proton exchange technology, or by adding hydrogen gas to the water or simply inhaling the gas form, has been found to exert several beneficial effects on mitochondria. Molecular hydrogen could be increasing mitochondrial membrane potential and ATP levels, maintaining integrity and function while alleviating mitochondrial dysfunction. Although the mechanism at the mitochondrial level is not fully understood, molecular hydrogen has been found beneficial for cardiovascular disease, Parkinson's disease, respiratory disease, cerebral infarction, diabetes, and rheumatoid arthritis.

As you've read, there are many ways to support mitochondria. Morning sunlight, red and infrared light while avoiding artificial light at night that blocks melatonin release, deep sleep, and repair mechanisms all support mitochondrial health. Exercise, cold exposure, and heat exposure in saunas or warm baths are wonderful ways to support mitochondria.

Balancing mitochondria support and uncoupling mitochondria with polyphenols, cold and heat exposure, strategic ketogenic diets, and fatty acids is important for healthy mitochondria, as well as nutrients like CoQ10, magnesium, and true hydration to build the liquid crystalline EZ water within.

There are things that damage mitochondrial function and health. Blue light like that found in modern LED lighting, toxins like glyphosate, herbicides, pesticides, processed foods, and stress all disrupt healthy mitochondrial function. Excessive alcohol consumption and medications like NSAIDs, antibiotics, and statins can also damage mitochondria. Even noise pollution and loud sounds have been found to upset healthy mitochondria whereas soothing music can boost mitochondrial function. Our thoughts influence mitochondria. Chronic stress can increase oxidative damage and cause dysfunction in mitochondria. Research has found that a mediative state of mind can boost ATP production and mitochondria health. Avoiding things that damage mitochondria is another great way to support mitochondrial health and function.

ELECTRIC EARTH

From the micro to the macro, we live in a sea of electrical current. Our relationship with the Earth beneath our feet is a source of maintaining this electrical charge. The surface of the Earth maintains a negative charge.

How the Earth Gets Its Charge

More than 30 miles (48.3 km) above Earth's surface, the ionosphere begins. The ionosphere is a region of our atmosphere where ions are formed from incoming solar radiation. The ionosphere spans 100 to 600 miles (160.9 to 965.6 km) in height with the capacity to let electricity flow right through it. This flow of electrons travels down the ionosphere to the lower levels of the atmosphere where clouds are formed. As a cloud is formed, it creates a battery, or separation in charge, between positive charges and negative charges within the cloud. As the charge builds, it is dissipated toward Earth in a bolt of lightning. The negative charge of Earth's surface is maintained by the negative charge of lightning. This creates a slight negative charge covering Earth's surface that is believed to be responsible for the benefits of the phenomenon called *earthing*.

Earthing

Earthing is the practice of coming in direct contact with Earth's surface, such as by placing our bare feet on the ground or bare hands on a tree or in garden soil. Research suggests that the sea of electrons that lines Earth can be absorbed by our biology when we come into direct contact with it. We are electrically conductive and can collect free electrons from Earth's surface and from those things embedded in Earth's energy field, such as trees, rocks, sand, grass, even animals standing on the ground, offer the benefit of free electrons. This conduction happens immediately upon contact and builds as we spend more time in contact with it.

This phenomenon was first researched independently by Clint Ober in the United States and a pair of father and son medical doctors, Karol Sokal and his son, Pawel Sokal. From his experience working with cable TV, Ober knew the benefits of grounding cable and wondered if it could benefit humans. He experimented with himself first by creating a rudimentary conductive system for the bed—a grounding mat for the bed. He used metallic duct tape connected by wire to a ground rod he planted in the soil outside to connect the grounding pad to Earth's energy. He found this supported sleep and significantly reduced his chronic pain.

In 2000, he designed a group experiment to test whether earthing was truly beneficial. Ober installed a version of his grounding mat in the beds of sixty volunteers. For half of the volunteers, Ober inserted a block in the cable so that the grounding mat was not actually grounded. The "grounded" volunteers experienced more restful and longer sleep with less muscle stiffness and pain. Karol and Pawel Sokal came to similar conclusions with their research, finding that earthing provides a sense of general well-being, better sleep, and reduced pain.

There are more than fifty research studies and reviews on the benefits of earthing, and the research has revealed some fascinating aspects of our biology and how it fits perfectly in Earth's hands. Scientists propose that we absorb and utilize the vast sea of electrons that lines Earth for physiological advantage. Evidence continues to show benefits for pain, inflammation, immune health, and sleep. The evidence surrounding earthing and cardiovascular health is also exciting, with research showing that earthing can decrease blood pressure and improve circulation. Our red blood cells' electrical charge increases during earthing, which helps prevents clumping. When red blood cells clump, the risk for clotting and clot-associated conditions like heart attacks and strokes increases. Our biology seems to thrive by being held within the energy of Earth.

The Electric Cardiovascular System

There is an electrical perspective of the cardiovascular system. Cardiovascular system disorders include atherosclerosis, heart attacks, and strokes. Heart attacks and strokes are caused by the formation of clots that block blood circulation. There is mounting evidence that atherosclerosis is also a result of clotting. Clotting tissue and fibrogen have been found in large amounts in atherosclerotic plaques that rupture, suggesting something more is happening than the current model of cholesterol deposition on the lining of the arteries. Damage to the endothelial lining of the body's vasculature could lead to clotting in that area and the beginnings of a plaque. Conventional medicine approaches treat these conditions from the viewpoint of diet and exercise, which are important. The additional perspective of electrical charge offers even more understanding of cardiovascular health and new options to support it.

The surface of red blood cells is covered with a negatively charged electrical potential called *the zeta potential*, which is increased when exposed to Earth's surface. Increase in zeta potential repels the red bloods cells, like charge repels like charge, which leads to less clumping of cells and better circulation, reducing the risk of clotting issues.

Coupled with research showing that infrared energy can increase the EZ liquid crystalline water within blood vessels helping drive blood flow, cardiovascular health starts to look different from a quantum biological perspective. The heart is one band of muscle that wraps in a helical fashion. This creates a vortexed flow of blood as the heart pumps that would be ideal for creating liquid crystalline water.

The lining of the vessels, the glycocalyx, is a layer of bound water against the interior surface of the vessel that can protect the vessel from damage. The research of Gerald Pollack and Zheng Li found that the blood in the body will continue to flow after stopping the heart if infrared energy is present, implying a role of EZ liquid crystalline water in the cardiovascular system. The EZ water could be acting as a battery to help drive the circulation of blood throughout the body. That liquid crystalline water battery lining the vessels that is stimulated by infrared energy could be a major player in cardiovascular health.

Rather than focusing solely on diet and exercise, adding earthing to increase the zeta potential of red blood cells and decrease clotting along with the building of liquid crystalline water to protect the lining of the vessels from damage while forming a water battery to help propel the circulation of blood could help the epidemic of cardiovascular disease that is rampant right now.

Research found that one hour of earthing also significantly improves pleasant and positive moods, more so than relaxation alone. It has been shown to increase vagal tone, an indicator of healthy parasympathetic function and a balanced nervous system. Earthing's beneficial impacts on mood also help balance stress hormones and even reduce anxiety in research with mice. It has even been found to balance the nervous system overall.

Scientists worked with infants in the neonatal intensive care unit, using grounding mats in their incubators. They observed an increase in vagal tone as measured by heart rate variability. A similar benefit in heart rate variability was seen in a group of healthy adults utilizing grounding patches.

Wearing conductive clothing made from linen, cotton, hemp, wool, and silk when sitting on the ground or near a tree allows electrical conduction to occur. Grounding shoes, mats, and sheets can also be helpful, although nothing can take the place of direct contact with Earth. Grounding works best on wet ground, but any contact with Earth's surface works. Even concrete allows for some electrical conduction.

When outside, we often encounter electrically charged negative ions in the wind, rainfall, ocean spray, and waterfalls. Negative ions support immune system, nervous system, and mental health. Being cradled in the energy of Earth has multiple benefits for our nervous system, vagal tone, and resilience to stress.

NONNATIVE ELECTROMAGNETIC FIELDS

Robert Becker's pioneering work on bioelectricity led him to propose that there were negative side effects of human-made electromagnetic fields. Becker warned against nonnatural electromagnetic fields, such as power lines, radio waves, and electronic devices, and suggested that prolonged exposure to nonnatural fields might increase the risk of cancer, immune dysfunction, and nervous system disorders.

A small research study found a potential link between childhood leukemia and extremely low-frequency electromagnetic fields like those found in power lines, electrical wiring, and electric appliances. Martin Pall, professor and researcher at the University of Washington, suggests that nonnative electromagnetic fields can activate calcium channels in the cells, causing oxidative damage. Research has found that electromagnetic field exposure produced significant changes in blood antioxidant levels and an increase in oxidative stress, which can lead to cellular damage. Recent research out of China found an association between poor sleep, cell phone use, and cardiovascular issues. Gerald Pollack and his team from the University of Washington have done research showing that Wi-Fi radiation emitted by a wireless router can diminish EZ liquid crystalline water. The International Agency for Research on Cancer (IARC) has classified radiofrequency electromagnetic fields as possibly carcinogenic. This limited and preliminary research needs more attention and funding. If the body runs on electromagnetic energy and information, it makes sense that nonnative electromagnetic fields could interfere with this.

Taking precautions such as unplugging the wireless router when not in use and during sleep, moving to wired options for the computer, phone, and entertainment system, turning off electrical breakers, sleeping with your phone on airplane mode and in another room, utilizing electromagnetic fields shielding products, and avoiding direct physical contact such as putting a computer in your lap or a cell phone to your ear, are all ways to help mitigate the sea of Wi-Fi we currently live in.

The law of inverse square states that the intensity of exposure drops dramatically the farther you are from the source. But the exposure becomes more intense the closer you are like holding a cell phone to your ear or putting wireless earbuds in your ears. A general rule is to keep Wi-Fi devices from coming into direct contact with the body.

And a daily grounding practice can help restore the natural electrical influence on the body. We are inundated with electromagnetic fields in modern life, but there are steps we can take to avoid and minimize our exposure.

ELECTRIC BREATH

Breath has traditionally been thought to carry energy. The idea that vital energy in the world around us can be summoned into the body via breath is not new to ancient Indigenous cultures. Qi, in Chinese medicine, and prana, in Ayurvedic medicine, describe this universal energy that exists within us and in the universe around us. Both have an intimate connection with breath. Similar to the idea of aether as the life force of the universe, Qi and prana also represent this all-pervading energy that can be connected to with breath.

A recent study looked at traditional yoga breaths and found an incredible relationship with energy in the body. This study used a specific system to evaluate changes in spinal energy levels across cervical, thoracic, lumbar, sacral, and coccygeal regions. They found that slow, deep breathing and alternate-nostril breathing increased spinal energy. Though a small study, it is wonderful to see traditional breath connected to metrics of bioenergetics.

Gerald Pollack recently published a paper on the idea that we are breathing in electrons with oxygen to power the bioenergetics of the body. Pollack proposes that oxygen's high electronegativity allows it to deliver electrons throughout the body. He cites several issues with the current model of respiration, including the size of the oxygen molecule in comparison to the areas it needs to diffuse through, the spacing of the capillaries to the lungs, the size of the respiratory capillaries, and more. He argues that the electron can diffuse through these small areas and across the space between the lungs and the capillaries. It's a fascinating argument for the idea that we breathe in energy that brings us back full circle to what the ancients spoke of.

In different research, breath supports mitochondrial function. Oxygen is the final electron acceptor in the mitochondria's electron transport chain. The presence of oxygen allows the mitochondria to efficiently generate ATP through oxidative phosphorylation, yielding significantly more ATP than glycolysis alone. Optimal oxygen levels ensure optimal mitochondrial function. This has a downstream effect of enhancing metabolism, cellular repair, and overall health.

Research has shown an association between emotions and different breathing patterns. Not only did the study participants display similar respiratory patterns while experiencing certain emotions, but they also produced emotions while performing different breathing patterns.

Slowing our breath can stimulate the vagus nerve and the relaxation mode of the parasympathetic nervous system, decreasing feelings of anxiety. Slowing our breath triggers a decrease in heart rate and stress hormones via the vagus nerve. Research with Afghanistan War veterans who experienced post-traumatic stress found that breathwork not only decreased anxiety in the short term, but also had a lasting effect, decreasing anxiety over a year's period. This makes sense when we see how breath can both regulate our nervous system and help our mitochondrial function.

Using your diaphragm to draw in breath, expanding both your belly and your chest, can transform your breath. Letting the air you breathe fill your lower abdomen, creates what many call *belly breathing*. Diaphragmatic breathing lowers blood pressure and heart rate. You can practice breathing like this sitting or lying down to explore a new way to lower stress and increase resonance.

Other breathwork styles can help further this practice:

- Box breathing creates an imaginary box of breath: Take one inhale in for four seconds, hold the breath for four seconds, exhale for four seconds, and hold the breath for four seconds before repeating the process. You can begin by counting four seconds at each interval. Later, you can substitute a four-word mantra, such as I am very safe, I am so loved, I'm healthy and strong, or whatever you choose, for counting.

- A different interval of breath, 4/7/8, is where you inhale for four counts, hold the breath for seven counts, and exhale for eight counts.

- Pursed-lip breathing is an effective way to reset the nervous system within a few breaths. I describe it as exhaling through a straw: Breathe in through the nose and exhale through pursed lips, letting the breath part the lips.

- Yogic breathing, like alternate-nostril breathing, is where you breath in through one nostril while blocking the other and exhale through the other nostril while blocking the previously open nostril.

- Practicing lion's breath involves exhaling while sticking out the tongue and saying "haaaa."

- Holotrophic breathwork is a fast-paced breath that allows for a shift in both the nervous system and perception of the world.

Breathwork is an easy and accessible way to tend to our resonance.

TENDING TO YOUR ELECTRIC BODY

We are electric beings. We can maintain our valuable electrical charge by supporting our mitochondrial, cellular, and fascial health while cultivating our relationship with Earth's surface.

Ground as often as possible. Get outside: Put your bare feet on the ground, touch a tree or a plant embedded in Earth's surface, or place your bare hands in soil, like when gardening. Wear conductive clothing when sitting on the ground or a tree to allow electrical conduction. Consider grounding shoes, mats, and sheets. Getting outside also allows us to encounter negative ions. Grounding can help bring the natural electrical charge back to the body.

Support mitochondrial function. Utilize red, infrared, and natural light to fuel the mitochondria while avoiding excessive artificial light and light at night, which can deplete mitochondria. Cold exposure, polyphenols, ketogenic diets, omega-3 fatty acids, and long chain fatty acids all promote mitochondrial uncoupling, which can help produce new mitochondria while preserving the life span of existing mitochondria. Movement and exercise help support mitochondrial function and growth. Supporting overall gut and microbiome health can help support mitochondrial health. Avoid unnecessary stress, utilize stress management techniques, and cultivate meditative practices such as journaling, gratitude, heart coherence, mindfulness, and meditation to support mitochondrial health. Consider molecular hydrogen to support mitochondrial function. Pleasant sound can help promote efficient mitochondrial function. Whenever possible, avoid toxins, processed foods, excessive alcohol, and noise pollution that can decrease mitochondrial function.

Utilize breath to increase electrical charge in the body. There are many breathwork styles to explore. Simply focusing on a longer exhale than inhale while breathing into the diaphragm can calm the nervous system while increasing energy in the body.

Use electrical therapies when needed. Pulsed electromagnetic field therapy has been found helpful for inflammation, mitochondrial function, and fascial health. There are also units available to help with pain or vagus nerve tone. Electroceuticals offer another option for health.

Avoid nonnative electromagnetic fields when possible. We're surrounded by them in our modern world, and we must mitigate some of that exposure.

Support the liquid crystal structures of DNA, cell membranes, and fascia. A diet rich in omega-3 fatty acids, phospholipids, and colorful fruits and vegetables helps maintain the strength and flexibility of the liquid crystalline structures in the body. Grounding, circadian rhythm alignment, and stress management are all important in nourishing the liquid crystal structures (see chapter 3 for more information).

Build the water battery within. As mentioned throughout this chapter, we must remember the electrical charge that the water lining cells and tissues carry (see chapter 2 for more information).

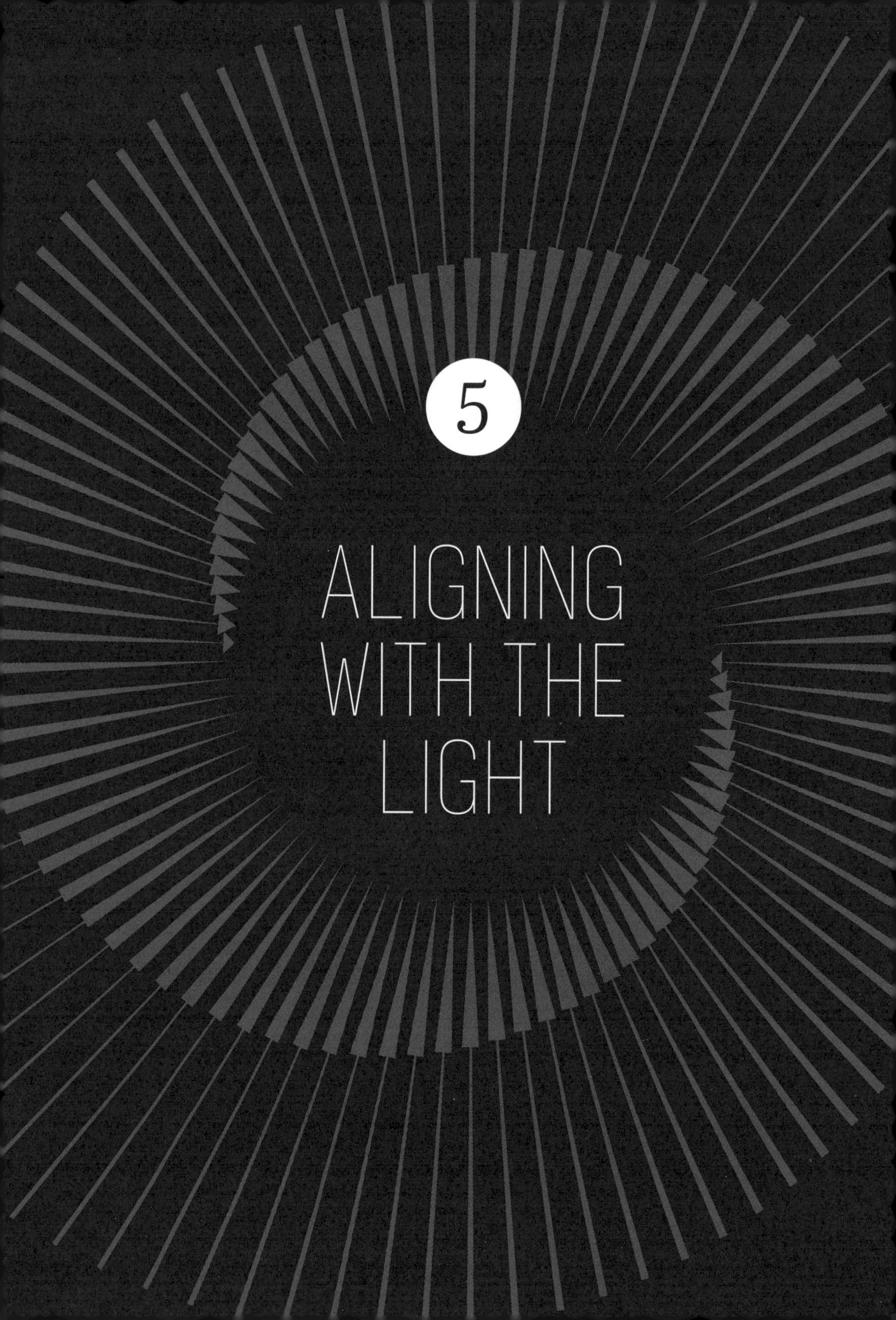

5

ALIGNING WITH THE LIGHT

We are tuned to the frequencies in our environment. Whether we are talking about our internal terrain or our external environment, we are receivers of this vast sea of frequency, and it shapes our biology. Light is one of those frequencies. Light pervades this universe, and our body is no exception.

We are light beings. The light in the world around us molds our physiology—from our cardiovascular system to our immune system to our digestive system. Light touches almost every cell in the body, guiding how the body functions, and it's not only the external light that shapes our biology. We have an immense communication network of light that operates continually throughout the body. This internally generated light seems to serve as a biological signal that also deserves attention. Let's explore light, how it affects our health, and how we can align with the light for better vitality and longevity.

THE NATURE OF LIGHT

Light is a form of electromagnetic radiation, able to store and emit information. Light is a mixture of perpendicular oscillating electric and magnetic fields that create a flow of energy that carries information throughout our body. This information educates and instructs our biology, guiding our nervous system, hormonal balance, mental emotional health, immune system, and metabolic function. The benzene ring in melanin, the aromatic amino acids of neurotransmitters, and in light-sensitive proteins like opsins and cryptochromes can capture, store, and transmit the energy of light from our environment into energy the body can use.

We often think of light in a segmental fashion, envisioning light functioning as it would out of a flashlight—as a single beam of light illuminating everything in its path but leaving the rest of the vicinity in darkness. But this isn't the whole picture. As photons of light enter our atmosphere, they are constantly bouncing off objects, reflecting off surfaces and scattering about. This is how light behaves when it strikes the leaves of a plant. It is not immediately absorbed. It bounces throughout the thin leaf until it is absorbed and travels to the photosynthetic reaction center for photosynthesis to occur.

This is how light works around us. There are photons of light bounding about, even in indirect light. This is also how light works in our body, photons of light ricocheting around until they are absorbed. The light in our environment is ever present, like the water surrounding a fish in the sea. It's all around us and within us, yet we perceive that it exists only in visible beams and rays.

We have lived through millennia in an intimate relationship with the sun. Ancient Indigenous cultures had rituals to honor this relationship. From the sun gods of Egypt and Africa to the wisdom of the Vedic texts, South American cosmology, Northern European Celtic traditions, and Asian cultures, our relationship with light has always been primary. The Indigenous People of Mongolia built their yurts with east-facing doors, just as the Navajo built their hogans with doors that faced the rising sun. Greeting the morning sun was a practice that highlighted devotion to the sun—not just as a life-giving force, but as a sacred entity and relationship. In modern times, many of us have turned away from that relationship. Recent research helps our understanding of this primordial force on our biology, and our health and beckons us back into a relationship with the light.

LIGHT GUIDES OUR BIOLOGY

We now know that every cell in our body has a circadian clock. "Circadian" refers to a rhythm that lasts about twenty-four hours. Our circadian rhythm is intimately connected with the body's function and its overall health. In 2017, three scientists, Jeffery Hall, Michael Rosbash, and Michael Young, won the Nobel Prize in Physiology for their work with circadian clock genes. In the 1980s, these three researchers isolated and started studying a gene in fruit flies that they named "period." Light programs this protein that accumulates each night and breaks down the next day. The idea that light drives a diurnal rhythm within our cellular function was something previously unknown. Their discoveries led to chronobiology, or the study of how light effects our biology.

We now know that light and circadian rhythm play a foundational part in our overall health. If we have circadian clocks in almost every cell, that means our cardiovascular, digestive, and respiratory systems, our detoxification organs, our reproductive organs, our inflammatory state, our hormonal state, our neurological function, and mood are all shaped by the light in our environment. Light has a powerful influence on our neurological state affecting depression, cognitive dysfunction, chronic pain, and sleep disorders. Light governs our inner workings on every level.

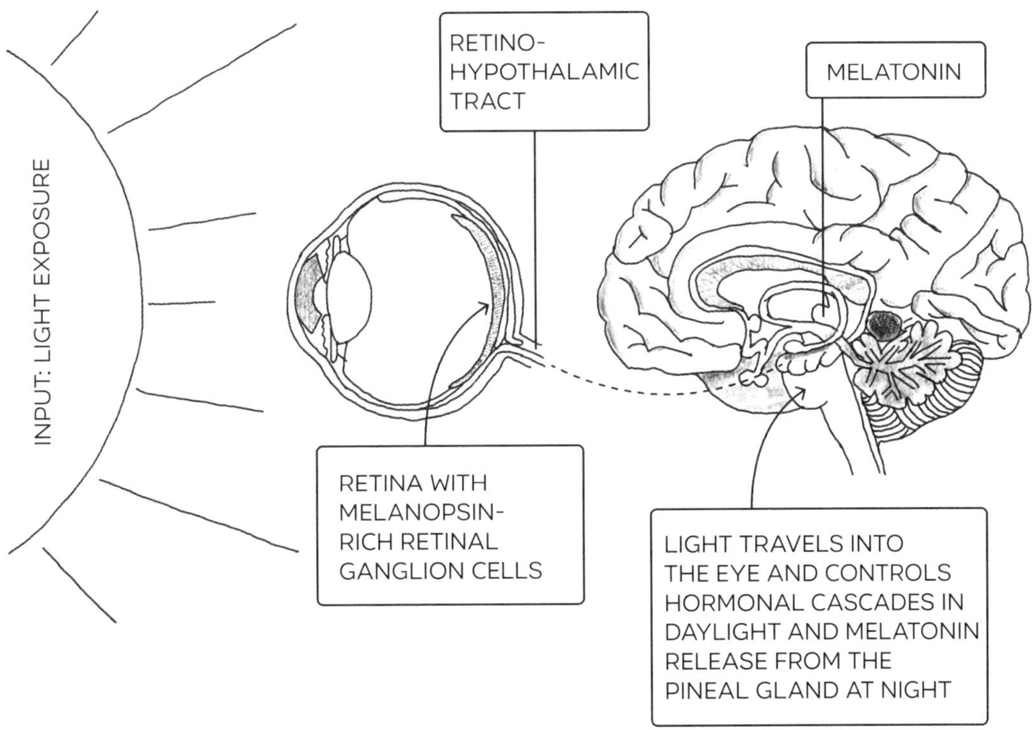

Light entering the eye is focused on the thin layer of cells at the back of the eye, the retina. The retina's light-sensitive cells sense the amount of blue and ultraviolet light and turn that into an electrical signal that travels to the suprachiasmatic nucleus in the hypothalamus, the body's master circadian clock. The suprachiasmatic nucleus then sends an electrical signal to all the peripheral circadian clocks throughout the body to align the body with the light in the environment.

One of the ways light guides our biology is through our eyes. As light enters our eyes, it travels to the retina, the thin layer of cells at the back of the eye that transform light entering the eye into electrical signals for the optic nerve. This light travels along a dedicated pathway in the optic nerve called *the retinohypothalamic tract*. Melanospin is a light-sensitive protein that exists in various parts of our body, especially in the retina. The light-sensitive cells in the retina, called *intrinsically photosensitive retinal ganglion cells*, detect light in the environment and send electrical signals along the retinohypothalamic tract to the suprachiasmatic nucleus in the hypothalamus at the center of the brain. The suprachiasmatic nucleus is our master circadian clock that synchronizes all the cells throughout the body to the light in our surroundings. As the light enters our eyes, it travels via electrical signals to our central clock in the brain, which then sends out signals to align all our peripheral clocks in the body to the light in our environment. This completes a beautiful dance of entrainment that aligns us with the light in our environment.

Our circadian rhythm is governed by several sophisticated and interconnected feedback loops. The two positive gene regulators, CLOCK and BMAL1, and the negative gene repressors belonging to the cryptochrome (CRY1 and CRY2) and period (PER1, PER2, PER3) families lead to circadian oscillations. The rising and falling of these feedback loops give us our circadian rhythm. These feedback loops work to set the circadian rhythm of our cells while directing our metabolism, our immune system, inflammatory system, and many other biological functions. The circadian clocks in our cells dictate the function of that cell and thus the health of that corresponding organ. Our chronobiology is paramount to health, influencing immune system conditions, metabolic issues like obesity and diabetes, hormonal pathways related to fertility and libido, and mental emotional states like depression and anxiety. This is why tending to our light environment is so important for vitality.

CIRCADIAN APPETITE

Meal timing also reinforces our circadian rhythm. Eating a breakfast balanced in protein, fiber, and fat within thirty to sixty minutes of waking helps set our circadian rhythm and metabolic rhythm. Eating outside is a wonderful tool for balancing that rhythm as well. Eating seasonal foods rich in nutrients such as vitamin B12 helps reinforce our infradian seasonal rhythm and bolster our circadian enzymes, which play an invaluable role in stabilizing our rhythms. Eat before or as close to sunset as possible to support the rest and repair cycle of the day and help maintain those valuable rhythms. Avoid alcohol, food, and blue light three hours before bed.

We have a circadian rhythm of calorie burning, too. We burn more calories in the morning and at midday. We are more sensitive to insulin at this time, too. As the day progresses, our metabolism slows, our digestive system slows the release of enzymes for digestion, and we have higher insulin resistance. Eating the bulk of calories earlier in the day with dinner before sunset, and eating seasonally, can help bolster our metabolism and improve insulin sensitivity and our ability to maintain an ideal weight. The seasons also have an impact on our metabolism. We are less insulin resistant in summer and more insulin resistant in winter. We are meant to align with the circadian rhythm of light and the seasonal rhythms.

OUR LIGHT ENVIRONMENT

Our light environment in our modern life consists of light from natural and artificial sources. The electromagnetic spectrum encompasses a wide range of energy and visible light is only a small sliver of that spectrum.

As shown in the graphic, the electromagnetic radiation spectrum of waves ranges from shorter to longer. The shortest waves on the spectrum are gamma rays, then X-rays, followed by the ultraviolet light range, and the visible spectrum of light we see with our eyes. After the visible spectrum of light, the light continues to grow in wavelength to the longer infrared spectrum, then microwaves, and ending with radio waves. Light in the ultraviolet, visible, and infrared spectrums have powerful effects on our biology.

THE ELECTROMAGNETIC SPECTRUM

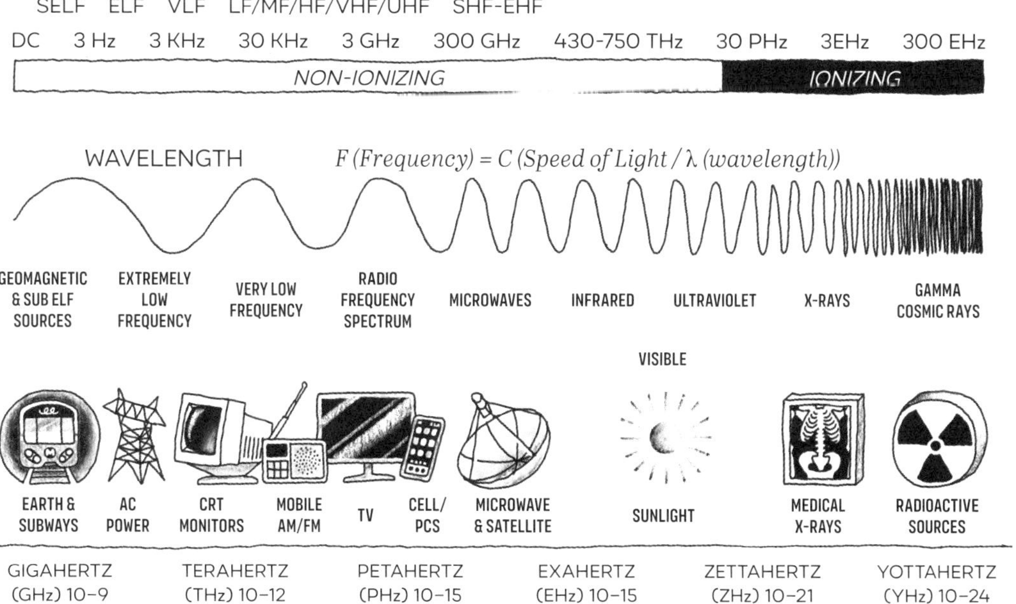

The electromagnetic spectrum is the range of all electromagnetic radiation. It is organized by frequency, or wavelength, from the highest intensity and shortest wavelengths in gamma rays to X-rays to ultraviolet to visible light to infrared to microwave to radio waves.

We are tuned to pick up the frequencies of light in our environment with the largest source of light coming from the sun. Sunlight offers a spectrum of ultraviolet light from ultraviolet C, which is filtered out of our atmosphere, to ultraviolet B, which we commonly associate with sun damage to the skin. Ultraviolet A is always present when the sun is up, even on cloudy days.

Sunlight also carries the visible spectrum of light we can see with our eyes, from violet to indigo to blue to green to yellow to orange to red, and all the blends in between. Sunlight also supplies an abundance of infrared light. As the sun begins to rise each morning, our eyes are exposed to a range of light dominant in the red light and infrared light spectrum. As the sun climbs, usually at about 10 degrees above the horizon, we see more blue and ultraviolet A light. As the sun climbs to solar noon, we see ultraviolet B at its peak around the hour of noon, depending on the given latitude and season. We don't need to look directly at the sun. These light spectrums are abundant in the ambient light outside. We just need natural exposure without sunglasses to gather these light signals.

Our body depends on these light cues for a multitude of biological actions such as hormonal cascades in adrenal and sex hormones, neurotransmitters like dopamine and serotonin, and metabolic cues. Melanopsin in the retinal cells detects the morning mix of ultraviolet A and visible light (especially blue light) and activates a variety of biological cascades. Early morning sunlight hits the melanopsin in our retina and in our skin stimulating the pro-opiomelanocortin (POMC) gene. Blue and ultraviolet light entering the eye are the strongest stimulators of our circadian rhythm. In the presence of ultraviolet light, POMC in the brain gets cleaved into adrenocorticotropic hormone, beta-endorphins, as well as melanin-stimulating hormone and lipotropins, which help burn fat. Melanin-stimulating hormone produced with morning light not only stimulates melanin production, but it also has an anti-inflammatory effect in the immune system. It also helps thyroid hormones become active during the day, which is crucial for our metabolism. Melanin-stimulating hormone controls hypothalamic production of melatonin and endorphins while modulating the immune system and our nerve function. Getting morning light is the foundation of a long and healthy life.

Ultraviolet light received through our eyes in the morning also energizes the conversion of aromatic amino acids (AAAs) into serotonin, dopamine, epinephrine, and norepinephrine. Tyrosine is an AAA, meaning the benzene ring in its molecular structure can capture light. When that light enters our eyes, it stimulates the conversion of tyrosine into serotonin, the neurotransmitter that helps us feel calm and content. It also triggers the conversion of tyrosine into dopamine, epinephrine, norepinephrine, and thyroid hormones, which help us feel energized, motivated, and focused. Tyrosine can also be converted by light into L-dopa, which can be transformed into melanin (more on that shortly).

CIRCADIAN RHYTHM OF THE SUN

SUNRISE
0° TO 10° ABOVE HORIZON
INFRARED, RED LIGHT RICH

MORNING ULTRAVIOLET A
10° TO 30° ABOVE HORIZON
BLUE RICH

RISING ULTRAVIOLET B
55° TO 90° ABOVE HORIZON

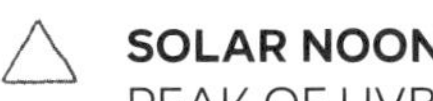

SOLAR NOON
PEAK OF UVB

SUNSET
10° TO 0° ABOVE EASTERN HORIZON
INFRARED, RED LIGHT

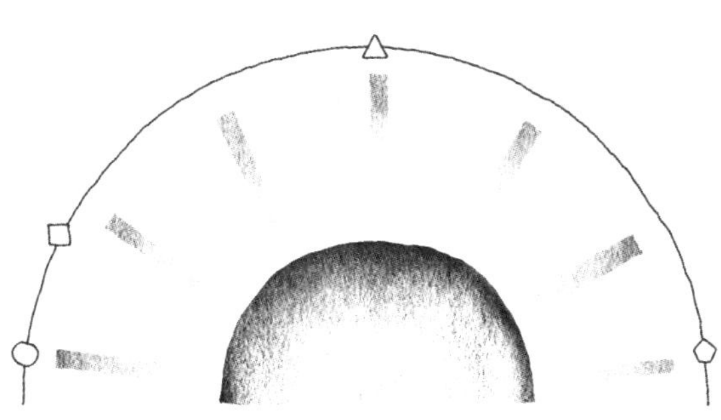

Each day, the sun cycles through the sky with predictable effects on our biology. Sunrise, until the sun is 10 degrees above the horizon, and sunset are times rich in red and infrared light. As the sun rises from 10 to 30 degrees above the horizon, the sun's light becomes abundant in ultraviolet A and blue light that signals various biological pathways in the body. The sun climbs farther in the sky and ultraviolet B light is present. As the sun leaves the peak of solar noon, it begins to lose ultraviolet B first, then ultraviolet A and blue light until it reaches sunset. This prepares the body for the nighttime release of melatonin for sleep and repair.

The adrenocorticotropic hormone from cleaved POMC signals the release of cholesterol from the adrenal glands so mitochondria can make pregnenolone, which is then further converted into cortisol and our sex hormones, such as progesterone, estrogen, and testosterone. The beta-endorphins released with morning light help our mood, pain levels, neurological function, and inflammation.

Natural morning light is critical for the hormone production that affects so much of our biology. It balances our natural release of sex hormones. Natural morning light is the perfect blend to signal healthy hormones, metabolic signals, inflammatory balance, pain modulation, and a properly functioning immune system. Something as simple as exposure to morning sunlight can have such a huge influence on our health and longevity.

Cortisol regulates the body's stress response, controls the metabolism of fats, proteins, and carbohydrates, controls blood pressure and blood sugar, and suppresses inflammation. We have a burst of cortisol from our adrenal glands once every twenty-four hours influencing our wake and sleep cycles. It helps us wake up and stay alert during the day while lowering at night for a restful sleep. We want this burst of cortisol to build over the first sixty to ninety minutes after waking. Causing a spike in cortisol first thing in the morning can set up a dysfunctional rhythm of cortisol secretion from the adrenal glands. These days, many of us grab our phones upon waking, causing an instant cortisol spike from the artificial bright blue band of light coming from the phone. Postponing phone time until after natural morning light exposure allows the body to build that cortisol burst in the morning gradually and avoid artificial spikes that can lead to issues with blood sugar, inflammation, stress, and energy issues.

Simply put, the light that hits our eyes in the morning regulates our hormonal state, appetite, libido, fertility, metabolism, pain, and inflammatory state. This makes aligning our rhythm with the sun an essential piece of health. Short bouts of exposure are enough to initiate these pathways: Five to ten minutes of morning light on sunny days and fifteen to twenty minutes of natural morning light on cloudy days is enough to signal safety to the nervous system and slowly raise cortisol. This benefits metabolism, stress response, and inflammation. Earthing (see page 135) at this time is also beneficial.

Sunlight also induces different brainwave states. Sunlight exposure regulates melatonin and serotonin, inducing beta waves with morning light and delta waves in darkness. Morning sunlight stimulates gamma and beta waves, enhancing alertness and cognitive function. Evening sunset triggers alpha and theta waves, preparing the brain for sleep. The darkness of night prompts delta brainwaves of deep sleep.

The Colors of Light

The rainbow of visible light has a profound effect on our biology, including from our skin to our gut microbiome, a concept long appreciated by ancient Indigenous cultures. The ancient Egyptian, Chinese, Indian, and Greek healers all used light and color as medicine.

- Egyptian mythology speaks of color therapy being discovered by the god Thoth.
- Traditional Chinese medicine assigns color to each of the five elements (wood, fire, earth, metal, and water) to assist healing.
- Ayurvedic medicine associates various colors with each chakra, or energy center, in the body.
- We see the same thing with Greek medicine and the healing attributes of color in the humors.
- In more modern times, heliotherapy, or using the sun as medicine, was in use as a treatment for tuberculosis and for the wounds and casualties of the First World War. Patients were cared for outside where they could be exposed to the healing light of the sun.

Each wavelength of color holds a specific information pattern for our body to receive:

- Yellow light on the skin has been shown to induce anti-inflammatory and antioxidant effects on fibroblasts, giving our skin relief from UVB damage.
- Green light radiance on the skin has shown myriad benefits, from proliferation and migration of mesenchymal stem cells (cells that can turn into any cell in the body, to serve as an internal repair system), wound healing in diabetic patients, anti-aging effects in vitro, alleviation of headaches and migraines, a decrease in pain in people who have fibromyalgia, a decrease in postsurgical pain, and as an effective treatment of seasonal affective disorder.
- Orange light shows benefits in pediatric burn healing as well as improved pain and health outcomes during chemotherapy.
- Purple or violet light helps reduce acne, assists in evening skin tone, and reducing hyperpigmentation and skin inflammation. Animal studies have found that violet light helps prevent the progression of myopia or nearsightedness.

(continued on page 112)

Red and Infrared Light Panels

Red and infrared light panels emit specific frequencies of red light and infrared light. Sometimes the red and infrared light spectrums are combined in one device. These panels are used for pain relief, healing wounds and injuries, preventing wrinkles, and improving blood sugar and mitochondrial function, which impacts almost every condition out there.

There is considerable research on specific wavelengths of red and infrared light and the benefits they offer for human health. These wavelengths are measured in nanometers, with the majority of research showing health benefits focused on the specific wavelengths of 630 nm, 660 nm, 808 nm, and 850 nm (ranges from 620 nm to 900 nm have shown benefits).

These specific wavelengths have been incorporated into red light panels with remarkable success, and the devices on the market usually utilize these wavelengths, but there can be a wide range of variation. So what should you look for when purchasing a red and/infrared light device?

- The specific light frequencies emitted from the device. You want a device that has researched wavelengths clearly labeled.
- The amount of electromagnetic frequency emitted by the device. You want low to no emissions. Devices that plug into the wall will always emit some electromagnetic field (EMF), but you want that to be a low amount. Devices that plug into an electrical socket will emit more EMF than rechargeable or battery-operated devices, so you also want some distance between you and a wired device.
- A low flicker. Even though the light may appear steady, there is always a certain amount of flicker, which refers to the number of times the light flickers on and off. It acts as a stressor on the body and can cause stress, anxiety, and seizures, which is why you want a device that is low flicker. This should be clearly labeled on the device or something the company can provide.

Red light has a powerful effect on our blood sugar levels. Researcher Glen Jeffery has done wonderful research on the power of red light. In one study, Jeffery and his colleagues had people drink a solution that was very high in sugar, which led to an inevitable spike in blood sugar. However, when the participants were exposed to red light, the blood sugar levels decreased by 27 percent. This significant result demonstrates how red light can decrease blood sugar and improve insulin sensitivity by signaling the mitochondria to utilize the sugar in the blood, which decreases blood sugar. This is a meaningful result that addresses one of the main health crises we face today. Every age is grappling with metabolic issues—from children to the elderly. In fact, Alzheimer's disease, a devastating disease to an entire generation and their families, is now being referred to as type 3 diabetes in research contexts because of its connection to insulin resistance. Our light environment could offer a powerful tool for addressing this health epidemic.

Research has also determined profound effects of red and infrared light on eye health. Researchers looked at people between the ages of thirty-five and seventy. A single three-minute exposure to low-intensity red light produced a 17 percent increase in visual acuity for the study's participants. Low-intensity red light is different from many of the red light devices on the market that can damage the eyes when looked at directly because of their high intensity. The study also showed a decrease in reactive oxygen species yet an increase in mitochondrial function. Millions of people are struggling with declining eyesight as they age. What an astounding intervention for maturing eyes.

Infrared light also increases our mitochondrial output of ATP, similar to red light. It can penetrate deep into the body, even down to the bone. Infrared light can improve wound healing; help prepare the skin for sun with less damage; relieve pain, stiffness, and the fatigue of rheumatoid arthritis; treat ophthalmic, neurological, and psychiatric disorders; and stimulate the proliferation of mesenchymal and cardiac stem cells. Anytime we go outside when the sun is up, we are surrounded by infrared energy.

We've seen the advantages of natural blue light received through the eyes in the morning, but blue light also has benefits when applied to the skin. Blue light has been used successfully to treat acne, atopic dermatitis, eczema, and psoriasis. Blue light has been found to have a beneficial relationship with our immune system. The blue light in sunlight increases lymphocytes, a vital part of the immune system, so they can communicate faster within the body.

Red light is the most explored light frequency by researchers. There are more than 6,000 studies on the effects of red light, which has a multitude of effects on our body, ranging from pain relief to lowering blood sugar. It affects light-sensitive proteins in the body and mitochondria. We've learned that improving mitochondria has specific and overall health benefits. They act as a collective so when one group of mitochondria is improved they can share that increased function to mitochondria in other areas of the body. This makes red and infrared light therapy helpful locally, when the body is exposed to light, but also systemically throughout the body in areas that are not exposed.

Red light also helps fibroblasts heal wounds and deposit collagen to prevent wrinkles.

Red and infrared light effects the ability of mitochondria to make ATP and melatonin efficiently. Melatonin, a major antioxidant involved in hundreds of biological actions, isn't secreted just by our pineal gland when the sun goes down at night. It's also made in our mitochondria and acts on many biological pathways and enzymes. Melatonin is a wonderful intervention for aging bones because melatonin increases bone density. Combined with red and infrared light's ability to increase anti-inflammatory cytokines in the body, we see why these spectrums of light are so anti-inflammatory.

DARKNESS CAN HEAL, TOO

The twenty-four-hour cycling of cortisol and melatonin is a foundational rhythm in our health. That circadian burst of cortisol should happen in the morning with the rising of the sun, which lowers the pineal production of melatonin. Cortisol helps us feel awake, energized, and alert throughout the day whereas melatonin helps us feel calm and ready for sleep at night. Cortisol blocks the secretion of melatonin from the pineal gland; if cortisol is high, melatonin is not released. As the sun goes down, our cortisol should drop as our melatonin rises, preparing us for the rest and repair of a good night's sleep.

Light at night negatively affects our melatonin release, disrupting our sleep and the rhythm of these necessary hormones and biological functions. Artificial light at night can keep cortisol levels high and inhibit the release of melatonin. Even small amounts of light while sleeping worsens cardiometabolic function and increases insulin resistance. Our sleep cycle also directs our growth hormone, insulin, and thyroid hormone cascades. Leptin, our body's energy storage signal, communicates with the hypothalamus at night, telling the brain whether we have enough energy to make hormones tied to fertility, or whether we have too much energy stored and need to upregulate metabolism, or whether we have too little energy storage and need to store more energy the next day. Melatonin helps leptin communicate this information to the brain while cortisol blocks it. Simply put, we need melatonin levels to rise at sundown to have properly functioning metabolism, fertility, immune system, and growth and repair routine.

Protecting the vital biological signals that happen in darkness means lowering the light at night. This can look like using red light filters on our devices to minimize the artificial blue light. Often, you can add timers to these filters to automatically turn them on at a certain time of day. You can utilize blue-blocking eye wear if you are exposed to artificial light at night. As the sun sets, switching off the overhead lights and turning on softer lights that are lower in height to mimic the setting sun can be helpful. I love salt lamps because of the soft orange glow they give off. There are light bulbs available that emit infrared and red light as well, such as incandescent lights and specially made lights, for use at night that do not disrupt the release of melatonin.

Sleeping in complete darkness and in a cool room helps reinforce circadian rhythm. Blackout curtains, tape over the light-emitting parts of appliances, and lowering the heat at night are also helpful. Having the place where you sleep at 1 lux or lower helps preserve that secretion of melatonin and initiate a good night's sleep. I talk more about lux on page 115, but there are free photography apps that measure lux to give you an idea of the intensity of light in a given setting. A decrease in body temperature is another circadian cue, so sleeping in a cool room supports our circadian rhythm. We truly are light beings, fine-tuned to light in our environment, but we need darkness just as much as light. It is the rhythm of the sun that allows for this intricate flux of biological function.

ARTIFICIAL LIGHT IN OUR ENVIRONMENT

Although the light from the sun provides a multitude of biological cues, artificial light in our environment also informs our body. Urbanization and industrialization in the late 1880s ushered in a new era of life the majority of Americans had never experienced. Technological advances in the 1880s, such as the electrical grid and Henry Ford's assembly line, dramatically changed life in America. Powerful machines that could work 24/7, electrical lighting to allow for such hours, and the demand for a workforce to fulfill production created a massive influx into cities. As people moved into the cities, the electrical grid grew to accommodate the demand for more electricity. Of course, running factories 24/7 was the main impetus for increasing the electrical grid, which grew from 2,250 electricity-generating stations in 1902 to 4,000 generating stations in 1920. The resultant exposure to artificial light and maintaining hours opposite our natural circadian rhythms had, and continues to have, a massive impact on our health and the health of our children. Being out of sync with the natural rhythm of the sun negatively affects our immune system, metabolic state, gut microbiome, mitochondrial health, and mental emotional wellness.

Our lighting has continued to change. Blue light from screens and LED lights emits a narrow band of blue light, not the full band of blue light from the sun that is balanced with the other visible colors and the infrared spectrum. Exposing ourselves to the blue light from LEDs and screens can disrupt our circadian rhythm as we discussed previously.

Remember, the spectrum of electromagnetic frequencies is in order of wavelength. Blue light has a shorter and more intense wavelength than the other colors of light. Melanopsin in our retinas has an absorption peak at the same level as blue light, making them especially vulnerable to the effects of blue light. Blue light from our screens penetrates our retinas' mitochondria, causing oxidative damage that can cause injury and cell death. Blue light can also deform the structures within the mitochondria, causing degeneration within the mitochondria, which harms their ability to make water, heat, and ATP. This is one reason we need to balance artificial light exposure with natural light exposure from the sun or more balanced light options. Mitochondria are paramount to our health and longevity so protecting and supporting them is a priority.

This artificial blue light that is the predominant spectrum of light shining from our cell phones, TVs, and computer screens is wreaking havoc on our metabolism. Blue light causes a spike in blood sugar and insulin. With repeated and prolonged exposure, this could lead to metabolic issues such as insulin resistance, diabetes, and obesity. There's a way to look at light as blue light putting the brakes on mitochondrial function and red light enhancing mitochondrial function. Balancing exposure to artificial light and natural light throughout the day is helpful. This can look like taking some calls outside, eating lunch outside, or taking a few breaks outside. Whatever the routine, it requires being outside.

Research has found that blue light increases blood glucose and insulin resistance after a meal. This means blue light exposure after a meal, especially in the evening, leads to even more dramatic increases in blood sugar, setting up a dangerous pathway to increased blood sugar, insulin resistance, and metabolic issues like diabetes and obesity. Artificial blue light exposure at night has also been associated with depression. Metabolic issues, depression, and environments laden with narrow-band blue light from LED lighting, sound familiar? The modern workplace and our indoor spaces have created a potentially massive obstacle to health.

Lux is the measurement of light that falls on a surface. We spend the vast majority of our time indoors surrounded by artificial lighting—a well-lit office space has about 500 lux, for example. In comparison, a bright summer day has about 50,000 lux whereas an overcast day has 1,000 to 5,000 lux. This natural light is dramatically richer in the different spectrums of light. As the sun sets, we enter a time of darkness that our biology depends on to regulate various functions. A moonlit night has about 1 lux whereas a night without moonlight has around 0.01 lux. These are the natural intensities of light our body has evolved with. A streetlight has an average of 15 lux, and a computer screen ranges from 10 to 37 lux.

Exposure to light at night or too little full-spectrum light throughout the day can dramatically affect our metabolic, immune, hormonal, cardiovascular, and mental emotional health. After sunset, moving to incandescent lights, specialized low blue light lighting, and low-intensity orange/red lights to avoid the continued secretion of cortisol and blocking the conversion of melatonin is helpful. Switching to lighting that is at a lower height, at hip level, to mimic the setting sun also helps protect the vital functions that rely on the signals of darkness. Use night mode, red light filters on devices, or blue light–blocking glasses to block the blue light that stops the conversion of serotonin into melatonin and disrupts our circadian rhythm.

Even Our Skin Sees Light

It is not just the eyes that are informed by the light in our environment. There are many benefits of sunlight on our skin, but it can also cause damage. Too much sun exposure is associated with aging, damage, and certain autoimmune conditions. On the other hand, research published in *Photochemical & Photobiological Sciences* found that avoiding sun exposure was associated with a higher risk of all-cause mortality, especially cardiovascular disease. Another study involving over 395,000 participants of European ancestry showed that individuals with higher ultraviolet exposure had lower risks of all-cause, cardiovascular, and cancer mortality. We need to find a balance of healthy sun exposure without risking the damage that can come from the sun.

Our skin has several light-sensitive proteins that allow us to reap the many benefits of the sun. Melanin, opsins, heme in the blood, and chromophores in the skin can catch photons from the sun to use for biological information and action. By grabbing photons of light, our skin acts as a receiver for light information from the world around us.

Ultraviolet B light stimulates vitamin D conversion. We know that vitamin D is important for regulating our immune system, inflammatory state, autoimmune conditions, and metabolic illnesses such as diabetes, obesity, and cardiovascular disease. A deficiency has been associated with diseases such as multiple sclerosis, asthma, cardiovascular disease, and autoimmune conditions such as rheumatoid arthritis. Ultraviolet light on our skin also triggers the release of nitric oxide, which dilates our blood vessels, and this mechanism has been shown to decrease blood pressure. Red and infrared light can also produce nitric oxide when they strike our skin. Safe ultraviolet light exposure has been shown to help decrease allergic rhinitis, psoriasis, dermatitis, vitiligo, and atopic eczema.

Interestingly, vitamin D and melatonin have an intimate relationship. Adequate sun exposure in the spring and summer months builds our vitamin D stores in the body. In latitudes where the sun becomes less intense in winter, if we align with this season of darkness and get more rest, increasing our melatonin, those summer stores of vitamin D carry longer through winter. Connecting with the seasons, the natural light, and the darkness has multiple benefits. We are designed to live with the interconnected cycles of nature, light, and energy.

Many don't think of skin as an endocrine gland, but it can be thought of as our biggest endocrine organ. Under the influence of sunlight and visible light, skin is a major player in the endocrine system. The skin participates in regulation and production of adrenal and thyroid hormones. The skin produces neuropeptides. It can produce and metabolize histamine, serotonin, dopamine, norepinephrine, and epinephrine. Ultraviolet light can trigger the skin to produce corticotropin-releasing hormone and adrenocorticotropic hormone, initiating an adrenal-like stress response. Ultraviolet light also increases the release of beta-endorphins, which help manage pain, support mood, and help manage stress response. Ultraviolet light also triggers the release of cytokines in the skin, making it a prominent player in regulating the immune system and inflammatory pathways.

Safe sun exposure means getting the benefits of the sun without the damage it can cause. When we get exposure to springtime or morning sunshine, we are able to build our melanin and vitamin D stores while stimulating vital immune and hormonal cascades when the ultraviolet index is low. The UV index tells us how intense the ultraviolet light from the sun is at a particular time. Locations close to the equator and during times in late spring and summer have more intense ultraviolet light and a higher UV index. This has a higher risk of causing DNA and skin damage. Many people wait until the peak sun of summer to go out in the sunshine without building up a tolerance. Melanin is the pigment that colors our skin, eyes, and hair, but it is also present in our internal organs. Melanin is a powerful protective mechanism against harmful UV radiation.

Does Sunscreen Block Sunlight's Benefits?

Sunscreens are designed to block the sun's ultraviolet rays. They generally block most of the UVA spectrum and some of the UVB spectrum. Most sunscreens are filled with toxic ingredients, such as phalates, oxybenzone, homosalate, benzophenone, and many others that cause harm in the human body and to marine life. These chemicals have been shown to increase the risk of cancer and act as a hormone disruptor in the body. Fortunately, there are nontoxic sunscreens when necessary.

There are many benefits to being exposed to the sun, such as decreasing all-cause mortality, bolstering the immune system, regulating metabolic pathways, stimulating hormonal cascades, producing neurotransmitters, and balancing inflammatory pathways. Sunscreen will block exposure to the spectrums of light and the benefits they produce, including interfering with the conversion of vitamin D in the body. On the other hand, the sun's ultraviolet rays can damage our skin if we aren't careful. Here are some tips:

- Wear protective clothing and sunhats when you have had enough sun; find shade during peak times of ultraviolet exposure when needed; learn to recognize the signs that you have had enough sun (which varies by skin type, melanin content, and tolerance to sun exposure) and seek shade or protection.
- Build protective melanin with safe sun exposure when the UV index is lower in spring and morning hours.
- Eat foods rich in omega-3 fatty acids, polyphenols, and phytochemicals, which can help us be in the sun longer without damage.
- Use an app to determine the amount and type of ultraviolet light in your environment as well as the amount of exposure you need to make vitamin D, or the amount of time you can spend in the sun without damage according to your location, the UV index, and skin type.
- Use nontoxic sunscreen during times when sun exposure can cause skin damage.

Eating colorful foods, like fruits and vegetables high in polyphenols, lycopene, and flavonoids, has been shown to increase the amount of time we can spend in the sun without damage. Omega-3 fatty acids from seafood have a similar effect. Eating processed foods containing processed seed oils and alcohol is thought to increase our susceptibility to sun damage by decreasing the available antioxidants in the skin. Maintaining our circadian rhythm also helps protect us from sun damage. Healthy levels of melatonin have been found to be photoprotective and help prevent damage from the sun, which makes circadian rhythm and mitochondria health important. As a fair-skinned woman, I must carry a hat and retreat to the shade when I have been in the sun long enough.

Light Dances with Water

Infrared light is the main builder of that liquid crystal cell-bound water battery within the body. The water that comes up against our cells, DNA, fascia, and tissues takes on a different structure. EZ water is negatively charged and produces a positively charged zone of water directly outside of it, creating a water battery. Infrared light is a powerful tool that has the ability to organize and build EZ water within us, which can act as potential energy within the body. Infrared light, especially mid and far infrared light, builds that special EZ water.

Ultraviolet light excites this liquid crystalline EZ water, creating a plasma of free electrons that could be used where energy or antioxidant action is needed in the body. That negative charge of the water lining our cells and the positive charge that builds right outside of the liquid crystalline water also potentially create a source of energy.

Although there are many sources of infrared light, the sun is the most abundant source of infrared energy on our planet—and it doesn't have to be direct sunlight to be beneficial. We are enveloped in infrared light even on cloudy days. Infrared light is reflected off the leaves of a tree and the grass on the ground, meaning sitting in the shade of a tree can be a rich source of energy for us any time of year.

A RESERVOIR OF ENERGY

It's not just protection from the sun that melanin provides. Melanin can scavenge free radicals that can cause oxidative damage in the body. It can also absorb heavy metals, acting as a source of detoxification in the body.

Melanin also offers a source of cellular energy. It is a quantum bioelectronic material. Melanin is completely surrounded by liquid crystalline EZ water. When the sun hits the melanin in our body, it has the capacity to split water into molecular oxygen and molecular hydrogen, which could have several roles in the body:

- Molecular oxygen is reduced to water in the mitochondria's electron transport chain, providing a valuable source of cellular hydration.
- Molecular hydrogen has a robust number of studies validating its health benefits. It acts as a selective antioxidant, donating electrons where needed yet not blocking the sophisticated communication network of the body. The current research focuses on inhaled hydrogen gas or water infused with hydrogen, but we are born with the ability to make molecular hydrogen.

The dance between sunlight, melanin, and water creates cellular energy and signals.

We should remember that melanin isn't just in our skin. It can be found internally in our brain, ears, eyes, nose, and internal organs. Melanin is an organic semiconductor and photoconductor, which is rare in biological systems. It can store and transmit electrical signals. When struck by light, it has the potential to release free electrons to be used throughout the body. Simply put, melanin could produce energy for the body when exposed to light. A decrease or inability for melanin to create this free energy has been associated with Alzheimer's disease and Parkinson's disease. There are two ways in which melanin produces energy for the body: One is the ability to split water and form free electrons when exposed to ultraviolet light, creating a source of electrons. The other comes from melanin's semiconductor nature that can turn external light, frequency, and vibration into electrons or energy.

Melanin also transforms sound into light and heat. It also does the reverse, turning heat and light into sound. Melanin not only can split water when exposed to ultraviolet light, but it also has the capacity to reform those components back into water. This could be a renewable reservoir of energy for the body to use. The molecular hydrogen and oxygen from the split water could act as electron donors able to reduce oxidation and inflammation in the body. When molecular hydrogen and oxygen donate their electrons, they don't become inflammatory free radicals as we might expect. Melanin has a special property to reform the hydrogen and oxygen back into water. Then the cycle can begin again. What a magnificent body we have.

Melanin is not the only component that can use light to communicate. The benzene ring found in so many of our neurotransmitters, like tryptophan and serotonin, can capture, store, and emit light throughout the body. The foods we eat, like polyphenols in fruits and vegetables, also have that benzene ring that can communicate with light. Each benzene ring has six pi electrons that can become excited by an electrical, magnetic, or electromagnetic charge. This excitement causes the electrons to dislocate and travel freely throughout the molecule and even be donated to other molecules. This allows for quantum states and almost instantaneous transmission of energy and information.

We have the internal hardware for a quantum messaging system centered on light, electricity, and magnetism. This can redefine our perspective of biology and what it takes to heal. Ignoring this puts us at a disadvantage when it comes to health and longevity. We should have access to all the tools known to truly thrive.

OUR INTERNAL LIGHT

Why would our body need an internal communication network for light?

There seems to be communication within the body based on light, and we are not just sensitive to external light. We also have an extensive and sophisticated light network within us. The light emissions of the body are coherent, suggesting it as a mode of communication. Although there is no research on this, internal melanin, opsins, and light-sensitive proteins could communicate with the light that our cells shine internally.

First discovered by Russian scientist Alexander G. Gurwitsch in the 1920s, cells can communicate with light. Gurwitsch set up a series of experiments with an onion root, which he pointed toward a second onion root. These onion samples were separated by quartz. The control was set up the same way, but the roots were separated by an opaque barrier. The quartz container can transmit light whereas the opaque barrier blocks light. The onion roots separated by quartz displayed a higher growth rate, suggesting nonchemical light mediated communication between the roots. Some continued this work on light communication, but it wasn't until 1984 that the term *biophoton* was established by Fritz-Albert Popp as a way to describe the unique biological phenomenon of light emission from living cells.

For decades, Popp researched our cellular light emission that he termed "biophotons." Biophotons are the weak photon emissions that come from all living systems—plants, animals, microbes, and human beings. These light emissions come from our DNA and the production of reactive species when our mitochondria make ATP. Healthy mitochondria produce coherent biophoton communication. Popp's research found that biophoton emissions were coherent, not random. This suggests a form of communication.

Biophotons seem to emit light signals in a Goldilocks zone: Too high of a light emission and too little emission both signify an inflamed, stressed, or diseased cell. Between these two extremes indicates a healthy cell. Biophotons are used currently to access reactive oxygen species, a measure of inflammation in the body. Biophoton emissions in the extremes of too high or too low have been associated with cancer, rheumatoid arthritis, and multiple sclerosis. Supporting mitochondrial function and managing stress levels can balance the light we shine within. We truly are light beings.

TENDING TO OUR LIGHT BEINGS

Align your circadian rhythm: Go outside at sunrise to signal safety to the nervous system and slowly raise cortisol levels. This benefits metabolism, stress response, and inflammation. Earthing at this time is also beneficial.

Get morning light when the sun is between ten and thirty degrees above the horizon, usually one to two hours after sunrise. This is the most valuable time to be exposed to sunlight as it is the primary circadian cue and should be the priority for natural light exposure throughout the day. It improves hormonal balance, metabolism, neurotransmitters, and mood as well circadian function throughout the body. Earthing at the same time is also beneficial.

Eat a protein-rich breakfast that includes quality fat and fiber within thirty to sixty minutes of waking to reinforce the circadian rhythm.

Take natural light breaks throughout the day. This reinforces the circadian rhythm and all the functions of the body that depend on it. It also exposes us to nourishing green, yellow, and blue colors.

Lower the lights as the sun sets. Exposure to sunset light signals safety to the nervous system and signals the body that it is time to switch to the functions that dominate the night. Change the color, intensity, and height of evening indoor lighting. Utilize blocking glasses and apps on devices if necessary. Avoid eating, drinking alcohol, and blue light three hours before bed. Sleep in a completely dark and cool room for optimal sleep and circadian rhythm.

Using red and infrared light devices is another way to help support overall health.

Safe sun exposure can be a wonderful tool for health. Exposing the skin to sun can activate hormonal and metabolic pathways and build protective melanin. Eating a diet rich in omega-3 fatty acids and colorful fruits and vegetables that is low in processed foods and alcohol can help protect against skin damage. Melanin is a photoconductor and semiconductor so it can turn light into energy, playing an important role in bioenergetics.

Support mitochondrial health to optimize healthy biophoton emission (see chapter 4 for more information).

Tend to the EZ cell-bound water inside. It is vital to health and our light body. Exposure to infrared energy has the potential to build that water battery within us. Infrared energy comes from the sun and devices, but it also comes from other places. We are exposed to infrared energy when we lie on rocks or sand that has been heated by the sun. Infrared saunas emit infrared energy but so do warm baths, beverages, and food. Movement is a way to build infrared energy in the body. One of my favorites ways to build infrared energy is to cuddle under a blanket with a pet or person I love. The world is filled with infrared energy; we only need to connect to it.

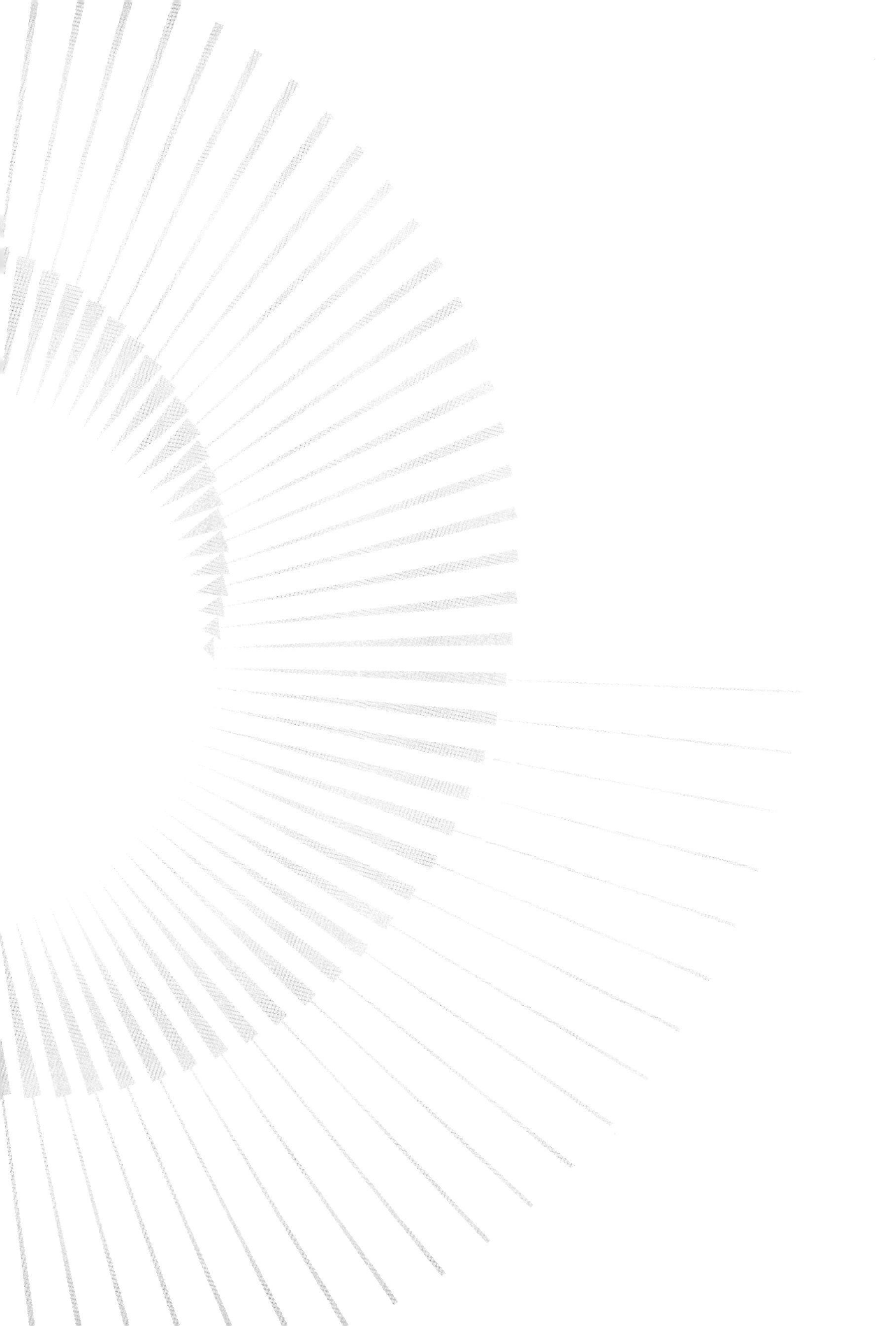

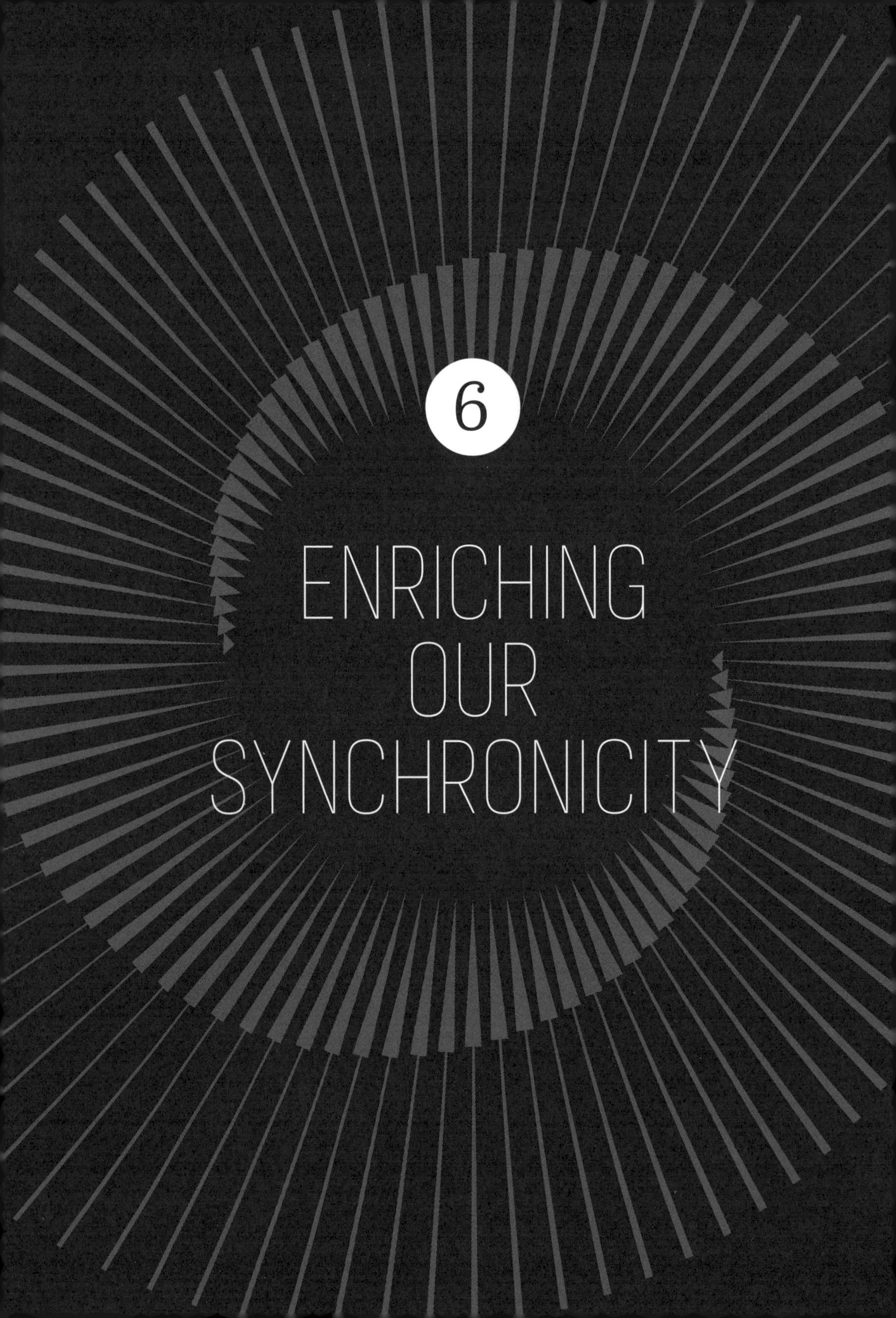

6

ENRICHING OUR SYNCHRONICITY

You've learned how electricity and light guide our biology, but it's not just electricity and light that educates our biological function. We orchestrate with all the frequencies around us. Like two people walking together whose footsteps eventually fall into sync, we synchronize with the rhythms around us. We are receivers of information in a beautiful choreography with the ecosystem we belong to. Getting in sync with our ecosystem leads to better health and vitality because it informs our neurological function, inflammatory state, immune system, and cardiovascular and nervous systems.

We are entrained with the rhythm of nature. Like two people dancing the tango, we dance with the world around us. The unseen order of nature informs, educates, and directs our biological action. We are magnetic beings responding to the pushes and pulls within us and from the world around us. It's not just our batteries and generators that have magnets inside them. Everything in our body, such as our cells, tissues, and organs, has a magnetic field. Our mitochondria have magnetic fields that guide the pull of protons and the creation of ATP, our energy currency. Our body also *responds* to magnetic fields. The biggest magnetic field known is the Earth we live on, and we're tuned to react to it as well as the sights and sounds of nature.

We have lived over millennia in sync with the rhythms and energetic fields of the natural world. Born into this realm of frequencies and information, we are meant to align with the environment we evolved with. Although science has recently begun to study the benefits of being in nature, the majority of that research has yet to sway our daily life. On average, we spend less than 9 percent of our time outside. A study out of the United Kingdom found that children spend less time outdoors than prison inmates do. Returning to a relationship with nature offers such healing in our nervous system, neurological function, immune system, inflammatory pathways, and hormonal balance.

FOREST HEALING

Just the act of being in nature has profound effects on our biology. The Japanese have a practice called *shinrin-yoku*, or forest bathing, which is the act of being immersed in a forest with the space to appreciate the sounds and sights while breathing in the air of the forest biome. Forest bathing began in Japan in the 1980s as a form of ecotherapy in response to the increase in stress-related illnesses.

Forest bathing has shown consistent benefits for the cardiovascular, immune, and nervous systems. In a 2021 study, researchers explored the seasonal effects of forest bathing during spring and winter, looking at twelve healthy volunteers who participated in a two-hour leisurely forest walking program. Systolic blood pressure decreased after the trips both in late spring and in winter. In research published in October 2018, scientists showed improvements in heart rate variability in 485 male participants while walking in a forest for just fifteen minutes. A study conducted in semi-ancient woodland, in Derbyshire, also produced improvements in heart rate variability in 57 percent of the study participants and reduced anxiety by 29 percent. Remember, heart rate variability is a measure of resilience in the nervous system and is associated with cardiovascular health, resistance to stress, overall well-being, and longevity. You want a high heart rate variability and being in nature can do that.

Decades of research has found that shinrin-yoku increases vital components of the immune system. It increases the anti-cancer human natural killer (NK) activity, the number of NK cells, and the intracellular levels of anticancer proteins, suggesting a preventive effect on cancers. The research also found reductions in blood pressure and heart rate, showing a preventive effect on hypertension and heart disease. Forest bathing reduces stress hormones, such as urinary adrenaline and noradrenaline and salivary/serum cortisol, which contributes to stress management. Time in the forest landscape increases the activity of parasympathetic nerves and reduces the activity of sympathetic nerves to stabilize the balance of autonomic nervous system inducing a calming, relaxing effect.

Forest bathing improves sleep. In the Profile of Mood States test (POMS), shinrin-yoku reduces the scores for anxiety, depression, anger, fatigue, and confusion and increases the score for vigor, showing preventive effects on depression.

While many forest bathing studies looked at long durations of exposure, from five- to one-day retreats into the forest, recent research found that just two hours a week can have profound effects on health and well-being. Research also confirms that our brain structure and mood improve when we spend time outdoors, likely influencing concentration, working memory, and the mind overall.

Although being held in the awe of the outdoors has shown considerable benefit to our health, we also know there are individual components to the outdoors that affect our biology. The microbes in nature offer a powerful education for our immune system as well as our nervous system. The recently discovered soil-derived microbe *Mycobacterium vaccae* was found to decrease stress-related inflammation and build resilience to future stressors. Research on the exposure to the essential oils of the trees encountered in forest bathing also increased NK cells that rid the body of dysfunctional cells while decreasing stress hormones. Scientists investigated whether inhaling plant-emitted biogenic volatile compounds, namely monoterpenes, had effects on anxiety symptoms. Information from 505 participants in 39 structured forest therapy sessions at different Italian sites found that exposure to high monoterpene concentrations during forest therapy did indeed decrease anxiety symptoms.

COLORS OF NATURE

The frequencies of the sights and sounds in nature also guide our biology in a beneficial way. The melanin in our eyes and ears serves as a guardian and receiver to the visual and audible signals around us. As we discussed in chapter 1, our senses are governed by quantum biology, and sight and sound are no exception. Viewing the green spaces of nature has a specific effect on our health. Patients in hospital settings had faster healing times and took fewer pain medications when able to view nature through a window versus viewing a concrete wall. Further research found that it was not just live nature; viewing nature videos or photos evokes a similar effect. Looking at photos, 3D images, virtual reality, and videos of natural landscapes led to a decrease in stress responses. Visual contact with flowers, green plants, and wooden materials had positive effects on cerebral and autonomic nervous activities, demonstrating how the frequencies of nature through our sense of sight influence our nervous system and stress-related illness for the better.

The same positive effects were found when viewing blue spaces, like rivers, lakes, and the ocean. In the book *Blue Mind*, Wallace Nichols discusses a robust collection of research showing how watching the ocean improves our mood through changes in the prefrontal cortex, amygdala, and neuron functioning. It makes sense that being in nature and close to water sends powerful signals of safety throughout our biology. We have evolved over millennia embedded in nature, living by waterways for survival. We're wired to be a part of the greater ecosystem around us.

The safety signal of blue isn't just from the water. We can gain an immense amount of safety by viewing the sky. Recent research found that viewing the blue sky has benefits for the cardiovascular system. Even looking at the nighttime sky has its benefits. Research participants found that stargazing increased their sense of well-being and happiness.

DANCING TO THE SOUNDS OF NATURE

Of course, it is not just the sight of nature that sends these safety cues. The sounds of nature and water ways also provide frequency information that benefits our biology. The terms *white noise*, *brown noise*, and *pink noise* have become popular in the last decade:

- White noise refers to a mixture of sound waves extending over a wide frequency range, like the sound from fans or radio static, and is usually used to drown out sounds that might interrupt sleep, like doors slamming and cars honking.
- Brown noise refers to noise that produces a bass-heavy rumbling sound that many find relaxing.
- Pink noise refers to a lower-pitched noise than white or brown noise and has some research on it that shows it benefits sleep by lowering the brainwaves to a state that is more conducive to sleep.

As is often the case, we replace nature with a technological substitute for convenience and assumed superiority as in the case of creating machines to mimic these noise ranges. In fact, one study found that although pink noise helps people attain a deeper sleep more readily, it also negatively affects the higher cognitive functions that occur during sleep. While these white, brown, and pink noise machines may be beneficial for sleep and relaxation in some cases, our body craves the sounds we have evolved with—natural sounds. Sound affects our body on several quantum biological levels, such as oxygenation levels and nervous system support, as we'll see in the next chapter. It is so much more than drowning out the sounds of modern life. Our body is tuned to the sounds of nature.

And, a sound isn't just a sound. It structures our water body within. It creates a unique cymatic or geometric pattern distinctive to that sound, and that pattern is imprinted on the fluid surrounding the cell or tissue. It makes perfect sense that sounds from nature do this in a way our body is familiar with and craves.

Entrained Brain Waves

Our brain waves are synced with our environment and have different frequency bands correlated with different brain functions.

Delta waves: The lowest frequency brainwave at 0.5 Hz to 4 Hz are related to deep sleep, healing, memory consolidation, and immune function. Deficient delta brain activity can cause poor sleep and cognitive decline. **Epsilon waves** refer to the lowest level of delta brainwaves and are associated with times of high states of consciousness, ecstatic states, and spiritual experiences.

Theta waves: From 4 Hz to 8 Hz, these brainwaves are associated with deep relaxation, deep meditation, and emotional healing.

Sounds of a crackling fire and heartbeat rhythms can entrain theta states of deep relaxation and delta waves, which promote sleep.

Alpha waves: Ranging from 8 Hz to 12 Hz , these brainwaves are related to relaxation, calmness, and creativity.

Ocean waves, rain, and flowing water sounds can entrain with alpha and theta waves, promoting relaxation and stress reduction. Additionally, forest surroundings contain natural low-frequency vibrations that match alpha and theta waves.

Beta waves: Spanning from 12 Hz to 30 Hz, these brainwaves are linked to alertness, active thinking, and decision making. High beta levels are associated with stress, anxiety, and overthinking whereas low beta levels can lead to lack of focus and mental fatigue.

Birdsong and natural soundscapes enhance relaxing alpha waves and lower beta waves. Studies suggest that morning birdsong increases cognitive alertness while reducing stress, promoting a balanced mental state.

Gamma waves: Around 30 Hz to 100+ Hz, these brainwaves are associated with high levels of cognition, information processing, focused thought, and consciousness. Disruptions in gamma waves may be related to cognitive decline and Alzheimer's disease.

Our body also craves silence. Carving out some time for silence is important to health, both mental and physical. Research has found that silence reduces heart rate and blood pressure. It can decrease cortisol and anxiety while boosting the ability to focus. In research with mice, two hours of silence induced growth in the hippocampus, the region of the brain associated with memory and emotion. Noise has adverse effects on our mental state, nervous system, cardiovascular health, metabolic disease, cancer, and respiratory disease. Just as we reap benefits from light and darkness, there are benefits to sound and silence. Silence offers the space for our nervous system to settle and our mind to open.

The sounds of nature are particularly beneficial for our biology. A new study from Carleton University, Michigan State University, and Colorado State University, in conjunction with the US National Park Service, found that the sounds of nature can have a variety of health benefits for humans. Researchers looked at sound recordings from 251 sites at 66 US national parks and discovered that regions with high levels of nature sounds and low levels of human-made noise improved health in research participants by decreasing pain, improving mood, enhancing cognitive performance, increasing positive emotions, and lowering stress and annoyance.

Researchers also found that different sounds had different effects. Water sounds improved positive emotions and health outcomes for the participants, whereas bird sounds decreased stress and annoyance. Additional research produced similar findings with birdsong having a beneficial impact on our health by reducing anxiety and paranoia while boosting mood and overall sense of well-being.

Looking into the mechanism behind the benefits of nature sounds, scientists found that these natural sounds help regulate the nervous system and brain connectivity. It only makes sense that our biology is meant to dance to the tunes of nature.

BUILDING NEGATIVE CHARGE

We also sync with the negative ions in our environment. Negative ions are a form of ionic antioxidants our body can utilize. Formed when ions gain an extra electron, negative ions also offer electrons for our body to use as antioxidants. Like a plasma of free energy, the negative ions in our environment give us a good source of energy. Negative ions are created from radiant or cosmic rays in the atmosphere, sunlight, and corona discharge, including thunder and lightning as well as plants releasing negative ions during photosynthesis and in response to touch.

Negative ions are also created by the shearing forces of water, called *the Lenard effect*, and are usually dispersed from waterways such as rivers, waterfalls, ocean spray, and rainfall.

Research has found that negative ions are picked up by the wind from plants such as trees and fields of grass as well as other members of the plant kingdom, so time spent outside near these also exposes us to negative ions. The measurement of these negative ions is being used as a measurement of air quality, with more negative ions indicating better air quality.

Just as negative ions are vital to air health, they also play an important role in *our* health. Research has found that these negative ions formed from water are associated with an increase in NK cells and an inhibition in cancer growth in mice. Water-formed negative ions also improved the ability of red blood cells to squeeze through smaller vessels and increased aerobic metabolism in humans after one hour of exposure. Research has also found that negative ion exposure decreases blood pressure.

Exposure to negative ions has profound impacts on our mental function and health. Research has found that negative ion exposure dramatically increased performance in mental tasks and neurological function. Negative ion exposure has been found to alleviate symptoms of seasonal affective disorder and depression, with one study finding negative ion exposure similar in effect to antidepressant medications.

Researchers have hypothesized that negative ions positively affect our health in a variety of ways, including by altering amino acid metabolism, which reduces inflammation, increases antioxidation, promotes energy production in the mitochondria, affects the expression of c-Fos (a protein associated with many biological functions and its overexpression is found in cancer growth), and regulates serotonin levels.

A handful of studies found no benefit from negative ion exposure, but these studies do not account for the redox state of the participants, which is important when assessing the benefit of negative ions. The redox state refers to whether a person has an abundance of electrons to quench inflammation or whether the body is in a state of deficiency. It's possible that these studies found no benefit from negative ions because the person's redox was rich and didn't need the extra redox potential from the negative ions. Or it could be the opposite—that the participant's redox was so poor it was hard to see any benefit because so many more were needed.

Our daily dance with the quantum particles in the air surrounding us can have such powerful impacts on our health.

THE EARTH'S RESONANCE

The Earth's Schumann resonance also seems to inform our biology. Schumann resonance refers to the Earth's unique electromagnetic waves that oscillate between the surface of Earth and the charged ionosphere in the atmosphere. It's named after Winfried Otto Schumann, who first mathematically predicted the electromagnetic waves, or Schumann resonance, of Earth in 1952. Some of these electromagnetic waves can combine and strengthen to create a repeating atmospheric heartbeat. This heartbeat, or Schumann resonance, has been recorded at the frequency of about 7.83 Hz, with a circadian variation of about ±0.5 Hz. This matches our brain waves in the alpha state, which is associated with relaxation and creativity.

The other Schumann resonance frequencies are approximately 14 Hz, 20 Hz, 26 Hz, 33 Hz, 39 Hz, and 45 Hz, which closely overlap with human brainwaves, such as alpha (8 Hz to 12 Hz), beta (12 Hz to 30 Hz), and gamma (30 Hz to 100+ Hz).

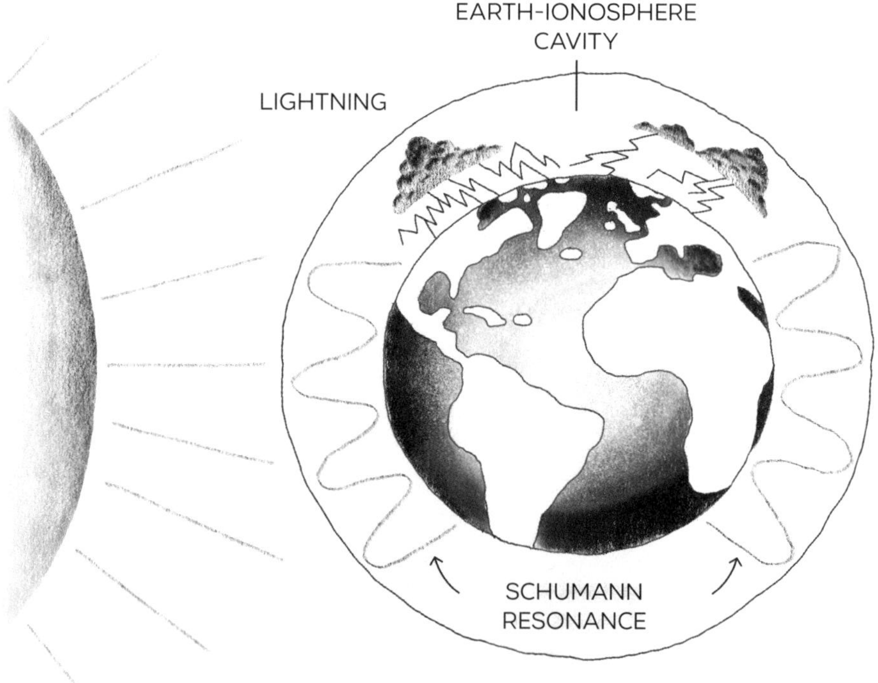

The Schumann resonance is a set of global electromagnetic resonances that happen between Earth's surface and the ionosphere.

Continued research shows the frequencies produced by the brain and the Schumann resonances seem to synchronize, as evidenced by the propensity of EEG rhythms to sync with Schumann resonance fluctuation. This implies a connection between the Schumann resonance and our brain state. Scientists have recorded changes in the Schumann resonance correlated with changes in the EEG of study participants. Researchers verified that several of the Schumann resonance frequencies are mirrored in the spectral profiles of human brain activity. They discovered that the EEGs had repeated and reliable periods of coherence with the Schumann resonance frequencies of 7 Hz to 8 Hz, 13 Hz to 14 Hz, and 19 Hz to 20 Hz in real time, implying a relationship between our brain activity and the resonance of the Earth.

The reliable similarity of the Schumann resonance and the measured human brain activity suggest the potential for an information interaction between the two. Remember, coherence can enable long-range information transfer and sharing. Similar research found that a group could synchronize their heart rate variability with Earth's local magnetic field, with more synchronization found in those with more heart coherence. Again, this implies a connection and possible information sharing between the Earth's magnetic field and the magnetic field of the human heart.

Researchers also found that this coherence between the Schumann resonances and brain activity could be associated with processes linked to consciousness, short-term memory, and perception. Not only that, but the measurements of the quantitative electroencephalography (QEEG) and Schumann resonance found that this information exchange might be quantum in nature with nonlocal effects. Further research found that the information transferred during this quantum coherence could come from our own biophoton emission. A potential quantum communication between the fields of the Earth and our biology changes our perspective. Once thought of as two separate things, this research suggests what ancient cultures always spoke of—an undeniable relationship with the Earth we live on. It calls for a deeper acknowledgment and respect for the planet we inhabit. It introduces a new paradigm of medicine, emphasizing the importance of nurturing our relationship with Earth.

MAGNETICALLY ALIGNED

We seem to be fine-tuned to Earth's magnetic field as well. Research on the geomagnetic effects on human neurological function has found some astounding results.

Researchers have examined the impacts of the geomagnetic field on humans' brainwaves that showed changes in participants' alpha brain waves in conjunction with the direction of the geomagnetic field of Earth. This is an amazing discovery. To find that humans are responsive to Earth's magnetic field is completely new. It brings more understanding to the effects of magnetic fields on human health. Weak magnetic fields influence a variety of actions in the body, including genetic expression and damage, cancer progression, immune system function, blood flow, pain, and metabolism.

Mayer waves are low frequency oscillations in blood pressure and blood flow. Slow-paced breathing, around six breaths per minute, or 0.1 Hz, can entrain Mayer waves, meaning that rhythmic breath synchronizes these natural blood flow oscillations. Slow-paced breathing also regulates heart rate variability and baroreflex sensitivity, the reflex that helps regulate blood pressure. The Earth's geomagnetic field is 0.1 Hz and has been linked to blood pressure and heart rate variability. So slow-paced breath can synch up with the oscillations in blood pressure and flow while improving heart rate variability and the resilience of the nervous system. The entrainment of all three—the breath, the flow of blood, and Earth's magnetic field—highlight how interconnected we are to this planet we live on.

In different but related research, scientists examined the relationships between solar and geomagnetic activity and human nervous system function as reflected in heart rate variability. There is no way to separate us from the Earth's environment where we live and the sun we orbit. In a small study, researchers continuously monitored the heart rate variability of ten people over a thirty-one-day period and found that the daily activity of the nervous system is sensitive to changes in solar and geomagnetic activity. The nervous system can sync with the magnetic fields associated with geomagnetic field-line resonances and Schumann resonances, both of which change according to the influence of the sun and solar wind. In an extension of this research, scientists found that the heart rate variability of one hundred people across the globe synchronized with the Schumann resonance and ultralow frequency waves emitted by the field lines of Earth's magnetic field. Further research demonstrated that we can synchronize our heart coherence as measured through heart rate variability across the globe, and this coherence seems to be associated with a synchronization with the local magnetic field. This offers an understanding that even though we can be influenced by changes in solar and geomagnetic activity, we can navigate these uncontrollable changes though the relationship between our heart and Earth's magnetic field.

The vibrating magnetic field of Earth and the amplitude of the Schumann resonances influence the nervous system, cardiovascular system, and brain function. Not only that, but researchers from HeartMath Institute propose that the coherence of our nervous system can influence Earth's magnetic field. Scientists hypothesize that Earth's geomagnetic field acts as a carrier wave of information. Further, when we collectively feel the state of heart coherence, it can instruct the global information in Earth's magnetic field. HeartMath's Global Coherence Initiative investigates the relationship between the heart coherence of an individual and a group, the geomagnetic variation of Earth, and Schumann resonances. The goal of the initiative is to validate this theory of a global information field contained in Earth's magnetic field and our ability to affect this field via our state of heart coherence. They point to evidence of a global effect when large groups experience similar states of coherence to substantiate the theory that when people intentionally generate positive emotions or heart coherence, they can change Earth's energetic and geomagnetic fields. It's thrilling to think that science is on the doorstep of illuminating the interconnections between the universal, global, and individual energy fields. The invisible connection has united us for millennia, and its acknowledgment by modern science is overdue.

CONNECTING WITH THE CONTOURS OF EARTH

Even the natural contours of Earth intertwine with our biology for our benefit. When we move on natural surfaces, uneven surfaces, we improve our neural function as well as our physical fitness. In today's world, much of our activity takes place on even surfaces, as a result we have little side-to-side swing in our gait. With movement on an uneven, natural surface, however, we must accommodate both physically and mentally for the different angles and textures of the terrain. This means more muscular exertion and tissue movement is required to navigate natural terrain. This also improves our awareness of the body's position and movement and, in theory, forms new neurological pathways as evidenced by growth in the region of the brain called the *hippocampus.*

Walking barefoot is an ancient practice in Asia, Europe, and the Americas. Reflexology is the practice of utilizing the acupressure points on the bottom of the foot to help balance and maintain health. Reflexology paths refer to paths made of smooth rocks on which people walk barefoot to stimulate different acupressure points on the feet. This differs from earthing where the benefit comes from coming in contact with the sea of electrons that lines Earth.

When traveling to China, researchers noticed that adults of all ages reported improvements in pain relief, sleep, and physical and mental well-being from walking thirty minutes a day on cobblestones. Researchers from Oregon Research Institute expanded on these studies using plastic replicas of the cobblestone paths in China. They found significant decreases in blood pressure and improvements in balance and physical performance in adults ages sixty and over from walking on the uneven surface of cobblestones.

SEASONAL BEINGS

Even the frequencies of the seasons hold sway on our biology. We have infradian seasonal rhythms informed by exposure to the seasonal changes in temperature and light. The decrease of infrared energy and sunlight hours in winter ushers in a time when we can focus on melatonin production, rest, and repair. The colder temperatures signal our biology to burn our summer and fall energy stores. Like a fasting cycle, summer and fall would be our feasting time whereas winter and spring represent our fasting mode.

Exposure to cold in the form of exposed skin on a winter day or a direct cold plunge into a cold lake or river has profound effects on our biology. Hormesis, a stressor like plunging into that cold water, enhances function rather than decreases it. Our body has evolved over millennia living in exposure to the cold whereas modern living has created a false and narrowed temperature range from our constantly humming heat or air-conditioning units. We go from a 70-degree Fahrenheit (21 degrees Celsius) house to a 70-degree car to a 70-degree office without exposure to the range of seasonal temperatures. Research into cold exposure in the air found that this cold acts as a stimulant to our metabolism and could help increase our energy-burning brown fat, and that cold exposure increases mitochondrial function efficiency as well as the number of mitochondria in a cell. This, in turn, would enhance our quantum biology by creating more cellular water, infrared energy, and ATP for our body to utilize as energy.

Cold exposure was also found to increase several important neurotransmitters. Research demonstrated increased levels of dopamine, serotonin, and endorphins after cold exposure. Cold exposure from water or air was found to increase adiponectin in adipose tissue through the process of thermogenesis to stay warm, which improves insulin sensitivity and fat burning. Since adiponectin is associated with longevity, cold exposure could have a positive effect on life span. Cold exposure also has the benefits of creating new mitochondria as we discussed in chapter 4.

Exposure to infrared energy in the form of sunlight and heat also benefits our health. The heat we are exposed to can act as a hormetic stressor, making us more resilient. Heat exposure has been found to increase mitochondrial function and efficiency by increasing the flow of electrons in the electron transport chain and by reducing reactive oxygen species. Heat exposure in the form of sauna use was found to protect against cardiovascular disease and decrease overall mortality from all causes in males.

Of course, one's response to cold or heat depends on the landscape of their internal resilience, with cold or heat exposure being problematic for some with cardiovascular issues and the elderly, and it can cause damage to mitochondria, proteins, and cell membranes in cases of extreme heat exposure/shock. Cold exposure doses also seem to be different for women and men, with women needing less temperature difference. The research seems to point to gentle exposure with the adaptation to cold or heat exposure holding the key to hormonal or mitochondrial health.

We have evolved in an intimate dance with the energetic signals of the weather, the seasons, and the light rhythms. We are meant to be exposed to seasonal cycles of light and temperature.

EATING WITH THE RHYTHM

Our relationship with the energetics of plants also has a powerful influence on our health. In addition to the protein, carbohydrate, and fat macronutrients we require, we also need the micronutrition that plants provide to thrive. A diet rich in fruits and vegetables offers us fiber and resistant starches. These resistant starches reach the colon undigested, and the gut microbiome ferments them into short chain fatty acids. These fatty acids serve as biological signals informing our immune system and inflammatory state. Butyrate is a short chain fatty acid derived from the fermentation of resistant starches. This butyrate goes directly into the cells lining the gut and feeds the mitochondria present there. This supports mitochondrial health and function, which is vital for health.

In their own right, fruits and vegetables provide a variety of phytochemicals, from flavonoids to polyphenols to sulfur to aromatic compounds. As Albert Szent-Györgyi claimed, they help electrical flow in the body. These flavonoids and polyphenols have influence in the mitochondria's electron transport chain, which produces the ATP energy we need to function, survive, and thrive. Polyphenols have been found to play an important part in mitochondrial uncoupling, helping create new mitochondria, preserve the life span of existing mitochondria, and inducing heat production in the body.

Eating plants in season provides more nutrition and phytochemicals for our body to utilize. Eating seasonally provides a variety of antioxidants, flavonoids, polyphenols, and aromatic compounds that our mitochondria can use. Seasonal, fresh, organic foods have a higher concentration of biophotons that seem to participate in communication throughout the body. While more research is needed, it stands to reason that eating food higher in biophotons has its own influence on this communication network and cellular signaling.

We evolved eating more carbohydrates in summer and more protein and fat in winter. Eating seasonally means eating foods local to your area and season. This means eating fresh fruits and vegetables when available and moving toward the seasonal vegetables of fall and winter when the seasons change.

RELATIONSHIPS HEAL

Simply by spending more time outside, we can reap the benefits of the abundant frequency information nature provides. The negative charge of Earth, the magnetic field of Earth, the negative ions in nature, and the sounds and sights of nature all effect our quantum biology. The influence of nature improves our cardiovascular function, immune system, mood, nervous system, neurological function, and hormonal balance. We have lived over millennia within the context of nature. It has so many benefits. It can help heal us if we let it.

We'd be remiss to think that nature is just a list of benefits that can be harvested. It is our relationship with nature that guides our health. We stand firmly in the cosmic flow of energy and information that comes into our atmosphere and travels through every plant, animal, and human on this planet. This universal flow of intelligence guides, informs, and educates our biology. When we are disconnected from this flow of energy, our health suffers.

TENDING TO YOUR SYNCHRONOUS BEING

When we realize we don't end at the barriers of our skin, that we are intimately and inseparably interconnected with the world around us, we can inhabit our true place in the greater ecosystem. We are held by this incredible ecosystem that we belong to, and it requires a relationship to maintain it properly. The invisible order present in nature is also present in us. We need only to connect with it.

Spend time outside. Get sun in the morning and throughout the day to sync your circadian rhythm with the rhythm of the sun. Get outside and look at your surroundings. So often we go out into nature without truly looking at our surroundings. A walk in a natural location provides exposure to the green and blue colors of nature that are so beneficial to health. Time outside can expose you to negative ions that improve immune function, mood, neurological function, and support sleep and energy levels.

Go outside and listen. Many of us listen to music or our favorite podcast while taking a walk or spending time outdoors. Make it a habit to go outside and notice the sounds of nature—the birdsong, the wind through the leaves, the babbling of a brook, or crash of the ocean surf. These sounds can improve our neurological function, stress levels, and mood and lower blood pressure.

Earth often. Put your feet on the ground. Connect to Earth's geomagnetic pull while also experiencing the natural contours of the ground. Just like the research on walking on cobblestones, walking barefoot can expose you to varying surfaces, which benefits your neurological function, lowers blood pressure, and improves balance and proprioception. Even walking with shoes on, but upon natural and varying surfaces, holds benefit. Get off the beaten path and feel better for it.

Eat a seasonal diet. Let the nutrients, phytochemicals, and the biphotonic light of the season help improve your microbiome, which is associated with better health and a longer life. It also improves neurological, cardiovascular, mitochondrial, and immune functions. Make it a goal to eat the rainbow and a diversity of seasonal plants each week. Our eating habits should reflect the seasonal influence.

Expose yourself to the weather of the season. Safe exposure to the heat of summer, the rain of fall and spring, or the cold of winter harvests energy and information for better health and vitality. It improves mitochondrial function, which is paramount to overall health and wellness. It can also improve insulin resistance and fat burning, which can help with metabolic issues that plague many adults and the elderly today. Aligning with the rhythm of the seasons can support overall health and longevity.

Cultivate a practice of stillness, of mindfulness, of meditation, or heart coherence. This creates the space to connect with the world around you.

And while all of this can sound like another to-do list, it's an invitation into awe and a relationship with nature. It offers you safety where it might be hard to come by. It offers unconditional acceptance and belonging in a time when rates of loneliness are skyrocketing. Cultivate your relationship with the sun, the moon, the plants, and the seasons. They hold the ability to heal. Nature offers us an unconditional relationship of acceptance, reminding us that we truly belong in this ecosystem.

7

CULTIVATING COHERENCE

Our universe is a symphony of resonant information waves. Everything, living and nonliving, has a unique vibration and a resonant frequency. Resonance occurs when something is exposed to its matching natural frequency and begins to vibrate at a higher rate—like a swing that gets pushed at the right rhythm to make it swing higher. Resonance is when a system is able to pick up a frequency, electrical signal, or vibration and reverberate it at a greater amplitude. We are resonant beings. We resonate with the energy of the people, sounds, vibrations, and energy fields around us. The invisible order of quantum biology is ever present and available to improve health.

We resonate with our environment, but conventional medicine has yet to apply that understanding. As humans, our physiology allows for a deeper coherence within ourselves and to each other. We have an immense power to regulate our emotions and thoughts, which has a profound influence on our overall health. We entrain with the energies of the world we live in and have the capacity to match and increase those frequencies within our biology and with the world at large. We can learn to cultivate this resonance for better mental, emotional, physical, and relationship health.

We can also resonate with thoughts, emotions, or sounds that cause an imbalance in the body. Chronic stress, trauma, ruminating thoughts, disempowering subconscious thoughts, incoherent energy, and noise all wreak havoc on our biology. These discordant energies degrade overall health and longevity. The body is like a symphony, each cell with its own beautiful frequency like an instrument in the orchestra. Without a coherent resonance within the body, it's like a symphony with each instrument out of tune and playing a different song. The result is chaos. Tending to our resonance allows the body to work in sync as a coherent whole. This is an essential piece of a long and healthy life.

We've learned how we resonate with the light in our environment and the same is true of the frequencies around us. We resonate with the sights, sounds, and energy in our environment, like two tuning forks set at the same frequency. When one fork is struck, it sings out a tune. The second fork can pick up that tune and amplify it even louder in resonance. We can amplify our natural resonance of energy with the natural world around us.

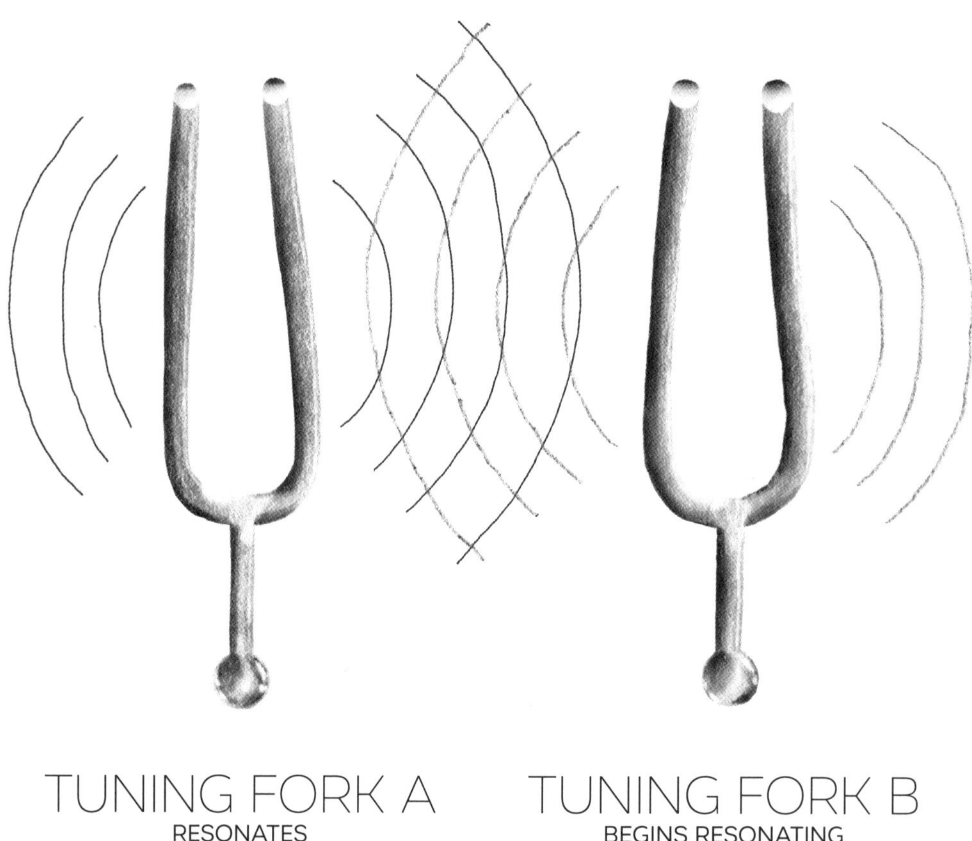

Tuning forks are a good example of resonance. If two tuning forks are tuned to the same frequency, when one is struck it will ring out a tune that will entrain the second fork to sing the same note.

THE POWER OF THOUGHT

Research into psychoneuroimmunology has found that the resonance between our thoughts, our brain, our hormonal state, and our immune system has a profound influence over our health. Our emotional state has a predictable influence over our biology. Psychological stress affects our immune system, our gut microbiome, our endocrine system, and our neurological function. The resonance of our thoughts is potent. Many today are chronically stressed or dealing with the effects of trauma. These conditions chip away at the body's homeostasis and can negatively affect health and longevity.

There are two main inputs that affect our psychoneuroimmunological state. One input is the intersection of the gut microbiota, the brain, the endocrine system, and the immune system. The gut microbiota produces metabolites, short chain fatty acids, and neurotransmitters that have a direct effect on our immune system and brain function. The other input comes from signals sent by the brain-hormone axis via the hypothalamic-pituitary-adrenal axis and autonomic nervous system, which sculpt the microbiome-gut-brain axis. The hormones we secrete in response to the stressors and environmental terrain inside and outside our body guide how the microbiome, gut, immune system, and brain communicate and function. These relationships are what constitutes the field of psychoneuroimmunology.

There are two branches of the nervous system. One is the parasympathetic rest, digest, and safety branch of the nervous system. The other branch is the sympathetic fight, flight, or freeze part of the nervous system that is dominant in times of danger or stress. Chronic stress and the sustained nervous system activation seen in trauma can rewire the nervous system to stay in the hypervigilance of the fight, flight, or freeze sympathetic response. Early life stressors can reprogram our stress responses into hypervigilance for a lifetime if not addressed. Chronic stress and trauma can also derange the gut microbiome toward less diversity and a composition of less balanced microbes.

Chronic psychological stress and trauma suppress many functions in the body, including degrading and confusing the immune system's communication. T regulatory cells, the cells that inhibit and stop inflammatory responses, decrease with chronic stress and trauma, letting inflammation run wild, which affects everything from chronic disease to cardiovascular health to autoimmune conditions. These responses to trauma are not the body betraying us. The body is appropriately responding to signals of danger. To heal, we must replace the danger signals with signals of safety.

There is a feedback loop with psychological and physical pain. We feel the pain in a sensory pathway; for example, we stub our toe and that sends a signal through a sensory nerve to the brain. That signal is communicated first to the limbic centers of the brain that deal with emotions, as well as to the brain's prefrontal cortex where decisions are made. Have you ever felt an emotional reaction to pain? Hit your elbow on a door and find yourself angry with the door? There is an emotional component to pain.

This pathway can become so ingrained that the feedback loop can work in reverse. A state of sympathetic nervous system dominance with ruminating thoughts, stress, and worry can signal the emotional centers of the brain. This triggers the limbic centers and prefrontal cortex of the brain, which activate the sensory pathway of pain, and we feel pain. Rather than a sensory pain that activates the limbic emotional center of the brain and the prefrontal cortex, the signal starts in the emotional centers. After time, the pain triggers become emotional or mental rather than physical.

Psychological stress and trauma are associated with chronic inflammatory diseases, cancer, cardiovascular issues, acute and chronic viral infections, sepsis, asthma, and other disorders. At the same time, chronic peripheral inflammation influences brain function leading to fatigue and overt psychiatric and mental illness. There is ample evidence demonstrating that peripheral immune activity and inflammation in the brain affect behavior and mental health.

Healing Trauma

Tending to any trauma or chronic stress that lingers in the body both on a physical and emotional level is foundational for balanced resonance. Treating physical trauma usually involves the help of a professional with medical or chiropractic care, physical therapy, or craniosacral and myofascial release therapy. Massage and myofascial release are wonderful therapies for treating physical trauma and fascial adhesions or restrictions. Neural injection therapy from biological medicine can help with physical trauma, such as scars from accidents and surgery. Red light therapy, acupuncture, acupressure, mitochondrial support, and cupping are also valuable for recovering from physical trauma.

Emotional trauma can be addressed through traditional avenues such as talk therapy and neurofeedback. It can also be addressed by tending to our quantum biology. We know that stress decreases the metabolic water in the mitochondria as well as the overall mitochondrial function and ATP production. Depression and anxiety have traditionally been treated solely on a chemical level with selective serotonin reuptake inhibitors, SSRIs. Now medicine is recognizing the role mitochondrial energy plays in these conditions. To return to balance mentally and emotionally, we depend on the energy from mitochondria.

Mitochondrial energy is essential for the biological cascades that center on stress. It's hard to maintain the cellular function associated with mental and emotional health without it. Nourishing our mitochondria is foundational for mental health after trauma and chronic stress.

Emotional trauma misaligns our circadian rhythms, so paying special attention to getting morning sun, movement, a meal in the morning, and natural light breaks throughout the day and lowering the lights at night can help sync that circadian rhythm and help the emotional trauma unravel. Aligning with the rhythms of the sun and the moon as well as the seasons can be helpful for unwinding chronic stress and emotional trauma. The sun, the cold, the heat, and the circadian and infradian seasonal rhythms that guide life and increase mitochondrial function are essential for healing, even from trauma. Aligning with the natural rhythm of light in our environment and syncing with the world around us are foundational for returning the body to homeostasis after trauma.

The circadian rhythm of the sun, the seasonal flux of the weather, as well as the sights and sounds of nature serve as massive signals of safety to our biology. They let the body know where it is in the greater ecosystem around them. Not only do they bolster mitochondrial, hormonal, and immune system function, but they also cultivate a relationship of safety. So many of us live in an unsafe world. Our relationships are not safe. Our families are not safe. Our workplaces and communities are not safe. When we can find safety in the rising of the sun or a patch of grass beneath our feet or the flux of the seasons, we can enter true healing. If we continually stay in a state of fight, flight, or freeze, we send constant signals of danger to our cells. This inhibits true healing. We must be able to achieve a state of safety for healing to occur. Nature is always there to welcome us, to envelop us in a caress of safety without demands or judgment.

There are many somatic exercises that can restore resonance after psychological stress:

- Utilizing emotional freedom tapping (EFT), the practice of tapping on specific acupressure points while saying affirmations like, "I release this emotion of guilt/shame/worry/fear/despair," or, "I acknowledge my feelings and witness how strong I am," can be a powerful tool in healing chronic stress and trauma.

- Practice intentional body scans by lying down, slowing the breath, and scanning the body for tension or emotions. Breathing into the tension or emotion, releasing it, or lovingly accepting it completes the scan and helps regulate the nervous system.

- Neurofeedback, tension release exercise, biofeedback, and eye movement desensitization and reprocessing, or EMDR, therapy are also wonderful tools for addressing trauma.

A diet rich in protein, colorful fruits and vegetables, and omega-3 fatty acids supports inflammatory pathways, the gut microbiome, cell membranes, DNA, and mitochondria, which are important for unwinding emotional trauma. There is a study from 2015 that looked at infants in the neonatal intensive care unit. Researchers used the obviously traumatic, yet medically necessary, separation of the sick infant from their mother at birth to study the effects of trauma on the gut microbiome. The researchers saw the expected shift in the gut microbiome from more beneficial species to more harmful species because of the traumatic event.

This response to trauma was recreated in animal studies. When the researchers supplemented the infants with omega-3 fatty acids, they saw the gut microbiome resume its original balanced composition. It was not that the omega-3 fatty acids alleviated the trauma, the infant was still separated and experiencing trauma. The difference was that the infants' biology had a massive input of safety and coherence with the addition of the omega-3 fatty acids. These fatty acids act as anti-inflammatory mediators in the body, increasing the anti-inflammatory T regulatory cells. They also have profound quantum actions in our cell membranes.

The omega-3 fatty acid docosahexaenoic acid, or DHA, has free electrons that can travel and donate electrical charge to areas that are energy deficient. Pain, inflammation, and even trauma can be seen as a loss in negative electrical charge. Reestablishing that charge and decreasing inflammation with is a wonderful way to address trauma.

Earthing is another valuable tool when healing from trauma. Chronic stress and trauma increase inflammation in our gut, our brain, and throughout the body. The inflammation from trauma, especially that which occurred during early childhood, can last a lifetime if not addressed. Grounding or earthing helps maintain negative electrical charge within the body, helping decrease the resulting inflammation from chronic stress and trauma. It also cultivates a relationship of safety with the world around us. No matter what is happening in the world, the ground is always there to hold us, and we can depend on that support.

Interventions that address the psychoneuroimmunological state show benefits. Treatments such as yoga, meditation, Tai Chi, acupuncture, mindfulness, religious/spiritual practices, cognitive behavior therapy, coping skills, and gentle physical exercises decrease levels of stress-related hormones like cortisol, epinephrine, and norepinephrine.

Demonstrating the ability of our thoughts to change our biology, psychoneuroimmunology therapies intervene at the intersection of the mind, immune system, and neurological function. These interventions are also associated with reductions in inflammatory processes and levels of pro-inflammatory cytokines in cancer, HIV, depression, anxiety, wound healing, sleep disorder, cardiovascular diseases, and fibromyalgia, with one study revealing a significant effect on disease progression. Psychoneuroimmunology-focused interventions were found helpful in cancer, pediatric chronic illness, and even during the COVID-19 pandemic. Pairing that with support for the gut microbiome, gut lining, mitochondrial health, immersion in nature, and circadian alignment can help unravel the knots that chronic stress and trauma weave.

HEART COHERENCE

Our internal coherence has a powerful influence on our capacity to heal. Coherence refers to a harmonious relationship between two or more systems and occurs when these systems work together as one, like two people dancing the tango or the multiple individual molecules of water creating a wave that travels the ocean. HeartMath Institute has done extensive research on the heart's magnetic field and its influence on biological health.

The heart has its own intrinsic nervous system with fifty billion motor neurons, sensory neurons, and local neurons. This intrinsic nervous system sends more sensory signals to the brain than the brain sends to the heart. It is a guiding force in our body. It contributes to the vast electromagnetic field of the heart. The heart's electromagnetic field is one hundred times greater than that of the brain, with some estimates much higher. This electromagnetic information constructs a coherence field that entrains the brain and body into a more balanced, calmer biological state.

Heart coherence is a measurement gleaned from heart rate variability. The heart rate is not constant like a metronome. It can change. Heart rate variability is the measure of this inconsistency that comes from the heart being under the influence of both the danger fight or flight sympathetic nervous system and the safety parasympathetic nervous system. As the nervous system signals danger, the heart rate increases, and when the nervous system sends signals of safety, the heart rate decreases. This leads to heart rate variability. We are meant to vacillate between the two with a high degree of variability. The higher the heart rate variability, the higher the state of heart coherence. HeartMath has found that heart coherence leads to innervation of the frontal lobe, enabling calm, rational thought patterns and away from the reactionary amygdala where fear is processed. When in a state of heart coherence, we are calmer in our nervous system, our brain function is more rational than reactive, and our immune system is more balanced.

HeartMath has developed heart coherence exercises to train the body into a state of coherence. We have an incredible capacity to regulate our emotions and behaviors and thus our physiological health. That unseen energy that resonates between our biology and our emotions can be consciously directed. We can direct this invisible order to a state of coherence and better overall health.

Expanded Heart Coherence

Another type of coherence, social coherence, relates to the harmonious alignment between couples or pairs, family units, small groups, or larger organizations in which a network of relationships exists among individuals who share common interests and objectives. A high degree of social coherence is reflected by stable and harmonious relationships. When two or more people are coherent, they work together as a unit, interdependent and acting as one. Coherence refers to two or more quantum particles or systems vibrating at the same frequency, oscillating as the same resonance, even at long distances.

Social coherence between people explains how the more coherent the group is the easier and better the work will be. Social coherence requires that group members be attuned and emotionally connected with each other. The group's emotional energy must be organized and regulated by the group as a whole. The invisible tapestry of social coherence is something many of us have felt. Working, praying, dancing, singing, and socializing with a coherent group just feels different.

A number of studies have investigated various types of synchronization in infants, pairs, and groups. HeartMath Institute has expanded its research from our individual heart coherence to social coherence in groups. It's not just our own heart that can be in a state of coherence; our heart's coherence can entrain the magnetic fields and coherence of others around us.

HeartMath Institute has found the heart's electromagnetic field contains information that can influence others. Like wind through the trees that moves the leaves in sync, individual coherence can move the coherence of those around us into patterns. Researchers hypothesized and found that group coherence is associated with heart rate variability coherence and heart rhythm synchronization, leading to more prosocial behaviors like kindness and cooperation. They propose that the heart's biomagnetic field might be the mechanism by which pairs and groups synchronize heart coherence.

Researchers utilized signal-averaging techniques to detect signals that were synchronous with one subject's electrocardiogram heart reading to the recordings of another subject's electroencephalogram, or brain wave recording. They proposed and found evidence that these same rhythmic patterns can also transmit emotional information via the electromagnetic field into the environment, and these signals can be detected by others. Researchers looked at couples, groups, and our relationships with animals and found evidence that our state of heart coherence influences the energetic fields of others, including animals. They looked at people who were touching, those who had no physical contact, and people with dogs and horses. All showed an ability to influence the brain waves of those around them via the heart's magnetic field. This makes tending to our individual coherence extremely important.

Beautiful research surrounding group meditation suggests that this entrainment and synchronization can extend to the community around us. In 1993, a group of about 4,000 participants in the Transcendental Meditation and Transcendental Meditation–Sidhi programs of Maharishi Mahesh Yogi assembled in Washington, DC, from June 7 to July 30. It was thought that the coherence of the meditating group could affect community coherence, and this could be measured through crime rates. And that's what they found. Crime rates decreased during the period of active meditation and continued to decrease as the size of the meditating group increased.

A similar study was performed in the Middle East during wartime conflict with similar results. Wartime violence decreased in proportion to the size of the meditating group. Researchers could not explain the decrease in violence by other usual factors like temperature, holidays, and timing. The resonance of the group of meditators had a predictable and profound effect on the community around them. What's more, as the number of meditators grew, the effects on the community also grew. The larger the meditation group, the greater the decrease in violence, validating our intuitive sense that thoughts can ripple throughout a community. We are truly resonant beings, and it's time we used that for our health and the health of others.

THE RESONANT NERVOUS SYSTEM

This capacity for coherence isn't limited to our internal terrain, we can also co-regulate those around us. Often, we act and feel as if we are solitary beings when, in truth, we are intimately and inseparably connected with the people around us. Whether our family, our community, or people across the globe, there is an invisible connection that can span miles (kilometers).

Stephen Porges introduced the polyvagal theory in 1994. The vagus nerve houses our parasympathetic rest and digest branch of the nervous system. Polyvagal theory teaches that three states exist in the autonomic nervous system. The autonomic nervous system consists of the sympathetic and parasympathetic branches of the nervous system and controls the involuntary actions of the body, such as heart rate, breathing, and digestion. Polyvagal theory describes how a person's level of activation goes from the ventral vagal, or parasympathetic, to sympathetic, to dorsal vagal.

The ventral vagal helps us feel safe. It helps us feel a sense of belonging and ability to connect with the community around us. This is our homeostatic resting point where we want to spend most of our time. Our sympathetic nervous system is our fight or flight arm of the nervous system that is triggered by danger signals like a bear jumping into the room or a fight with a coworker. It helps us mobilize and prepare for danger. When we cannot get away from the danger signal that initially triggered the sympathetic fight or flight, we can go into the dorsal vagal response of shutting down, dissociation, and collapse.

Polyvagal theory describes how we are constantly scanning our environment to assess signals of safety and danger, or what Porges describes as "neuroception." This neuroception is concerned not only with signals of safety and danger from our external environment but also from the internal environment of the body and our perception of the people around us. Porges theorizes that the evolution of the vagus nerve paralleled the development of pathways that regulate the striated muscles of the face and head, while the visceromotor component involves the myelinated vagus nerve that regulates the heart and bronchi. This makes us hardwired to express and observe the state of the nervous system in the muscles of the face and in the heart rate. This creates an integrated system between the heart, the vagus nerve, and the muscles of the face and head where signals of safety are expressed and perceived during facial expression of emotion. This sense of safety governs our homeostatic balance of health, growth, and restoration. Although polyvagal theory is still a theory, it has been applied successfully in therapy for mental and emotional health in clinical practices for decades. Even though this mechanism of co-regulation remains elusive, the effect of co-regulation is clear. There is an unseen communication with those around us that extends throughout society.

The Resonance of Co-Regulation

Co-regulation is the bi-directional ability to match behavioral cues and arousal levels with others to regulate emotional states. When a young child cannot regulate their emotions, a caregiver can help influence them through co-regulation. As the caregiver models loving behaviors and calm intonations, the child mirrors this emotional regulation. The child picks up on the energy of the caregiver and is pulled into its flow. Research has shown the benefits of co-regulation as a parenting tool with children, infants, and children on the autism spectrum. How disconnected we've become to require research that our emotions bleed out to the world around us and can have profound effects on the health of our children.

This collective connection extends to all our interactions. Not only can we emotionally resonate with our children, but we can also resonate with those around us. You've probably experienced this. Someone walks into the room fuming with anger and we can feel our own blood pressure and stress levels rise. Conversely, when someone enters the room radiating joy and love, we can feel our nervous system relax. We resonate emotionally in our relationships.

This emotional co-regulation has been documented between therapist and patient. After analyzing hundreds of audio sessions, researchers discovered that both therapist and patient co-regulate their emotional states. Simply put, the emotional state of the therapist influenced the biology of the patient, and the emotional state of the patient also influenced the biology of the therapist.

Recent research into mirror neurons adds another layer of understanding to the picture. Scientists have identified mirror neurons that mirror low-level body movements. These mirror neurons are motor neurons that seem to allow mimicking of small body movements in others—like when you watch someone stub their toe and it makes you cringe and feel a brief sense of discomfort. Mirror neurons could also help explain how we read intention in others.

Emotional resonance has also been demonstrated in online interactions. In a fascinating investigation, researchers examined data from millions of Facebook users, focusing on periods of rainfall. They found that rainfall directly influenced the emotional content of their status messages. It also affected the status messages of friends in other cities who were not experiencing rainfall. People who were directly emotionally affected by the rainfall altered the emotional expression of one or two other people, which then rippled out to the greater collective. Even without physical proximity or common experience, people experienced emotional entrainment simply by reading about the experience. Recent research found that emotional entrainment comes in a variety of forms via social media interactions. This invisible entrainment is not bound by our immediate surroundings.

SYNCING BRAINWAVES

It is not just our nervous systems and emotional states that can co-regulate and sync; our brain waves, heart rates, and rhythm of breathing can synchronize as well. A study looking at long-term couples found that not only could they influence each other's heart rates, but they could influence the synchronization in heart rate. The synchronization was more pronounced the closer in physical proximity they were. Heart rate and respiratory rate synchronization were found in young couples as well. Research confirms that heart and breathing rate synchronization also happens in social interactions, like conversations and rituals. We truly resonate with our community, and we can tend to this capacity for better health.

Brain wave synchronization has also been demonstrated in a variety of different situations. Brain wave synchronization was reported when two or more people participated in cooperative tasks and puzzle solving. Recent research found brain wave synchronization was not confined to people in physical proximity. It was observed in two people physically separated but playing an online video game. An interesting study looking at copilots also found that the copilots had high brain synchronization during parts of the flight when they needed to work together but less synchronization when they were completing separate tasks. We must be mindful of what and who we resonate with. It's not just when sharing tasks; we resonate through our relationships as well.

Studies have shown that when married couples hold hands, their brain waves synchronize, having a profound effect on pain sensation. The resonance of brain waves in married couples decreased pain. Researchers separated twenty-two paired couples into two rooms as well as seating the couples together but not touching and sitting together while holding hands. Researchers did this once and then repeated the scenarios while inflicting mild heat pain on the arm of one of the couple. They found that couples synced brainwaves with their partners and experienced decreased levels of pain when together, especially while holding hands. The heightened interbrain synchrony resulted in two distinct subjective experiences of pain: relief in one person and empathy in the other. As one person felt pain, it produced empathy in the other, which helped decrease pain in the person experiencing pain. Interestingly, the brain synchronization was not due to a shared task or experience but, rather, a synchronized response in relationship. What a beautiful example of the powerful resonance we have in connection with others.

This makes sense given the research that found emotions can be communicated via touch. In a fascinating study, scientists put up a barricade between two strangers. The first participant stuck their arm through the barricade. The second participant tried to convey emotion from a list of different emotions via a one-second touch to the stranger's forearm, while the stranger tried to guess the emotion. Statistically, the chance of guessing the correct emotion with the long list of emotions given hovered at 8 percent. The study participants, however, were able to correctly guess the emotion of compassion with 60 percent accuracy whereas the other emotions were correctly guessed 50 percent of the time. Our human capacity for resonance is incredible.

Fascinating research from Uri Hasson and his lab at Princeton University discovered some amazing things about brain entrainment and communication. Hasson studies brain-to-brain entrainment, or synchronization, during human communication. He and his team have found that during storytelling, soundwaves from the speaker entrain the listener's brain responses with the speaker's brain responses. This brain entrainment was dependent on a coherent idea or story. It was not present when the story was played backward, which created incoherent noises, nor was it present in a scrambled mix of words without meaning. It suggests that the entrainment comes in part from the intention of the speaker, not just the sounds and words. The speaker's conscious intention seemed to influence the resonance between speaker and listener.

Hasson recently hypothesized that brains synchronize according to rhythmic oscillation. Neurophysiological evidence suggests that interpersonal interaction between two or more people relies on continual communication between interacting brains and continual adjustments of these neuronal dynamic states between the brains. The hyper-brain cell assembly hypothesis suggests that hyper-brain cell assembly can occur not only within our brain but also among multiple brains. This communication between brain cells encompasses and integrates oscillatory brainwave activity within and between brains, and represents a temporary and shared hyper-brain unit, a superorganism of sorts, in relation to social behavior and interaction. Simply put, our life requires a resonance of frequencies within our brain and with the brains of those with whom we interact. Without this resonant coherence, our brains don't function properly. What an incredible example of an unseen connection linking our consciousness within us and with those around us.

THE BIOFIELD

This ability to affect each other's physical and mental state is the backdrop to the healing modalities termed *biofield therapies*. These therapies access the subtle energies of the biofield of the body to affect healing for the patient. Acupuncture, Reiki, healing touch, prana healing, Qigong, distant healing, and therapeutic touch are all examples of biofield therapies. Shamini Jain has done wonderful work elucidating the workings of the biofield in her book *Healing Ourselves* and in her nonprofit the Consciousness and Healing Initiative.

The term *biofield* was coined in 1992 during the US National Institutes of Health Conference. The biofield was defined as a field of energy that is not necessarily electromagnetic in nature. The biofield can be defined as the electromagnetic field of a cell, an organ, a tissue, or an organism, but it isn't limited to that. We are familiar with some biofield measurements, such as the electromagnetic biofield of the brain assessed with an electroencephalogram, or of the heart with an electrocardiogram. We measure the biofield of biophoton emission, or light emission, of the organelles and cells, and these energetic fields are generated by all kinds of living systems—organs, tissues, cells, organelles, atoms, and subatomic particles.

One aspect of the biofield is the light emission from living cells, or biophotons. In animal and human studies, biofield therapies have shown a marked increase in the biophoton emission from cells. Research with mice demonstrated how just ten minutes of Reiki applied to intervertebral disc cells dramatically increased those cells' biophoton emissions.

Biophoton emission has also been associated with intention. Research looked at biophoton emissions in both the trained biofield healing practitioner and the patient receiving treatment. Researchers Beverly Rubik and Harry Jabs found that biophoton emissions decreased significantly, by 11 percent, in the healer's hands after the healing session. The biophoton emission during energy healing displayed a unique emission pattern for each treatment. Interestingly, Rubik and Jabs also found that participants who engaged in bioenergetic practices emitted more biophotons from specific bodily regions, some in alignment with their intention. They came to the exciting conclusion that biophotons might be involved in quantum processes or quantum-like entanglement between humans and may play a role in energy healing and biocommunication. Though the study was small, it brought more validation to the idea that conscious intention can drive bioelectric change in the body.

Dr. William Bengston has made incredible inroads demonstrating the power of unseen intention on healing. Bengston developed the Bengston Energy Healing Method®, a form of intention-focused healing. He conducted extensive research on how this technique affects tumor growth in mice. Bengston found complete healing and remission in mice with cancer that typically would have a 100 percent fatality rate. Magnetic recordings of the Bengston Method applied to cancerous cells showed a significant decrease in tumor growth in breast cancer cells and no tumor growth in bladder cancer cells. Exposure to electromagnetic field recordings of the Bengston Method led to changes in 37 out of 167 genes tested, with 68 genes showing statistically significant alterations. What an astounding example of the power of intention in healing.

Morphogenic Fields

The biofield includes the subtler energies that surround and influence a cell as well. Many ancient Indigenous cultures spoke of this energetic field and had ways to measure and treat it. Some research points to the relationship between the organism's energy field and an all-inclusive, long-range coherent field. Researchers point to fields firmly rooted in classical and quantum physics, such as electrical fields, electromagnetic fields, and photonic fields like coherent biophoton emissions. Other researchers look at these fields as bridges between the material structures of life and the more esoteric fields of Chinese Qi, Hindu prana, Reich's orgone, Reichenbach's odic force, and health practitioners' bioenergy, etheric energy, or subtle field. Still others describe these fields as plasma. Plasma is a gas of charged particles that some researchers have found to be self-organizing, and able to display emergent intelligence and hold information—much like the concept of ether.

Rupert Sheldrake is a biologist in the field of developmental biology. Rupert has established his own take on the biofield. He refers to these mysterious fields of development as "morphic fields." Morphic fields are nonphysical fields that organize the form and behavior of an organism. These fields carry information, not energy. These morphic fields contain a collective memory so that once a species has learned a behavior it becomes easier for others in that species to learn it, even if they are far away. Morphic fields have a nonlocal influence and resonance across time so that current forms and behaviors are shaped by those who came before, and the resonance of the collective memory can influence future generations. It explains a causation that isn't material, like how dogs know when their owners are coming home, or how a person can learn a skill or break an athletic record and someone across the globe then learns the skill or breaks the record more easily.

Morphic fields enforce organization on otherwise random patterns of activity, giving life unique forms in development. It explains how we grow an arm or an ear from the same cells—the information in morphic fields guides the development of form. Furthermore, these fields evolve through a kind of nonlocal resonance, called *morphic resonance*, where two similar morphogenic fields can pass information and memory. Though controversial, these fields exemplify the invisible order quantum biology seeks to uncover.

THE FIELD

Ancient Indigenous cultures spoke of a universal field. In ancient Indian philosophy, Ayurveda, and Vedanta, the element Akasha, or ether, related to air, sound, vibration, intuition, and mental expansion. All actions, thoughts, and events are recorded vibrationally in the Akashic, or cosmic ether. The clearer the mind, the more information it can receive from the Akashic. The more resonance between mind, body, and spirit, the more we can connect with the cosmic intelligence.

With the ideas of the Akashic field, the unified field, or the zero-point field that holds all the information for living systems to access, we return again to an imperceptible blueprint that seems to guide life on this planet. Indigenous cultures and sages have long referred to a vast field that holds, maintains, and conveys information. The ancient Egyptians believed in the cosmic order of Ma'at. The ancient Chinese spoke of the Dao. The ideas of Pachamama, the Great Spirit, and Australian Aboriginal dreamtime all speak of a realm of universal consciousness and intelligence. The ancient Greeks described the logos, an ordering intelligence of the cosmos. Sufis speak of the Lawh al-Mahfuz, a divine record of everything. In the Jewish practice of Kabbalah, the Ein Sof represents the unknowable source of divine intelligence. The idea of a universal field of intelligence has been part of humanity for millennia.

Vacuum physics, or zero-point energy, shows that what we once thought was empty space is anything but empty. This empty space is filled with quantum fluctuations in the virtual photons that fill the so-called empty space, or vacuum. Max Planck first described zero-point energy, and now that energy can be measured at one-trillionth of an erg, a size so small it's hard to wrap our heads around. This zero-point energy has a demonstrable effect called *the Casimir effect*. In the Casimir effect, two plates are placed near each other in an absolute vacuum. Though they should stay in place, there is an attractive force pushing them together. There is some unaccounted attractive force between the two plates where nothing should be. This is the zero-point field. And the zero-point field has a demonstrable effect on the total energy, structure, and reactivity of benzene molecules, those six-sided rings found in the microtubules of our brains, the protein fibers of our fascia, melanin, and neurotransmitters. There is an undefined energy that exists that acts on matter in our world.

Ervin Laszlo's Akashic field theory creates the correlation between the ancient Vedic concept of the Akashic and the zero-point field that underlies space itself. The Akashic field theory speaks of a field of information that permeates the universe, accounting for a consciousness and intelligence that imbues all things. Laszlo relates this field to the zero-point field and suggests that quantum phenomena, like quantum entanglement, utilize this universal field. This echoes Chinese Qi, Hindu prana, Reich's orgone, Reichenbach's odic force, and health practitioners' bioenergy, etheric energy, or subtle field that describe this universal field of energy from which material life emerges.

Dean Radin has also done research into our connection to this universal field. In one study, Radin investigated whether human intention could influence the strength of entanglement between pairs of entangled photons. Participants attempted to increase the entanglement strength with their mental intention. The results showed a statistically significant increase in entanglement strength during the intentional periods. Radin also explored the power of intention to affect the behavior of photons in a double-slit apparatus. In this study, participants tried to use conscious intentions to influence the inference pattern of the photons as they hit the background wall. Again, the study showed a subtle difference in the quantum wavefunction during times of intention, suggesting consciousness can play a role in quantum phenomena.

In a pair of different studies, Radin collaborated with Masaru Emoto to explore how conscious intention could influence water crystallization. In one study, 2,500 participants in Japan directed their positive intentions toward water samples in electromagnetic-shielded rooms in California. Control group water samples were kept separate and not subjected to these intentions. The samples exposed to intentions had more aesthetically pleasing water crystal formations. They repeated this same experiment with 1,900 participants in Austria and Germany—with one difference. They took photos of the water crystals in both the intention-exposed water and the control water and showed them to 2,500 independent judges. This triple-blind experiment showed similar results. The water exposed to intentions was found to be more aesthetically pleasing. While these experiments faced scrutiny, they raise fascinating questions about what consciousness is and by what mechanism it can travel.

Although we have yet to understand the full extent of biofield therapies, we know that intentional interventions directed toward healing have shown therapeutic benefits in a range of modalities and disease states. One of the most extensive areas of biofield research is regarding pain. Two recent large research reviews looked at more than thirty studies with pain and found that biofield therapies had a beneficial effect on pain above placebo or sham treatments. Biofield therapy has been shown to decrease pain and fatigue as well as immune markers associated with tumor growth in patients. Cardiovascular conditions have also benefited from biofield therapies. Research has found that biofield therapies can decrease blood pressure while increasing heart rate variability. Recent research has even found that Reiki had a similar effect to that of propranolol, a commonly prescribed cardiovascular beta-blocker, after acute coronary syndrome. Research found biofield therapies beneficial in a wide range of conditions such as inflammatory bowel disease, Alzheimer's disease, fibromyalgia, dementia, and mental health issues, such as depression and anxiety. Although the exact mechanism remains unknown, the benefits of biofield therapies are too great to ignore.

What Is Quantum Consciousness?

Is consciousness a connection with universal energy or a product of biological actions? Ancient Indigenous cultures held the belief that consciousness was something running through all things in nature—people, plants, animals, planets, and the elements of water, earth, air, and fire—a connection to a cosmic intelligence. Some modern theories echo this idea.

The theory of quantum consciousness describes consciousness as a manifestation of quantum processes in the brain that rely on a connection to a universal field, rather than brain activity itself. This theory attempts to unravel the invisible order implicit in consciousness, although this idea is heavily debated in certain scientific circles.

Quantum brain dynamics, proposed by Hiroomi Umezawa and others, describes how long-range coherence and memory are maintained through quantum effects in water molecules and proteins in the brain. Researchers Mari Jibu and Kunio Yasue explain that the movement of particles along protein filaments of the cytoskeleton, extracellular matrices, and surrounding water fields of the brain is quantum information transmission and creates the formation of quantum coherent states in the cortex.

The holonomic brain theory put forward by Karl Pribram illustrates how brain functions work like the wave interferences of holograms, suggesting a possible nonlocal system of quantum entanglement.

In the book *Quantum Theory*, respected quantum physicist David Bohm claimed that the unseen implicate order could pertain to both the material world and consciousness, again connecting consciousness to a universal field of intelligence.

The orchestrated objective reduction theory was developed by physicist Roger Penrose and anesthesiologist Stuart Hameroff, who proposed that consciousness arises from quantum computations in microtubules in the brain. The theory suggests that quantum collapse of waves in the brain is the origin of consciousness. Tryptophan in the microtubules in our brains act as receivers of information for the universal intelligence, or zero-point field, which collapse into conscious thought. Others add that biophotons created by the microtubules in the brain could reflect quantum coherent states in the brain.

Panpsychism posits that consciousness is a fundamental property of the universe, present even in basic entities. Animism speaks of the idea that all things, living and nonliving, are conscious and have a soul or spirit. The power that organizes and animates the material universe is present in everything.

The debate on what consciousness is continues. Quantum consciousness suggests we resonate with a universal field of consciousness; consciousness is fundamental, woven into the fabric of the cosmic.

OUR CONNECTION TO THE FIELD

So how does our body interact with these biofields? By what mechanism does our body capture and utilize this subtle energy? Although we don't know, there are compelling ideas that paint a picture of how the biofields within us and external to us could interact with our body from a quantum biological perspective.

Our DNA, cell membranes, fascia, the tubulin within the neurons of our brains, and the water that lines them all have liquid crystalline properties. Liquid crystals are aligned and ordered. Liquid crystals can capture, store, and transmit light, electricity, sound, and frequency information. This would also make them potentially able to receive frequency information of all kinds.

These structures also contain benzene rings with pi electrons. These electrons, which can be thought of as waves of energy, can be excited by vibratory, frequency, or energy information. Pi electrons are free to move throughout the molecule and to other molecules. They can even pass information without being in direct physical contact, a process called *Förster resonance energy transfer*. There can be energy and information transmission from a distance—a form of energy and information transfer. Benzene's structure, total energy, and molecular reactivity seem to be influenced by zero-point energy. While there is no evidence or research on this yet, does the zero-point field excite or communicate with the benzene ring's pi electrons? It is certainly possible and is another candidate for how the biofield could be informing our biology.

DNA, proteins, fascia, and tubulin make perfect conduits for the vibratory information held in biofields and, potentially, in a universal energy field. And it seems that water is the first to receive this vibratory information.

This is seen in the Resonant Recognition Model we explored in chapter 3. Irena Cosic's work proposed and found evidence of a language of vibration and resonance in the water that lines the proteins within us. This model brings some validation to the idea of the body as an antenna. It focuses on living systems and their biomolecules. It describes how these biomolecules communicate and produce action via the resonant transfer of energy and information in various spectrums of electromagnetic frequency. These electromagnetic frequencies are generated and emitted by the biomolecules themselves. The Resonant Recognition Model focuses on biomolecules and electromagnetic frequency and evokes an understanding of how the body could pick up on frequencies outside of itself. The body doesn't have to use chemicals or mechanical force to induce action. Action can hinge on the vibrations of frequency.

The body's photoreceptive and liquid crystal structures, from our DNA to our proteins to our cell membranes and the liquid crystalline water that lines them, are potential sites of interaction with the field. Even the benzene ring and aromatic amino acids are candidates to receive information from the field.

Liquid crystalline water can act as a conduit between the unseen vibratory communication and the physical liquid crystal structures. Water is a bridge for frequency information. It can direct vibratory information to structures so they can potentially capture and utilize frequency information from light, sound, and the vibrations of energy. The ability of these structures to act as receivers, as antennae, to the vibratory information in the environment makes them well suited for extending that communication outside the body. Not only can they receive information, but they also communicate that information throughout the body. Our ability to act as receivers depends on our ability to resonate with the energies that surround us.

THE RESONANCE OF SOUND

Sound has profound effects on our biology and is a perfect example of resonance. Sound consists of pressure waves. As these pressure waves collide, they create inelastic collisions that produce infrared energy or light. The water that lines proteins can capture frequency and sound, which can initiate protein folding—the basis for biological action.

Research from the Niels Bohr Institute in Denmark has repeatedly found that sound seems to initiate nerve conduction, not electricity. This new theory states that sound acts upon the nerve; the pressure waves stimulate the piezoelectric conduction of the fascia within the nerve, turning the sound waves into electrical impulse. The body responds to sounds in extraordinary ways. While not often talked about, sound has a compelling influence on human biology. Working with sound can improve our health and vitality.

John Stuart Reid, an acoustic physicist, has done extensive research on sound and water and their effects on our biology. After a quite painful back injury, Reid was scheduled to conduct sound research in the sarcophagus in the King's Chamber of the Great Pyramid. To his surprise, after spending a few hours experimenting with low-frequency sounds in the King's Chamber, his back pain had disappeared.

This led him to research the effects of low-frequency sound on biology. He invented the CymaScope, a machine that creates cymatic patterns from the interaction of sound on fluid. Remember, the pressure waves of sound can arrange and order matter such as sand and fluids. This field of cymatics was pioneered by Hans Jenny, who completed numerous experiments on the cymatic patterns of water, sand, and other materials.

SOUND WAVE

INFRASOUND
(BELOW 16 HZ)

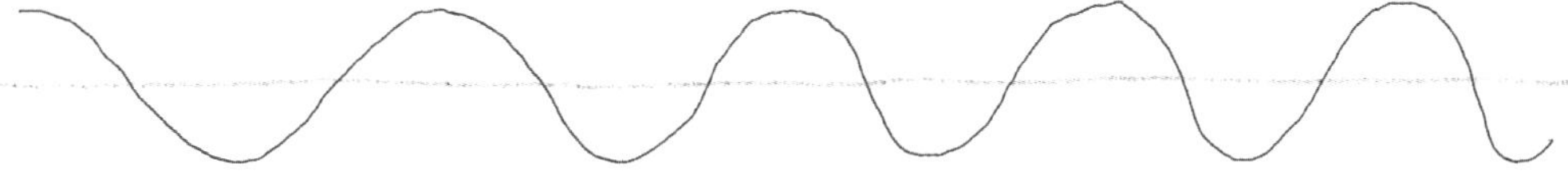

AUDIBLE FREQUENCIES
(16 HZ TO 20 KHZ)

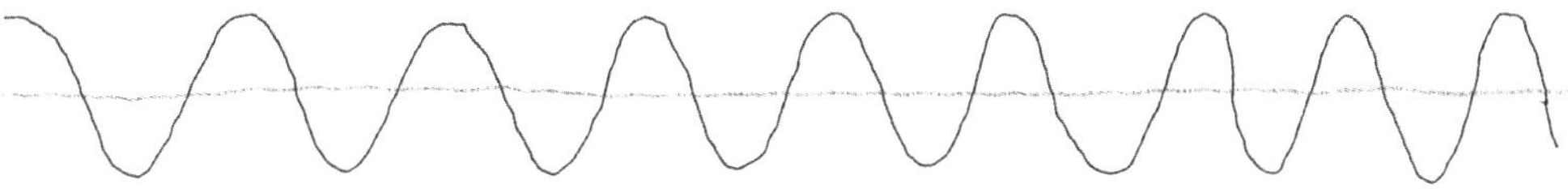

ULTRASOUND
(OVER 20 KHZ)

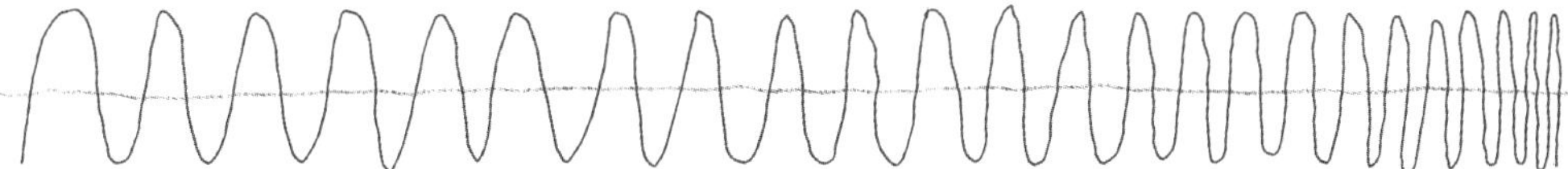

Sound waves are pressure waves that propagate through a medium. Infrasound, below 16 Hz, and ultrasound, above 20k Hz, cannot be heard but have reliable effects on the body and health.

John Stuart Reid has found that low-frequency sounds have profound effects on pain, vagal tone, and immune function. The leading theory on pain describes how pain is sent through sensory nerves into the brain. This continues until the inhibitory nerves are stimulated and the pain gate in the sensory nerve is closed. The pressure waves from sound are capable of closing these pain gates and alleviating pain. This could explain why sound has been helpful for those with chronic pain.

The vagus nerve leaves the brain and innervates the ear as well as the eyes, nose, throat, heart, lungs, and gastrointestinal tract and is associated with the body's inflammatory state. Sound waves through the tragus of the ear offer a novel way to decrease inflammation by stimulating the vagus nerve. Listening to sound through headphones, not earbuds, stimulates the vagus nerve as the pressure waves of sound hit the tragus of the ear. Vagus nerve stimulation has been used to treat conditions such as pain, depression, migraines, and epilepsy. Having a noninvasive way to treat pain and inflammation is truly needed, and sound has the potential to do so.

Reid teamed up with Professor Sungchul Ji for a series of experiments with sound and whole human blood. Derived from a blood bank, they tested several popular types of music and frequencies on the blood. They looked at classical music, popular music, rap music, heavy metal music, and music of lower frequency. What they found was shocking.

The low-frequency music, especially popular music, increased the oxygen binding capacity of the red blood cells by 20 to 30 percent. The oxygenation of the body is crucial to health. When examining donated blood under a microscope, you see that a percentage of the blood cells are healthy, some are damaged, and some are dead. Not only did the low-frequency sound increase the oxygen binding capacity of red blood cells, but it also increased the viability of the red blood cells, repairing some of the damaged cells and increasing their life span. This led Reid and Ji to postulate that the heart works not only as a pump but also as a provider of low-frequency sound that enables our red blood cells to repair and live longer as well as bind and deliver more oxygen throughout the body.

Reid and Ji repeated the experiments with white blood cells. Although the results were not as dramatic, only a 2 to 4 percent increase in life span, they did find that low-frequency sound increased the viability and life span of white blood cells. This is an incredible insight into the relationship between sound and our biology.

Sound immersion in the form of singing bowls, music, and tuning forks is an excellent way to tend to our resonate being. Most commercial speakers filter out the lower frequencies, but you can purchase headphones and speakers that play these lower frequencies, allowing you to reap their benefits.

Eileen McKusick, the founder of Biofield Tuning, explains that sound is electric, a form of acoustic electromagnetism. It moves charge and structures, and electrifies matter. Sound works to organize and construct matter from the ether or plasma. McKusick has even found that using sound to address health can be done at a distance. In the first-of-its-kind study, five certified Biofield Tuning Practitioners used tuning forks to deliver three healing sessions per week for four weeks to fifteen people with moderate to high generalized anxiety at a distance. Though separated by miles, these healing sessions revealed statistically significant decreases in anxiety as well as feasibility for studying Biofield Tuning virtually. A subsequent research study with 100 participants seeks to validate this idea even further.

Connecting with the sounds of nature is also a wonderful nervous system reset. The sound of water decreased cortisol, the hormone secreted during stressful events, by 60 percent, making this an effective option to relieve stress. A small study on nine participants found that the sound of 528 Hz increased oxytocin, the love hormone, by more than 90 percent and reduced cortisol, the stress hormone, by over 40 percent in study participants. In a different study, one hundred mice were exposed to Mozart's Sonata for Two Pianos in D Major, K.448 every night for sixty-three days. The mice exposed to the music had reduced gut inflammation, a balanced microbiome, and improved stress response via lowered cortisol. We should be utilizing the power of sound for healing.

Research at the Massachusetts Institute of Technology found that 40 Hz light flicker and 40 Hz auditory stimulation had powerful effects on neurological function—40 Hz is a key gamma frequency. After exposing mice to 40 Hz light or 40 Hz sound for an hour each day over the course of a week, the mice displayed significantly reduced amyloid-B plaques, the plaques found in Alzheimer's disease. The 40 Hz light stimulation decreased plaques in the visual cortex while the 40 Hz auditory stimulation decreased plaques in the auditory cortex and hippocampus. Exposure also activated microglia, the brain's immune cells that clear out plaques and debris. Exposed mice had better memory and cognitive function and showed increased coherence and better synaptic function. More recent research by the same group found that combining the 40 Hz light and sound had wider brain effects and long-term stimulation helped preserve neuronal health, synaptic density, and vascular function. Though not mentioned in this research, it would be interesting to see the effects 40 Hz light and sound had on the neuromelanin in the brain. Remember, melanin can split water when exposed to light and create electrons and protons that could decrease inflammation and support mitochondrial function.

Self-generated sound, such as toning, humming, or chanting, can increase our nitric oxide, which helps with circulation. It can increase our lymphatic flow. It can decrease our stress hormones and increase oxytocin, the hormone associated with feelings of love and safety. Self-initiated sound can increase melatonin, a master antioxidant, to help decrease inflammation and help with sleep. Self-generated sound can stimulate the release of serotonin and dopamine, leaving us feeling calm, focused, and happy. Nitric oxide produced by self-generated sound such as humming has been shown to block pain receptors at the level of the spinal cord. We can resonate with sound for better health and longevity.

THE ELEMENTS OF SOUND

Sound has an interesting connection to matter on this planet. The elements of the periodic table are the building blocks for every known thing on Earth. Each element has a unique resonant frequency, creating a symphony of vibration throughout our planet. Our cells also produce sounds, creating a symphony internal to the body. Not only do they produce vibrations, but they are also affected by the vibration of sound.

Fabien Maman and Joël Sternheimer were both interested in the effects of sound on living cells. Sternheimer had discovered the vibratory frequency of elementary atoms and was mapping certain molecular structures into musical patterns. Sternheimer took the music of the elements and created musical scores of the various tissues in our body. For example, he created a unique song for a protein in the electron transport chain. He even included warnings on the sheet music instructing not to play the music unless you knew exactly how the tissue would respond.

Fabien Maman also looked at the effect of music on cells. Maman found that the color and shape of cells changed when exposed to certain musical tones. He found that each cell had a vibratory resonance with a certain note that would create a mandala pattern. A unique geometric pattern appeared on the cell when exposed to that cell's individual vibratory resonance. Maman also found that when HeLa cancerous cells were exposed to discordant frequencies, they would explode.

Anthony Holland, music professor turned resonant frequency researcher, also studied the frequency of sound on human cells. He is the president of Novobiotronics Inc., a nonprofit scientific and educational research organization that focuses on the effects of frequency-specific oscillating pulsed electric fields (OPEF) on cancer cells and pathogenic organisms. Like the opera singer who breaks the wine glass by singing the resonant frequency of the wine glass, cancer cells can be eradicated by resonant frequencies. His research has shown that by using resonant frequencies, he can slow tumor growth by 65 percent and kill up to 60 percent of cancerous cells. Focused high-intensity ultrasound is now being used to eradicate traditionally hard-to-treat cancers, such as pancreatic and prostate cancer, by a similar method in select hospitals in the United States and across the globe.

In other research, James Gimzewski and Andrew Pelling found that cells make different sounds depending on the cell's health. They used an atomic force microscope to turn the vibrations of cells into audible music. Each cell displayed a unique sonic signature. Cancerous cells had a different cell membrane structure and should sound different from healthy cells. John Stuart Reid found similar results. He imaged the sounds of healthy brain cells and cancerous brain cells. The cymatic sound patterns in the healthy cells were intricate, beautiful mandalas that indicate a flexible, freely resonate cell structure. In contrast, the cancerous cells exhibited more chaotic patterns. It's incredible to think that our cells have their own sound pattern by which they can communicate health or disease.

TENDING TO OUR RESONANT BEING

We are resonant beings. We have the capacity to resonate with things that uplift our health, mood, and mind. We can resonate at higher levels of vitality if we simply connect with the healing energies around us.

Try heart coherence exercises. To resonate coherently, cultivate a state of heart coherence. A deep breath while connected with a sense of love and heart coherence induces a state of coherence. Using exercises that grow internal coherence is an ideal way to improve heart rate variability, heart coherence, and psychoneuroimmunology. There are several heart coherence videos on the Internet, including several videos you can find on my YouTube channel to build inner coherence.

Cultivate a meditation, gratitude, or mindfulness practice, which helps sync the body into a greater sense of resonance. Thoughts have a powerful effect on resonance, and learning to regulate thought processes and emotions leads to better health. Becoming aware of subconscious trains of thought can lead to less reactive emotions and a calmer approach to life. Listening to positive affirmations or recording your own voice speaking affirmations specific to your history and future to listen to can be healing and assist in uncoiling trauma and negative subconscious trains of thought. Remember, cells don't know the difference between the thought of danger or a real danger. When we stay in a state of stress and danger, we cannot heal.

Carve out time for silence. Silence allows the body to reset and access a deeper connection. The inputs of healthy sound are beneficial but so is silence. Silence brings a resonance that sound cannot. It is a vital part of health and longevity.

Explore different somatic exercises for addressing trauma and chronic stress.

Practice breathwork to regulate resonance. There are several ways to approach the breath (see more in chapter 4); simply breathing deeply into the diaphragm and exhaling longer than the inhale is a powerful tool for building internal resonance and signaling a sense of safety.

Connect to a safe community through dancing, singing, drumming, ecstatic dance, chanting, worship, and telling stories or having a good conversation, which can help tend to resonance within. Not only does this prime mitochondria with movement, help oxygen flow, and improve vagal tone with low-frequency music, but it also builds co-regulation with safe community so the body can enter into safety mode, away from danger mode, and begin to heal. Spending time with loved ones, whether biological family or found family, is a wonderful tool for tending to our resonant beings.

Biofield therapies such as Reiki, acupuncture, acupressure, sonicpuncture, craniosacral therapy, laying of hands, distant healing, tuning forks, and Qigong are powerful ways to tend to resonance.

From homeopathic remedies to herbs, the plant realm has many avenues for cultivating resonance, including a diet rich in quality protein, quality fats like omega-3 fatty acids, and colorful fruits and vegetables. This fuels the health and life span of the mitochondria, the gut microbiome, and supports inflammatory pathways affected by chronic stress and trauma. Mitochondrial health is crucial for overall health especially when creating balance after chronic stress and trauma (see chapter 4 for more information).

Align your circadian rhythm, which will send a ripple of resonance throughout the body. Get outside and resonate with the sights and sounds of nature. Incorporate grounding, a wonderful tool for building resonance after chronic stress and trauma, into your routine.

Utilize sound for health. Sound healing builds resonance in the body. Self-generated sound, such as humming, chanting, and toning, increases oxytocin, serotonin, dopamine, melatonin, and nitric oxide. Immersion in sound, such as sound baths, concerts, or tuning forks, can help with inflammation, ease pain, and bring us back into balance. The vibration of sound can help with better health and longevity.

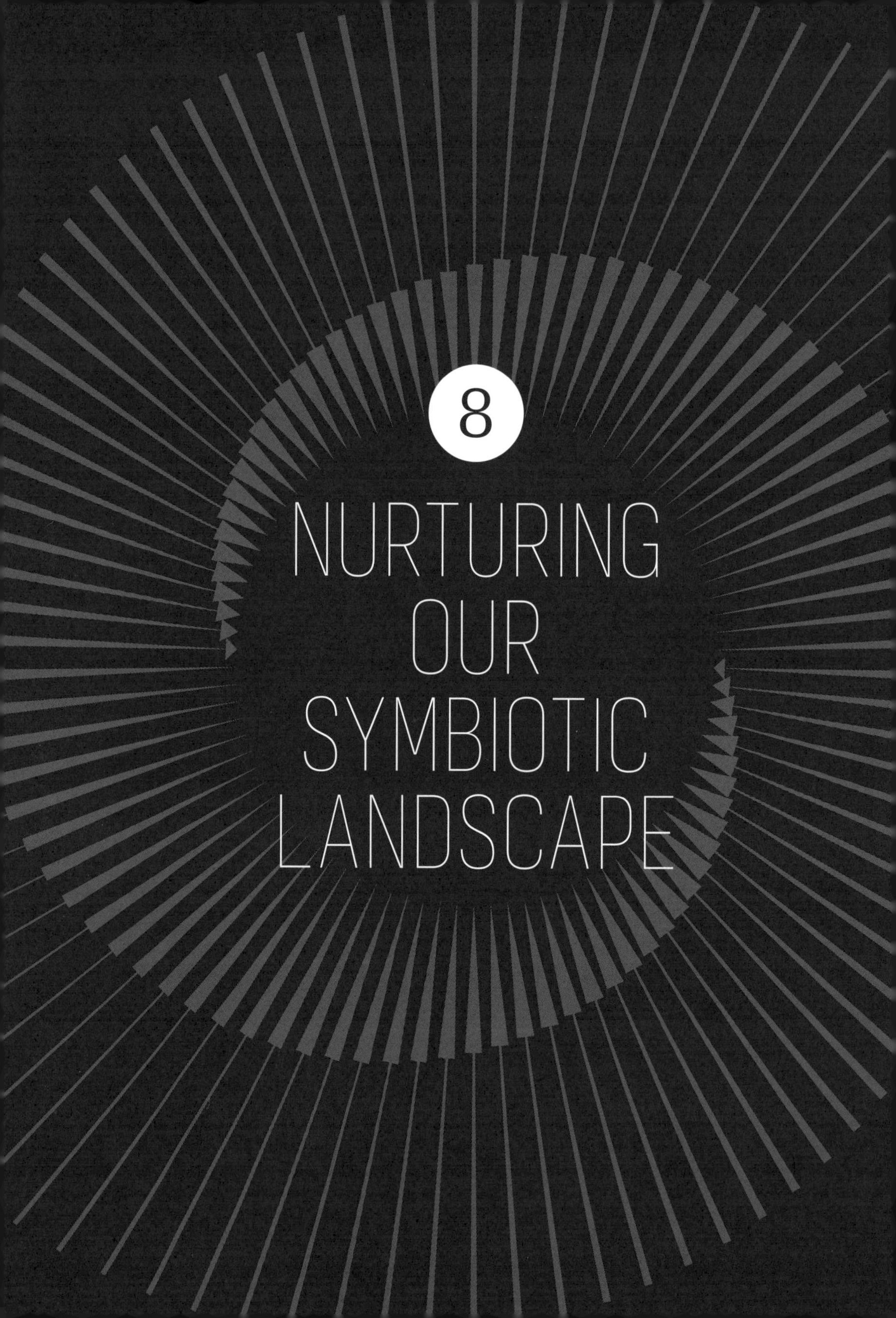

8

NURTURING OUR SYMBIOTIC LANDSCAPE

We live in a symbiotic landscape. We are intimately connected with the microbiotic world that lines our skin, digestive and respiratory tracts, and almost every system in the body. While conventional medicine frames this relationship in the cloak of good microbes and bad microbes, a quantum biological perspective offers a more interconnected view, a perspective where our relationship with the microbiome mirrors the interconnection we have with the world around us.

When we talk about the microbiome, we're referring to the mixture of bacteria, viruses, protists, archaea, and fungi that reside on our skin and throughout our body. These microbes have always been intertwined with life on Earth. Since the beginning, we've forged an intimate and inseparable relationship with microbes. The microbial community has a profound effect on health and longevity.

The discovery of this microscopic world continues to transform science and medicine. The deeper we dive into the research, the clearer the picture becomes. We have a bi-directional relationship with the microbes that reside within, and it extends past a chemical understanding. We are symbiotic beings. Our microbiome picks up signals from the world around it, both the external environment and the internal terrain of the body. The microbiome can interpret these signals and coordinate action in the body—a beautiful dance of light, electricity, sound, electromagnetics, and quantum building blocks that guide our overall vitality and life span.

From a quantum biological perspective, the microbiome is a transducer of the frequency information in the world that helps direct its behavior, dramatically influencing our health and longevity. The microbiome is like the transducer in a microphone: The soundwaves of the singer's voice hitting the microphone's diaphragm create movement that is converted into an electrical signal. Microbes contain cytoskeletons rich in tryptophan with the ability to communicate via superradiance or collective photon emission. The microbiome is rich in the benzene ring that can take the wave information from light, sound, chemical energy, or vibration and turn it into energy and information.

The microbiome can sense and communicate with light, sound, and electromagnetic fields. Recent research proposes that microbes communicate by nonlocal means as well, a form of quantum entanglement that does not need physical proximity to communicate. This paints a completely new perspective on the microbiome from that of the chemical-mechanical model, to one that isn't defined by the invader-defender perspective, and it offers new ways to support the microbiome.

Without a doubt, microbes in our microbiome have profound effects on our health. Our microbiome is associated with our overall inflammatory state, immune function, and mitochondrial health. The research shows that microbiome imbalance is associated with intestinal inflammation and permeability, cancer, cardiovascular disease of all kinds, autoimmune diseases like inflammatory bowel disease, multiple sclerosis, Parkinson's disease, rheumatoid arthritis, type 1 diabetes, and Alzheimer's disease as well as neurological conditions, autism spectrum disorder, depression, and anxiety. On the flipside, microbiome balance is associated with a beneficial influence on these disease states.

Our gut microbiome talks with our gastrointestinal tract, lungs, respiratory tract, kidneys, brain, heart, nervous system, immune system, liver, gallbladder, spleen, pancreas, uterus, vagina, genitourinary tract, bladder, and mitochondria, influencing health for better or worse depending on the composition of the microbes present in the microbiome. This composition is not a random occurrence either. The microbiome's composition reflects our internal terrain and the surrounding terrain outside of us. It's absolutely incredible. Medicine has concentrated solely on the chemical aspects of the microbiome, yet there is an emerging picture of the microbiome from a quantum biological perspective.

THE MICROBIAL WEB OF LIFE

Each organ system in the body has its own unique and specific microbiome. We see the same thing in the natural world. There is a microbial counterpart to everything—the air, water, dirt, plants, and animals that surround us. Our individual microbiome extends into a global microbiome that is shaped by the global environment. The air we breathe has a dramatic effect on the diversity of our gut microbiome. Not only is our microbiome part of a global microbial web, but the distinct microbiomes within us also communicate and influence each, creating an internal microbial tapestry.

Meet the Microbiome

The microbiome includes archaea, bacteria, fungi, protists, and viruses.

Archaea and Bacteria: The archaea microbes are said to be the ancestors of all eukaryote life, appearing on Earth more than 3.5 billion years ago. Both archaea and bacteria are single-cell prokaryotes, or organisms that lack a membrane-bound nucleus. Archaea are single-cell organisms that are structurally different from bacteria, making them particularly well suited for the harsher environments on Earth. Archaea make up only about 1.2 percent of the gut microbiome, but they have an important role in our health by regulating the microbiome composition and supporting bacterial growth and survival. Bacteria, on the other hand, are the most-studied and abundant microbes in the human gut microbiome. There are more than 2,000 known species living in the human intestinal tract, comprising more than one hundred times the genomic DNA of humans.

Fungi: Fungi are also foundational to our health but make up only a very small percentage of the overall microbes present in the gut microbiome. Our mycobiome plays a pivotal role in our microbiome. Just like the mycelia in the forest that support and guide the growth and health of the plant life around it, so too does the fungi in our microbiome. In healthy gut microbiomes, fungi play a pivotal role in our immune response and homeostasis. The composition of the fungi in our microbiome has been associated with cancer prognosis, autoimmune reactions, cardiovascular health, and type 2 diabetes.

Protists: Protists are another group of microbes that includes protozoa, unicellular algae, and slime molds. Protists are eukaryotes, meaning they do have a membrane-bound nucleus. They can be single-celled or multicellular. Protists have a major influence on our microbiome, modulating our immune system and gut ecology, even though they only account for 0.1 percent of the microbes present in the microbiome.

Viruses: Viruses are the final group of microbes in our microbiome. More than 40,000 viruses were recently discovered in our gut microbiome. Several classes of viruses, called *bacteriophages*, infect bacteria and offer substantial benefits to the gut microbiome by regulating the composition and thus health of the microbiome. Clearly, we are just beginning to understand the role of our microbiome and the microbes that constitute it.

MICROBIOME COMMUNICATION

Our microbiome reaches throughout our body, guiding and informing our physiology: chemically through metabolites and quantum biologically through gasotransmitters, electricity, sound, biofilm communication, oscillation, light, and infrared energy. Understanding the microbiome from a quantum biological perspective offers new ways to support the microbiome and overall health and longevity.

The Microbiome's Metabolite Communication

One of the ways microbes in our microbiome communicate with us is through metabolites. In the gut, there are three main types of metabolites: bile acids, short chain fatty acids, and a handful of other metabolites.

Bile acids work on our insulin levels and propensity toward insulin resistance and diabetes. They help us digest. Bile salts originate in the liver and then the gut microbiome metabolizes them into secondary bile acids. Short chain fatty acids, particularly acetate, propionate, and butyrate, also beneficially influence our insulin metabolic pathways as well as our immune system, nervous system, and endocrine or hormone-secreting system. Undigested starch reaches the colon, and the local microbiome ferments the starch into short chain fatty acids. Short chain fatty acids are also used as fuel by the mitochondria in the cells that line the gut. These fatty acids and bile salt metabolites are in constant communication with the major systems that govern our physiology, subtly guiding our biology at all times.

Our gut microbiome produces other metabolites that have a variety of effects on our physiology. The tryptophan we eat is converted by our enterocyte cells lining the gut and our gut microbiome into serotonin, kynurenine, and indole derivatives, which function as neurotransmitters and metabolic regulators. While serotonin made in the gut does not cross the blood-brain barrier, it influences our immune system, our inflammatory cytokine production, and our mood via the vagus nerve.

This sophisticated signaling communication is stimulated by the previously mentioned metabolites produced in the gut and has a direct effect on mental health. Normal levels of serotonin in the gut have a balancing effect on mental health whereas low serotonin levels have adverse effects on mental and emotional health. Indole derivatives have a direct impact on leaky gut—the more indole metabolites you have, the less intestinal permeability you have. Leaky gut is associated with an increase in inflammation, inflammatory bowel disease, celiac disease, irritable bowel syndrome, and autoimmune disorders like lupus and multiple sclerosis. In research with mice, we see the same thing with the blood-brain barrier. The balance of the microbial metabolites improves the integrity of the blood-brain barrier. This protects the brain and the prevents neurological conditions like Alzheimer's disease, multiple sclerosis, and Parkinson's disease.

The microbial metabolites of phenylalanine and tyrosine are precursors to dopamine, a key neurotransmitter that helps us focus and feel happy. Microbial metabolites also help control the enzymes that regulate DNA expression. In general, microbial metabolites help regulate our gene expression, central nervous system, and metabolic activity while affecting both immune cells and tissue cells. It's essential to expand our approach to supporting healthy microbiomes if we truly want to achieve balance and health, not only in the microbiome, but for overall health and longevity.

The Microbiome's Quantum Building Blocks and Communication

The gut microbiome creates building blocks for our quantum biology. It produces gasotransmitters, such as nitric oxide (NO), methane, and hydrogen sulfide (H_2S). These molecules have a direct effect on the function of the mitochondria. The microbiome seems to produce gasotransmitters in response to an imbalanced internal terrain.

Nitric oxide is an important signaling molecule involved in endothelial function, vasodilation, blood pressure, immune function, and glucose metabolism. The oral microbiome, specifically the nitrate-reducing bacteria, produces nitric oxide via the breakdown of salivary nitrates into nitrites. These nitrites are then swallowed, going throughout the body where they are converted into nitric oxide in the blood vessels and tissues. Our resident oral microbiome has the capacity to control distant events, such as blood pressure, immune function, and metabolism through nitric oxide production.

Compelling research shows that microbial production of nitric oxide controlled genetic expression in the host. Genes are influenced by the environment that surrounds them, and this research suggests that the microbiome's production of nitric oxide can do just that. While this research was performed on worms, the systems involved are akin to those in humans, and scientists believe the phenomenon exists in the human body as well. The microbiome makes nitric oxide, which can serve as part of a communication network as well as having a regulatory effect on vascular health, immune function, metabolism, and genetic expression.

Both methane and H_2S produced by the gut microbiome can support mitochondrial health. Methane has been researched to preserve mitochondria after injury. Methane acts as an antioxidant, anti-inflammatory, and anti-apoptosis, or protector against cell death. Hydrogen sulfide's beneficial effects on mitochondria include improving the mitochondrial function, biogenesis (producing new mitochondria), and ATP production while inhibiting cell death. In research with mice, H_2S was given for sixteen weeks, and it significantly inhibited the increase of serum triglyceride, blood glucose, and insulin levels while changing the composition of the microbiome. Simply put, hydrogen sulfide improved blood lipids and insulin levels while also creating more balance in the composition of the microbiome.

The production of H_2S also has a beneficial effect on exercise recovery, promotes tissue repair in the gastrointestinal tract, and helps control inflammation. There is a delicate balance regarding H_2S. At low levels, it is protective, but at higher levels, it can induce damage.

The production of methane and H_2S is often associated with small intestinal bacterial overgrowth (SIBO), which is considered excessive production of H_2S or methane from an overgrowth of more harmful bacteria. Patients who have SIBO are given antibiotics to eradicate the bacteria producing H_2S, methane, and the unwanted symptoms that accompany this dysbiosis.

Alzheimer's disease is an example of how the microbiome's seemingly harmful actions could be an attempt to help a dysfunctional biology. Studies have also found an association between SIBO and people with Alzheimer's disease, a neurological condition that robs people of their cognition and memories. Alzheimer's patients had a higher level of SIBO than the control group, a higher level of microbes that produce methane and H_2S. H_2S, however, has been found to be a successful therapy for Alzheimer's. Researchers suggest it acts as an anti-inflammatory agent, protecting the neurons from damage and death via apoptosis. Methane has also been used successfully in addressing neurological conditions. Research suggests it has anti-inflammatory and antioxidant influences while protecting neurons from death. Alzheimer's disease is associated with neuronal death and brain atrophy.

Is dysbiosis a microbial response to a biological cue? Maybe an increase in diabetic markers or decrease in mitochondrial function or neuronal health can elicit a response from the gut microbiome to increase H_2S, methane, or nitric oxide production to maintain balance. Microbes in nature can be seen as organisms responding to the environment around them. They maintain the delicate homeostasis of the organism in the greater order of cycling and recycling energy and matter. Why wouldn't this apply to the human microbiome as well?

Rather than approaching the microbiome from the perspective of good guys and bad guys and the need to eradicate the bad guys, we would be better served by finding the reason for the microbial shift and action. If we managed the gut microbiome's health by considering what the microbiome is responding to and in what manner, we would have a root cause to address as well as tools to support it. As with Alzheimer's disease, we see that blood sugar dysregulation, intestinal permeability, inflammation, and mitochondrial dysfunction are all associated with the disease. Alzheimer's disease is also associated with small intestinal bacterial overgrowth or an overgrowth of methane and H_2S-producing bacteria. H_2S and methane help support mitochondrial function, gut health, proper blood sugar levels, and inflammation—the very things compromised in Alzheimer's disease. What if the gut microbiome is producing H_2S and methane to help with the blood sugar dysregulation, intestinal permeability, inflammation, and mitochondrial dysfunction seen in Alzheimer's disease? If the gut microbiome is responding to these co-factors of disease, and we intervene at this level, think of the preventive effect this could have. An expanded approach for balance in the gut microbiome is worth considering.

THE MICROBIOME-MITOCHONDRIAL CONNECTION

The bi-directional mitochondrial microbiome communication, meaning the mitochondria communicate with the microbiome and the microbiome communicates back, is an important feature in approaching health through a quantum biological perspective. This means we must consider that the action we direct on either one will affect the other. We can improve the health of the mitochondria by tending to the microbiome and vice versa. They share an intimate relationship with each other and our overall health and longevity.

We've talked about the essential role mitochondria play in creating a bodywide communication system, a network of flowing electrons, protons, water, infrared heat, ATP, biophoton emissions, and reactive oxygen species. Mitochondria are a focal point of quantum biological action, as is the gut microbiome. They both act as antennae that receive and emit frequency information. Their relationship and influence on each other are important to understand when approaching health and longevity.

The mitochondria and the gut microbiome are believed to share common ancestors in bacteria. The short chain fatty acids and bile acids that the microbiome produces regulate redox balance and energy production within mitochondria. Bile acid metabolism by the microbiome might also directly modify mitochondrial biogenesis, inflammation, and intestinal barrier function. Recent research found that signals from the gut microbiome to mitochondria alter mitochondrial function, the integrity of the gut lining, and activate immune cells and inflammasome cytokines, which are associated with chronic gastrointestinal inflammation, inflammatory bowel disease, and colorectal cancer. Similar associations have been made between mitochondria and gut microbiome communication and brain health. It is imperative that we tend to the mitochondrial microbiome connection.

Microbiome metabolites help overall energy via mitochondrial ATP production while at the same time decreasing inflammation in the body. The short chain fatty acid, butyrate, is crucial for intestinal homeostasis and balance. Butyrate increases fatty acid oxidation and acts as a histone deacetylase inhibitor, upregulating Foxp3 (a crucial immune function regulator) expression, which increases T regulatory cells. T regulatory cells go throughout the body, stopping inflammatory reactions in infections, autoimmune conditions, and inflammation. They are essential in our ability to decrease and regulate inflammation.

In this essential bi-directional dance, mitochondria also influence the gut and the gut microbiota as well as our intestinal barrier health, such as the mucus layer of the intestinal tract and the mucosal immune response there. The mitochondrial production of reactive oxygen species has a direct impact on the composition of the gut microbiome as well. Increasing reactive oxygen species levels influence our health, the health of the cells lining the gut, and the gut's microbial diversity. In return, our intestinal microbiota influences reactive oxygen species levels, mitochondrial function, and overall health. This bi-directional relationship between the mitochondria and the microbiome has a direct effect on inflammation and the health of the gut and the mitochondria, which can influence conditions like cardiovascular disease, autoimmune conditions, cancer, and metabolic issues. This fascinating relationship between our mitochondria and gut microbiome illustrates how truly interconnected everything is within the body. But the impact of the microbiome doesn't end on a chemical level.

THE MICROBIOME AND LIGHT

The microbiome is a central hub of light communication in the body. It has an intimate relationship with circadian rhythm and the light in the surrounding environment. The microbiome produces, stores, and communicates with light. The gastrointestinal tract lining contains photoreceptors, or light-sensitive receptors, establishing potential light communication from the gut microbiome throughout the entire body.

Cultivating a healthy light environment and expression in the gut microbiome is an important step in supporting overall health and well-being. The gut microbiome contributes to and reinforces our primary relationship with the sun. Almost every cell in our body has a circadian clock. Emerging research shows we have a bi-directional relationship with our gut microbiome when it comes to circadian rhythm regulation. The disruption of the circadian signals through the retina and suprachiasmatic nucleus in the hypothalamus can influence the composition of our gut microbiome. If we are not aligned with the rhythm of the sun by waking around sunrise and sleeping at night, we change the species composition in our gut microbiome. In research with chronic jet lag, chronodisruption leads to changes in the gut microbiome, which predisposes changes and dysfunction in metabolic states. It's important to align our light environment with the seasonal rhythm of the sun to support the microbiome and overall health.

Conversely, our gut microbiota influences the rhythm of our biology. Our gut microbiome reinforces our relationship with the sun by way of their own circadian rhythm. Bacterial circadian rhythms are around twenty-four hours in length, like ours, and are influenced by melatonin and temperature. Our gut microbial community can regulate our circadian and metabolic homeostasis by way of their own diurnal oscillations. The circadian rhythm of our gut microbiome has an intimate relationship with our genes by directly influencing genetic expression. Recent research found that microbial circadian behavior drives our circadian genetic, epigenetic, and metabolite oscillations. The microbiome's circadian rhythm, or lack of it, can influence our genetic expression. Researchers found that chronodisruption in our gut microbiome dismantles normal chromatin and transcriptional oscillations in our genetic expression while stimulating genome-wide oscillations in both the intestine and liver, affecting our physiology and disease susceptibility.

It is amazing to think that the microbes in our gut under the influence of light in the environment communicate with our DNA, guiding our genetic expression for generations to come.

The third circadian pathway in the gut is the feeding input pathway; our cells are entrained to our meal timing because, as diurnal animals, we evolved to eat when the sun is up and fast when the sun is down. Fasting, or feeding restriction, changes the phase of circadian gene expression in peripheral tissues. Simply put, the timing of eating helps regulate circadian rhythm. Timing our meals to when the sun is up reinforces a healthy circadian rhythm whereas eating when the sun has set leads to chronodisruption, or misaligned circadian rhythm. This circadian regulation is highly conserved among plants, animals, and humans. Our digestion and metabolism of fats and carbohydrates is circadian and seasonally driven as well. It's all connected.

Interesting research has found that artificial light can negatively affect the gut microbiome. Research in mice found that exposure to artificial light has negative effects, such as promoting pathways in type 2 diabetes, obesity, and nonalcoholic fatty liver disease. Exploration into the microbiome of birds found that artificial light dramatically reduced bacterial diversity in the gut microbiome, which significantly impaired melatonin production. This has been demonstrated in human studies with jet lag as well. Artificial light at night disrupts the microbiome, which has several negative effects on our overall health and metabolism, such as systemic inflammation, metabolic disease, and cholesterol dysregulation. Conversely, red light has been found to support gut health by decreasing inflammation and promoting healing while balancing microbiome diversity.

A LANGUAGE OF LIGHT

Several microbes in the gut microbiome produce melanin. We have learned that melanin is a semiconductor as well as a transducer. It can take vibratory information, such as radiation, electromagnetic fields, or light, and turn that into energy. The melanin molecule in living systems is completely covered by liquid crystalline water and has the ability to create a source of free electrons. Under the exposure of ultraviolet light, researchers suggest that this water lining melanin splits into molecular hydrogen, H_2, and molecular oxygen, O_2, which are then able to donate energy or re-form into water for the whole process to begin anew. In the microbiome, melanin is produced to help protect the survival of the microbial community. Microbial melanin also helps certain species produce nanowires that conduct energy. So melanin in the microbiome could also be acting as a semiconductor, a transducer—both for the health of the microbiome and potentially our own health as well.

It is not just the external light environment that influences the gut microbiome. Remember biophoton research looking at ultralow photon emission from our cells (see page 154). Biophotons are ultra-weak ultraviolet light emissions from the cells of living systems. All living cells radiate biophotons. This light emission is not random. It is coherent and suggests a means of communication. Recent research found that specific microbes in the gut produce their own unique biophoton emission. Not only do individual microbes have their own unique light communication, but this communication spans to other microbes.

Scientists demonstrated bacterial biophoton emission at work in a series of experiments looking at the biophoton emission of *Escherichia coli* and *Serratia marcescens*. *E. coli* cultures were placed on a photomultiplier tube housed within a dark box; this is used to measure biophotons emission. A second bacterial culture, either *E. coli* or *S. marcescens*, was put in an identical dark box and received injections of hydrogen peroxide. Examination displayed significant differences in the emission of the biophoton signals of both samples depending on whether a peroxide injection occurred or not. Further, there were significant differences in the biophoton emission if the bacteria receiving the injection was *E. coli* or *S. marcescens*, suggesting that bacteria may communicate in a species-specific manner via biophotons in response to stress.

Simply put, the research suggests that each microbial species has its own unique biophoton emission. Biophoton emission is a form of communication with light and evidence of unique emission patterns is like saying each microbial species has its own voice. In addition, there is evidence of communication between the species. When one species was stressed, it affected the biophoton emission of the other species. Not only did the biophoton emission of the species being stressed with the hydrogen peroxide change, but the other species changed their biophoton communication as a result of the other's stress. This is a truly incredible example of light communication at a distance within the microbiome.

Our gut is lined with light-sensitive proteins, such as flavins, cryptochromes, and melanopsins. Microbes also have the capacity for superradiance, where quantum coherence between microbes allows them to coherently emit light as energy that is much brighter than if released by individuals. With photonic communication in place between cells and between microbes, is there communication occurring between microbes and our cells via light? Why would there be light-sensitive proteins in a place without light unless there is some kind of network of photonic messaging? Are melanin and melanin-producing microbes offering a solution to energy deficiencies in the microbiome and the body? Do biophotons interact with melanin to create a source of energy for the microbe and the body? Although more research is needed, these questions evoke an incredible picture that is much bigger than the chemical model we focus on now and breeds a respect that conventional medicine currently lacks when it comes to addressing microbiome health.

ELECTRIC MICROBIOME

Looking deeper into the quantum biology of the microbiome, we see microbes are also communicating with electricity and the movement of electrons. In 2010, Kenneth Nealson and team discovered that the gram-negative bacterium *Shewanella oneidensis* has a different way of cycling electrons by directly depositing electrons onto metal surfaces. Rather than keeping the flow of electrons internal, *Shewanella oneidensis* grows nanowire hairs to be able to transfer electrons to metal. Similar research on the bacterium *Geobacter*, and more recently on *Flexistipes sinusarabici*, *Calditerrivibrio nitroreducens*, and *Desulfurivibrio alkaliphilus*, have found similar nanowires used to conduct electrons, creating an electrical current.

These nanowires are composed of proteins, called chromophores, that act as light harvesters able to capture and transfer electrons. The process, termed the external electron transport chain, is where the microbe carries the electrons on the nanowire hairs as a small electrical current and gets rid of electrons by depositing them on metal. Extracellular electron transfer has been found to be spin selective, meaning the quantum spin of the electron determines the effectiveness of the electron transfer. Recent research found that this phenomenon of external electron transfer occurs in the gut microbiomes of mice, rats, and guinea pigs, making the case for its occurrence in our mammalian gut microbiome as well.

This flow of electrons through the microbe's nanowire hair was found through computational and experimental evidence to be quantum biologic in nature. The same researcher that first discovered quantum phenomena in photosynthetic bacteria in the early 2000s, Greg Engel, recently found that photosynthetic bacteria use a quantum mechanical effect called *vibronic mixing* to move energy between two different pathways, depending on whether there's oxygen in the environment. Vibronic mixing happens when vibrational and electronic characteristics in molecules couple, or quantum entangle to one another. The molecules' vibrations blend completely with the electronic states of the molecules, creating an inseparable entanglement that helps guide energy where it needs it to go. A much more elaborate and nuanced picture of our relationship with microbes appears as we look past the chemical model of signaling molecules into the realm of quantum coherence and frequency information.

In 2021, researchers made a fascinating discovery—that *Shewanella* wasn't just depositing electrons, it was consuming them, too. They found that *Shewanella* could live on electricity alone without the need for carbohydrates. Researchers tuned an electrode with a specific electrical emission and the microbes swam up to the electrode and started accepting, or eating, the electrons. In 2019, scientists successfully used this principle to harvest *Shewanella* by placing electrodes in bodies of water to attract and collect the microbes. The idea that life can flourish on electricity alone is something that had previously never been discovered.

Contrary to the thinking at the time, these electrical microbes are not just found in extreme environments. Fast-forward to 2018, when researchers found more than one hundred electricity-producing microbes in the human gut. These gram-positive bacteria residing in the human gut microbiome transfer over 100,000 electrons per second, creating an electrical current. Animals and plants transfer their electrons to oxygen via the electron transfer chain in the cell's mitochondria but bacteria in environments with no oxygen, like our gut, or during fermentation, must find a different electron acceptor. In this research, microbes transfer their electrons to flavin molecules in their environment. Flavins are blue light acceptors that possess unique quantum biological characteristics. The cells that line the gastrointestinal tract contain flavin molecules, acting as ready acceptors in this flow of energy. Although we don't have direct evidence that the flow of electricity through the microbiome is communicated to the flavins in the gut, all the hardware is there. Nature rarely puts unnecessary pieces into living systems. This could be a way to transfer energy in the form of electrons from the microbiome to our own body.

It gets even more interesting when we look at the biofilm communication that microbes use. When microbial populations hit a certain number, the microbial community starts acting as a quorum, or as a collective. As the collective rises in numbers, it can create what is called a *biofilm*. Biofilms are hard-to-remove films that grow as a protective mechanism to danger signals and create more social cohesion and cooperation in the microbiome. These biofilms are scaffold matrixes of polymers that provide habitat for microbes, like apartment buildings for our microbiota. Biofilms help microbes communicate, but they also seem to communicate with our cells.

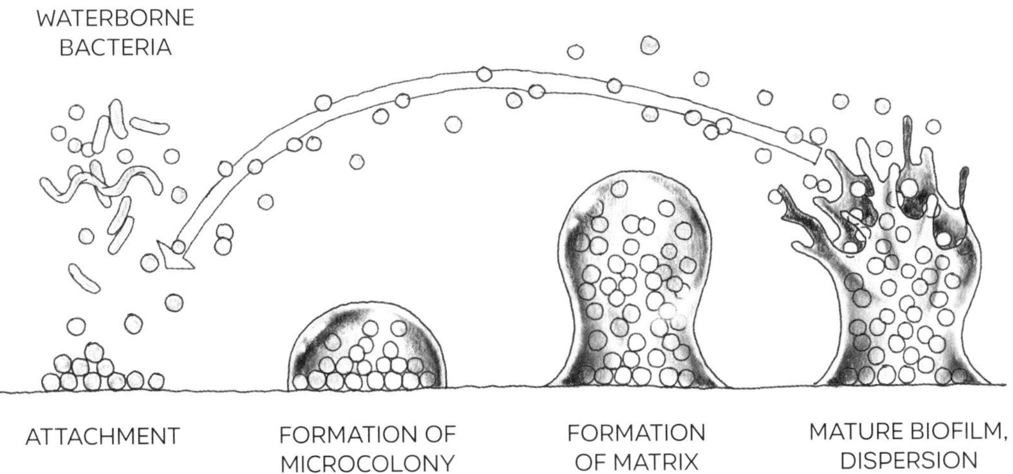

As microbial colonies are established, biofilms are created and eventually disperse. These biofilms can communicate with our cells.

Recent research found that when *Geobacter* is exposed to an electrical current, they form dense biofilms. These dense biofilms connected hundreds of microbes, sharing a gridwork to move electrons through. Living biofilms of *Geobacter* use nanowires of photoconducting cytochrome OmcS, which increase the flow of electrons a hundred-fold. These OmcZ nanowires conduct electricity 1,000 times more efficiently than the nanowires *Geobacter* creates in soil. When exposed to light, the current of electrons in the nanowire was sustained for hours.

What's more is these biofilms seem to be communicating with our cells as well. In research with mice, salmonella infection generated a directional electrical field. When that electrical field was reproduced in the lab, it attracted the mouse macrophages to the anode where the electrical field was being produced. When the macrophages engulfed the salmonella, their surface electrical properties changed, and they were directed by electrical guidance away from the initial electrical field that attracted them. Different research has found that our human macrophages are directed and controlled by electrical fields. This adds a completely new perspective to our relationship with microbes—a perspective that extends past the chemical model to include the flow of electricity and electrons as modes of communication with microbes.

THE MUSIC OF THE MICROBIOME

Interestingly, sound also plays a role in microbial communication. Researchers have discovered that bacteria emit and respond to sound waves. Scientists demonstrated that sound emitted from a speaker at frequencies of 6 kHz to 10 kHz, 18 kHz to 22 kHz, and 28 kHz to 38 kHz increased colony formation by *Bacillus carboniphilus*. Scientists discovered that a different species of bacteria, *Bacillus subtilis*, emitted frequencies at between 8 kHz and 43 kHz with broad peaks, at approximately 8.5 kHz, 19 kHz, 29 kHz, and 37 kHz. There was a similarity between the frequency of the sound created by *B. subtilis* and the frequencies that initiated a response in *B. carboniphilus*, implying that these sound waves function as a growth-regulatory signal between cells. The idea that microbes produce sound to influence the composition and health of the microbiome is mind-blowing.

Sound has been found to alter bacterial quorum communication as well. The effect of Indian classical music was investigated on microbial growth. Out of the ninety different microbes, only one displayed a negative response to growth under the influence of Indian classical music. The other eighty-nine microbes displayed increased growth, metabolism, and pigment production from the exposure to music. In more recent research, music was found to regulate the microbial pigments associated with quorum communication. Sound also enhanced microbial growth as well as the production of metabolites and pigments. Electromagnetic field stimulation was also correlated with the increase of microbial melanin specifically. Melanin is a microbial pigment, making a connection back to what we just explored with melanin and energy in the body. Melanin can convert, store, and release light and electromagnetic fields as bioelectric energy for the body to use. This is fascinating to explore in a system that contains microbes that communicate with light and electromagnetic fields while being able to produce their own melanin stores. Is microbial melanin production tied to a communication network of light and a transmission of energy, both in microbiome and with our cells?

Artificial noise also affects the microbiome. In research with white-crowned sparrows, scientists demonstrated that city noise acts to increase corticosterone and decrease food intake as well as directly effecting the gut microbiome diversity. Noise negatively altered the gut microbiome of mice, corresponding to an increase in overall inflammation. A similar finding was discovered in research with rats. Artificial noise changed the percentage of Proteobacteria and Actinobacteria in the gut, which is consistent with abnormalities in glucose and insulin regulation seen in diabetes progression. Modern life does an excellent job of inundating us with artificial light and sound. It's no wonder we are in the midst of an epidemic of metabolic diseases.

THE QUANTUM MICROBIOME IMMUNE SYSTEM CONNECTION

Health begins to look a lot different from a quantum perspective. The microbiome has a direct impact on our immune system. The immune system takes information from the microbiome, the external environment of light, electricity, and electromagnetic fields as well as the internal terrain of hormones, thoughts, and mitochondria and sends these messages throughout the body. It sorts these inputs and gets the messages where they need to be. A quantum biological view of the immune system highlights how interconnected our ecosystem is and guides us away from a solely invader-and-defense standpoint of the immune system.

The immune system responds to light signals. We've talked about the effects light has in driving different immune responses and cytokine patterns. The loss of the normal electrical charge of an immune cell alters the signals and cytokines that the cell releases. This causes chaos in the immune system. Certain immune cells, like macrophages, are guided by electrical fields. The immune system is influenced by electromagnetic fields, too. Nonnative electromagnetic fields have been found to disrupt the immune system. This research is in its infancy. We are just starting to understand the effects and implications of light, electricity, and electromagnetic fields on the immune system. The microbiome communicates with biophotons, electricity, and electromagnetic fields. Are the immune system and the microbiome communicating via light and electromagnetic fields? This certainly warrants more research.

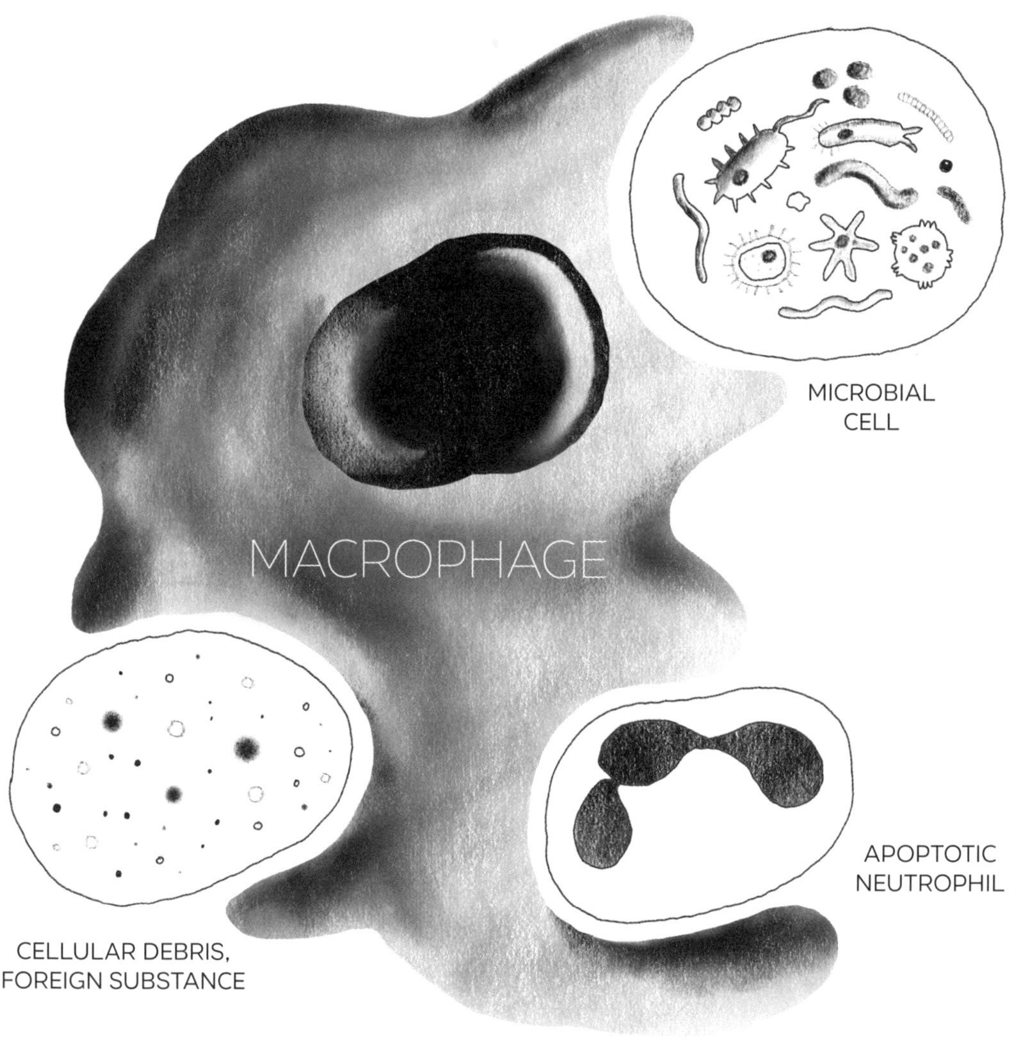

Macrophages are immune cells that help rid the body of diseased and dysfunctional cells and debris. They can be guided by an electrical field to migrate to an area and engulf a cell that needs to be cleared from the body.

It is possible to conceive of the immune system, in tandem with the liquid crystalline water network within us, as a communication network. There is research that demonstrates that cancerous cells have more bulk water and have diminished EZ liquid crystalline water lining them. There is also research showing that the loss of the negative electrical charge creates cellular changes associated with cancer that disappear when the negative charge is returned. Some researchers propose that the liquid crystalline water contributes to the cell's negative electrical charge and the loss of both is a contributing factor to cancer. It isn't just the cell's negative charge that supports healthy function; it's also how the electrical charge and the EZ liquid crystalline water serve as receiver and emitter of vibratory information. Without these, the immune system cannot function properly—the communication network breaks down.

Often looked at as a defensive mechanism against pathogens, mucus and fever could serve additional purposes. Fever increases infrared heat, aiding the building of liquid crystalline water in our body while enhancing mitochondrial function. Mucus is filled with liquid crystalline EZ water and could serve as an aid in communicating with electromagnetic fields, light, and frequency information from microbes. If this quantum network is intact, the microbes can more easily pass on their information, electromagnetic fields, electrons, gasotransmitters like nitric oxide, hydrogen sulfide, and methane, electricity, and light. We see that microbes do pass these things within our biology. What if microbes are increasing in the numbers we see in infections to communicate when the communication network has faltered? Like raising your voice when someone can't hear you. This would require that we focus on bolstering the communication system—the liquid crystalline water and the bioelectric network of the body.

Many things used traditionally to recover from an infection serve a different function from a quantum biological perspective. Propolis, a substance bees use to keep their hives clean, has a broad antimicrobial action against viruses, fungi, and bacteria that has gained a reputation for its use in infections. It also serves to create EZ water. Research has found that many traditional healing remedies support the building of liquid crystalline water, propolis being one of them. Propolis forms extensive EZ water. Similar results were found with health-promoting agents such as holy basil, turmeric, coconut water, acetaminophen, and aspirin. All these substances increased the EZ liquid crystalline water against a hydrophilic surface—remember, our cell walls are hydrophilic, and this includes our immune cells. What we have viewed as a combative invader-defender relationship could also be seen as a communication network that has faltered and is trying to rebuild the electrical charge and liquid crystal matrix with fever and mucus.

TENDING TO YOUR SYMBIOTIC NATURE

Our relationship with microbes mirrors the beautiful interconnection we have with the world around us. We don't end at the barriers of our skin. It's time we extend our view of the microbial world from the strict chemical perspective into an expanded quantum biological view—a view that recognizes the action of quantum gasotransmitters, light, electromagnetic fields, and sound of the microbiome and the role of the immune system as a communication network, working to get messages from the internal and external environment throughout the body. Tending to the microbiome and immune system with a quantum biological approach can bolster this relationship between the immune system and microbiome and thus our overall health and longevity. Read on for ways to accomplish this.

Consume a diet rich in resistant starches and colorful fruits and vegetables that can help support the health of the gut microbiome as well as the mitochondria of the cells that line the gut. Resistant starches are transformed into short chain fatty acids that support the health of both the gut microbiome and the mitochondria in the cells that line the gut.

Support the mitochondria. Tending to the mitochondria has a direct impact on the health, function, and vitality of the gut microbiome. Mitochondria and microbiomes have an intimate communication and influence on each other. It is hard to separate the health of one without discussing the other one (see chapter 4 for more information on supporting mitochondrial health).

Get outside. The microbiome reflects the terrain within us and external to us. The air we breathe seeds the respiratory microbiome, which influences the gut microbiome and feeds into the cardiovascular and vaginal microbiomes. Seek exposure to natural air, natural sounds, natural light, and the sea of electrons on Earth's surface as well as its magnetic field as often as possible to support the immune system and the microbiome.

Strengthen the nervous system. Prioritize rest, sleep, boundaries, and activities that are enjoyable and fulfilling. Cultivate stress management practices, whether a gratitude practice, meditation, mindfulness, or heart coherence practice to support the health of the microbiome and the immune system (see chapter 7 for more information).

Align your rhythm with the circadian rhythm of the sun. Gain exposure to natural light in the morning and throughout the day, and lower the lights at night to sync with the circadian rhythm of the sun to support both the microbiome and the immune system (see chapter 5 for more information). Additionally, red light therapy can be helpful to the overall health of the microbiome and the immune system. Experiment with red and infrared light to support the gut microbiome, the immune system, and the cells lining the gastrointestinal tract.

Nourish the microbiome with sound. Low-frequency sounds, soothing sounds of nature, and sounds that are personally enjoyable can help support the gut microbiome. Avoid noise, which can damage the balance of the microbiome.

Ever important, nurture the water network within. The microbes in the gastrointestinal tract are housed in a watery mucous layer. This liquid crystalline water is important for the health of the microbiome. In one preliminary research study, drinking energized coherent water was found beneficial for the diversity and health of the gut microbiome. Tending the liquid crystalline water within can also enhance the water lining our immune cells, which allows for better function and communication in the immune system. Build the liquid crystalline water within and include energized water in your daily routine (see chapter 2 for more information).

From a quantum biological perspective, the immune system needs certain quantum inputs to function properly and to serve as an antenna for all the frequency information that consistently streams in. Our microbiome and our immune system have a profound relationship that dictates the state of vitality in the body. Tending to both is crucial for our longevity and health.

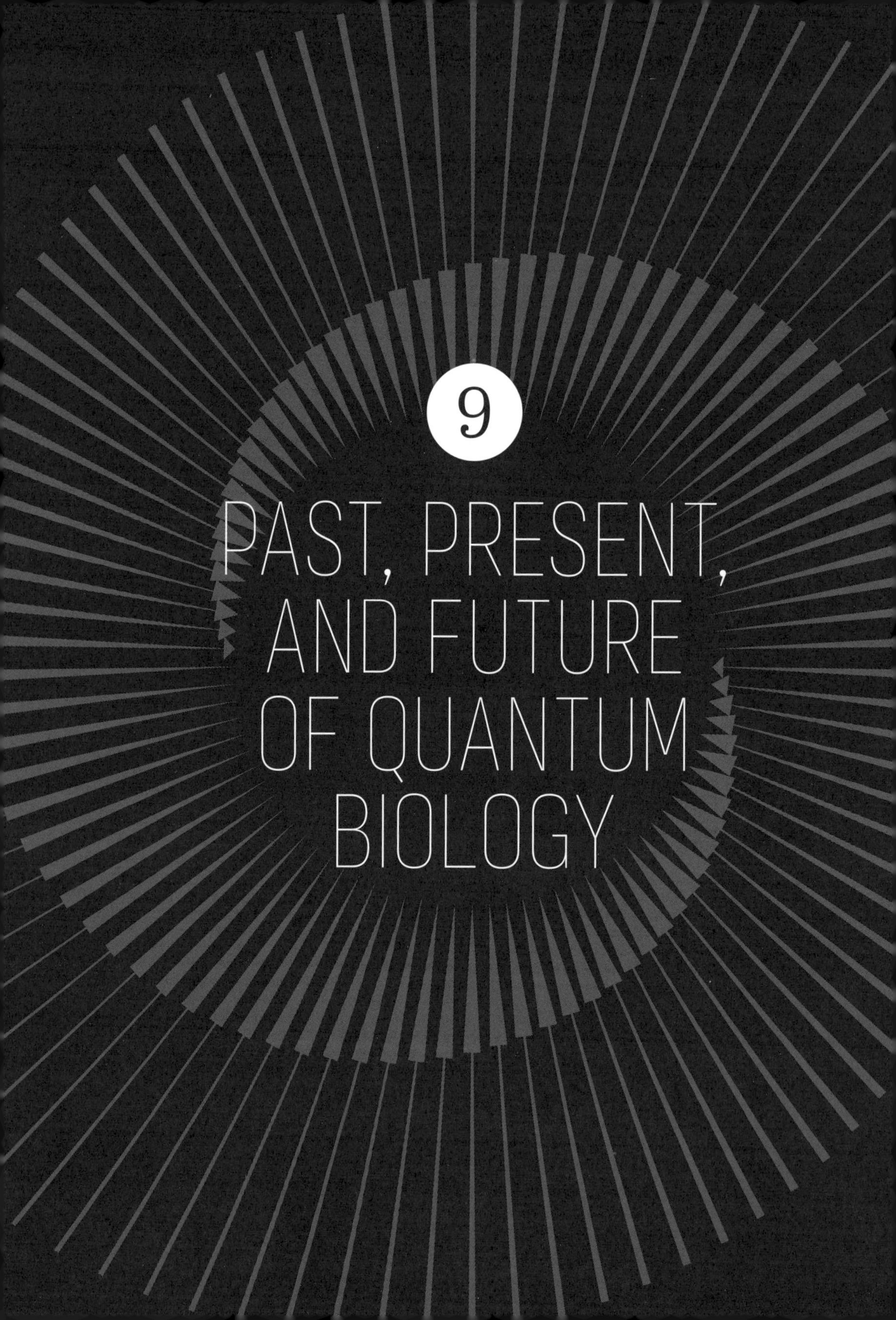

9

PAST, PRESENT, AND FUTURE OF QUANTUM BIOLOGY

What an incredible perspective quantum biology offers on the body and health. It doesn't require that we abandon the current perspective. It requires a reconciliation of the current perspective and the quantum biological perspective. A lot of what quantum biology explores brings us back to what the ancients always spoke of—that ancient wisdom was cast aside with the scientific revolution. The scientific revolution of the mid-1500s to the mid-1600s ushered in a new approach to science and health. It also relegated the vitalistic healing traditions of Indigenous cultures and beliefs to the sidelines.

PAST

We have been working under a chemical-mechanical (Newtonian) model of health from Sir Issac Newton for several centuries, which started by looking at the body as a machine—predictable and deterministic. As you now know, this model is reductionistic, breaking things down and separating them into parts. It is also deterministic. If you know the starting point, you know the end.

Rooted in seventeenth-century science, the Newtonian model provided a completely new approach to life. Before this model, life was thought to be governed by supernatural forces, such as gods, divinities, elemental forces, and beings. Science had been dominated by traditions that saw nature as a culmination of forces. From the Greek tradition of humors to the traditional Chinese medicine view of the elements to the Celtic tradition of nature imbued with life and healing to the Vedic perspective of the elements, there was a common belief that all of creation was infused with a vitality and intelligence.

Advances in technology with the advent of the telescope and the microscope caused science to shift its focus. The Newtonian model brought a new understanding of the solar system and the microscopic world, which ushered in a coordinated method for ascertaining scientific truth. Rather than relying on belief and subjective relationship, the Newtonian model depends on observation, where the observer is separate from the system being observed. Scientific consensus can come when observers can compare their observations and settle on a common truth.

The Newtonian model of science sees the universe as a clockwork mechanism. This mechanistic model was applied to biology, health, and medicine. The brain was seen as the body's computer. Consciousness is an emergent process of brain activity; it's a product of the neurons' activity. As neurons fire, conscious thoughts occur. DNA is the blueprint of life. Genes determine destiny. This model dictates that life is governed by chemical reactions and physical mechanisms only. Placebo is seen as an anomaly because there is a definite split between mind and body.

In the Newtonian model, healing is based on a chemical-mechanical approach. Drugs, surgery, and other physical interventions are the mainstay of medicine. The focus in biology is on biochemical pathways, genetic determinism, and mechanistic physiology. Health is defined as an absence of disease.

PRESENT

With the birth of quantum physics in the early 1900s, a new era dawned and the evidence for this perspective continues to grow. From a quantum outlook, life isn't just a mechanical or chemical interaction. A quantum biological model proposes that life is a matter of probability, not a strictly deterministic matter—not a matter of randomness but an array of possibilities where one action can have many outcomes depending on its relationship with the world around it. Systems can't always be reduced; entangled parts can act as one. Action isn't always a product of direct and physical contact. The almost instantaneous influence of vibration can travel across large distances. Outcomes aren't strictly determined. Observers are part of the equation, not separated and removed.

From a quantum biological perspective, life resembles a symphony more than a machine, with each cell, organ, and being playing its unique tune in the beautiful song of life. Consciousness isn't just about computation. It is not produced by the brain, rather the brain acts like a radio, receiving consciousness from the universal field of intelligence.

In this quantum paradigm, genes don't determine everything. Epigenetics shows how the environment and mind-set influence gene expression. Energy, intent, and information fields affect cell behavior. The mind-body connection takes center stage in a quantum biological model. Thoughts, beliefs, and intention have the power to influence health.

In the quantum biology model, health is about coherence. It's a balance between the mind, body, and energy systems. Disease can arise from disruptions in energy flow and a loss of coherence. Genes don't always dictate disease; it is the environment that influences how genes express themselves. The body has an intelligence to it that can be directed to healing.

From a quantum biological perspective, the body isn't just mechanical. It is directed by electrical charge, magnetic fields, and electromagnetic fields. Light and sound produce biological action. Water depends on relationships—what it encounters determines its organization and function. Water can capture, amplify, and transmit energy and information. Breathwork, grounding, Reiki, heart-brain coherence, and sound therapy can help bring unity to the body. We have the ability to co-create our own wellness.

Some ideas in quantum biology bring us back full circle to the traditions of ancient Indigenous cultures. Early explanations of health and disease rested on unseen forces and beliefs about the physical and metaphysical universe. Vitalism, the idea that the origin and workings of life require a force beyond chemical and mechanical forces, was something all Indigenous cultures shared. Cultures held deep reverence for a field of universal energy or information that was intimately tied to health. The rise of monotheistic religions held a similar reverence for the unseen will of God. It was the scientific revolution that ushered in a time when only the seen forces mattered—only those forces we could see with our eyes or under a microscope held validity.

Our technology has advanced to a never-before-seen level. We can observe, measure, and test life at the nanoscale. Life at the quantum level looks different than it does at a macroscopic level. What we're learning now adds another layer of understanding to our health. This new understanding of life at the quantum scale ties together seamlessly so much of what we have learned as well as what we have discarded.

We are advancing an understanding of what was once inconceivable. Quantum biology looks at the effects of the flow of electrons, protons, photons of light, and vibrations of sound. It explores the influence of fields of energy, whether electromagnetic, electrical, magnetic, scalar, or quantum. It highlights the importance of our relationship with light, sound, water, temperature, color, and vibrational energy from fields of frequency. While the explanation and the science behind the ideas are different, ancient cultures held the same importance for these relationships.

Modern quantum biology for health and ancient wisdom share several pillars of health and healing. Ancient Indigenous cultures had an active acknowledgment of a field of universal energy, or ether, that held information for the journey of life. We are beginning to explore the idea of the biofield in health, or the zero-point field in physics, but this was an accepted and integral part of Indigenous health and disease. Ancient cultures held that universal energy gave life to all things, even inanimate objects. Whether it was the animals or the plants or the rivers, each had its own contribution to the greater web of life and thus health. Health and vitality depended on a person's relationship to all things in this web. Indigenous cosmology reinforced this worldview, instilling a deep belief and reverence for the natural and the supernatural. This was the landscape of medicine for millennia.

As Gregory Cajete describes in his book *Native Science*, there are striking differences between the relational Indigenous science and the absolutism of Western science. In Native science, there is an inclusive definition of being alive. Everything is viewed as having energy and its own unique intelligence and creative process, not just the plants, animals, and microorganisms, but also rocks, mountains, rivers, and landscapes. Everything in nature has something to teach humans. As Cajete explains, the Indigenous physicist not only observes nature, but also participates in it. A relationship is cultivated with the natural world that is being investigated. A relationship of mutual respect and care is established.

A RETURN TO ANCIENT WISDOM

Every ancient culture had its own approach to health and disease. Tailored to the local region, the medicines and traditions varied from culture to culture, but there was a common perspective shared. The ancient cultures of India, Africa, China, Europe, and the Americas are beautiful examples of the wisdom present in Indigenous beliefs across the globe. Each explored an intricate flow of energy throughout the body that was dependent on our connection to the world around us. This flow of energy was essential and inseparable from their view of health, disease, and the workings of the universe. Their scientific explorations stemmed from a deep connection with the world around them, including their own body. Indigenous society afforded the space in life to observe and cultivate those relationships while learning how they relate to health and disease.

Modern quantum biology and ancient wisdom both share a respect for the modes of healing that extend past the chemical-mechanical model. Ancient cultures revered and respected the unseen aspects of healing. Sound, frequency, light, emotions, and the invisible field of energy that connected everything in life had a prominent role in these traditions.

Sound Healing

Sound was regarded as sacred in ancient cultures. The Maya have the story of Quetzalcoatl using the conch shell to create the first vibration of life. Indigenous Australians, the Aboriginals, thought the yidaki, or didgeridoo, creates a sound that connects us to dreamtime, the place we came from and will return to upon death. It is the place where our ancestors dwell. The yidaki was used, and continues to be used, for healing with a recent study finding its benefit for stress reduction, relaxation, and lowering blood pressure. Playing the yidaki has also shown benefits for sleep apnea and asthma.

The Mayan pyramids of Chichén Itzá have both acoustic and light effects that display a strong grasp of the laws of frequency. If you stand at the bottom of the 365 stairs that lead to the top of the Pyramid of Kukulkan and clap, you can hear something like the call of the quetzal bird echoed back, while a sound like a serpent's hiss reverberates off the Temple of the Warriors. Although there are no records to point to for their use, it seems too extraordinary to be coincidence.

Ancient Egyptians used vowel chanting and instruments to invoke healing in people. The vowels had healing properties. It's interesting to note that Egyptian hieroglyphics only use consonants, no vowels are written down. Sistrums were used for sound healing with records showing that these instruments were used for respiratory illnesses. The sistrum was applied to the nostril to help respiratory function and health. Some researchers even claim that the pyramids were used as resonate sound chambers for healing.

Greek physicians used flutes, lyres, and zithers to treat their patients. Vibrations of sound were used to aid digestion, treat mental disturbance, and induce sleep.

Indigenous Peoples in North America use drums and singing to evoke healing. Navajo singers, known as Diné Hataałii, the traditional healers of the community, use song and chants to evoke healing by bridging the physical realm with the spiritual realm.

Light Therapy

Many ancient Indigenous cultures have morning rituals of greeting the sun as a source of light and life. Native America traditions include welcoming the sun each morning in gratitude for the light. During the fall and spring equinoxes in Chichén Itzá, reflecting off the sides of the Pyramid of Kukulkan, you can see a light- and shadow-induced serpent—a visual representation of the reverence that Maya have for the power of the sun.

Heliotherapy, or the use of sunlight for healing, has been used for centuries. Hippocrates and the physicians who followed him used sunlight to treat all kinds of disease. Ancient Ayurvedic medicine incorporated sunlight to stimulate health. Ancient Egyptian, Greek, Roman, and Arab physicians also used sunlight to promote healing. There was a clear relationship between sunshine and collective health.

Water Remedy

Water was also revered as a healing medicine. The ancient cultures of the Egyptians, Greek, Celts, Romans, and the Hebrew people viewed water as medicine. It was part of their creation stories and connection to the Earth. Sacred wells throughout Europe and sacred bodies of water throughout the world were valued for their healing abilities. Water was used in hydrotherapy where different water temperatures conferred various health benefits. Water treatments, balneotherapy, or bathing in medicinal and thermal springs, aided specific and general health. Thalassotherapy, or the use of ocean water to heal, was commonplace. There was a respect for the different water sources, characteristics, and temperatures to provide both wisdom and healing.

A RELATIONSHIP WITH THE PLANTS, THE LAND, AND THE COSMOS

The vitalism and traditional medicine of ancient cultures held a different source of knowledge. These ancient cultures had a relationship with the sun, Earth, plants, animals, water, and the cosmos that could be used to heal. They held a deep reverence for this relationship with the world around them. It was all part of an intimate dance of life. There was a respect for wisdom gathered through the silent observation necessary to hear nature's lessons. Health and disease centered on being in balance with the world we live in.

Each culture also had precise healing modalities using plant and animal medicines as well as ways to treat the unseen energetic flow of the body. Indigenous cultures were all tied to the land. Nature was an intimate part of daily life.

China

In traditional Chinese medicine, the patient exists within a greater context. The five-element theory in Chinese medicine places the patient within the ecosystem of the universe. The five elements—water, wood, fire, earth, and metal—are physical representations of the universal elements. These five physical elements correspond with metaphysical elements as well and are reflections of the duality, or more precisely the polarity, of Earth. They represent the yin and yang energies of Earth. In Chinese medicine, we are reflections or extensions of the life that extends throughout the universe.

There is an unmistakable sense of connection with the world within Chinese medicine. Humans are intimately and inextricably intertwined with the greater ecosystem, never separate from it. There is careful consideration for the influences of the seasons, weather, and the universe at large, all having a profound impact on disease and health.

Ancient Egypt

This connection with nature and the universe was also present in ancient Egyptian medicine. Most of our knowledge of ancient Egyptian medicine is derived from the medical pharaonic papyri. The Ebers Papyrus dates back to about 1500 BCE with some accounts that it was copied from texts centuries older. It explains the relationship between health and disease and contains a vast variety of treatments using plants, animals, and minerals. Ancient Egyptians thought health and illness resulted from a person's relationship and connections with the universe, including its people, animals, and good and bad spirits. These connections to the universe were the deciding factors for health and disease. A person was never separate from the universe that held them.

The Celts

The ancient tribes of Europe, often referred to as the Celts, also viewed health and disease as intertwined with the world around them. Although diverse groups of people of varying regions and dialects, the Celts had a deep reverence for nature and the healing powers of plants, animals, and water.

Written history is sparse from this time, but recounts recorded later show a diverse culture of groups that held nature, the movements of the moon, stars, sun, planets, and our relationship to them as essential to health. These people had a deep respect for a relationship with the natural world. Celts and their ideas of health had a special connection to plants, the role of fire and water in healing, and how our health is tied to our alignment with the cycles of Earth, of the seasons, and of the cosmos.

The Maya

The Maya civilization also had a rich view of health, disease, and the cosmos. They had an intimate relationship with nature, believing that rivers, streams, forests, caves, and springs had guardians and must be maintained in a reciprocal relationship where the collective tends to the natural and supernatural world. The Maya calendar reflects the Mayas' view that humans are extensions of the vast energy that connects both the physical and the mystical world. Each day is aligned with the four cardinal directions and affected by an animal, a plant, and a deity. The same collection of forces that orients the days of the year also orients the human body. If you live out of alignment with these forces, illness can ensue.

Illness in the Maya culture could be from organic causes, like lifestyle or environmental change, or caused by supernatural beings. The Maya People understood illness to be a result of an imbalance in the intimate relationship between the person, the community, and the cosmos. They believed that all things were bound by a force—what we do affects the universe and everything in the universe reverberates through us.

India

Similarly, Ayurveda has its roots in a unified cosmovision. Dating back 5,000 years, the Vedas are the earliest record we have of ancient Indian civilization. The word *Ayurveda*, "the knowledge of life," is the combination of the Sanskrit words *ayur* ("life") and *veda* ("knowledge"). According to Ayurvedic medicine, matter is composed of five Mahābhūtas, or elements, that have the properties of space/ether (Akasha), air (Vayu), fire (Agni), water (Jala), and earth (Prithvi). These elements merge to form the three Doshas: Vata, Pitta, and Kapha. Vata is created from the lighter elements with characteristics of space and air. Pitta is shaped from the elements with properties of fire and water. The heavier elements form Kapha, with properties of water and earth. Each dosha regulates specific biological functions, and each person has a unique balance of Vata, Pitta, and Kapha.

Ancient Ayurveda viewed health as a balance between one's personal makeup of elements and the world around them. Meticulous care was taken to observe the person's relation to the stars, planets, and moons, to the seasons, the weather, the elements, as well as the community surrounding them. This allowed Ayurvedic physicians to advise the proper time to eat, exercise, and meditate as well as what to eat, how to engage with community, and what thoughts brought health to an individual's constitution.

Ancient Vedic knowledge viewed the cosmos as a changing dance between the order and impulses of nature. According to Vedic science, humans are comprised of two aspects: the never-changing pure consciousness and the ever-changing physical body. This same polarity is seen in the ancient Vedic view of the cosmos with the never-changing order and intelligence of the universe paired with the ever-changing manifestation of matter we see in the world around us.

UNIVERSAL ENERGY FLOW

Along with this connection to the earth and the cosmos came an understanding of the flow of energy in the universe, which was reflected within the body. Ancient Indigenous cultures around the globe acknowledged, utilized, and successfully treated disease by tending to an energetic flow within the body.

China

Traditional Chinese medicine has an intimate understanding of the idea of an energy flow that reflects the greater energy field of the universe. Beyond the five elements of Chinese medicine there are three vital essences:

1. The Qi, or energy
2. The Jing, or essence
3. The Shen, or spirit

Qi is the flow of vital energy in the body and keeping it flowing and balanced is the foundation of health. Energy flows through the human body like it flows through the universe. The ancient Chinese meridian system of energy flow, or Qi, guides diagnosis, herbal prescriptions, acupuncture, and acupressure. Acupuncture and acupressure use needles or pressure on acupuncture points that relate to the energetic meridians, or lines, of energy flow throughout the body. Placing a needle or applying pressure to these acupuncture points alters the flow of energy, which has a beneficial influence on health. Ultimately, the health and balance of the body lies in having sufficient energy within the body's governing energy systems.

Ancient Egypt

Ancient Egyptian medicine also understood the flow of energy throughout the body. The Ebers Papyrus explains that the body has twenty-two metu "vessels," which connect the body and carry vital substances such as blood, air, semen, mucus, and tears. These metu connect to form a network controlled by the heart. Although the metu are internal channels within the body, they are exposed to the external environment at several points. Egyptian healers assessed the health of metu by examination of the patient's pulse similar to the pulse readings of traditional Chinese medicine.

The papyrus compares the free movement of the metu vessels to the Nile, noting the balance of the flow in the metu vessels is essential to the health of the body, like the balance of the Nile flooding and irrigating the soil is vital for the land of Egypt. If the metu vessels are blocked or clogged by foreign or noxious matters (Wekhedu), then disease can occur.

Special care was taken to keep the metu channels clear and flowing. If the channels became dry, all sorts of maladies could ensue. The removal of toxins ensured the freedom of movement in the metu vessels needed for optimal health. Just like the meridians in Chinese medicine, the concept of energy flow throughout the body is essential to health.

Ancient Greece

Egyptian medicine was the foundation of Greek medicine, which also understood energy in the body. Greek doctors such as Melampus, Asclepius, and Hippocrates, who is often referred to as the father of modern medicine, received medical training in Egypt. The humoral tradition of Hippocrates's medicine was a direct lineage of Egyptian theory of health and disease. Hippocrates categorized the basic constituents of the human body as humors. The four humors were based on the four elements of the universe:

1. The liver excreted fire in the yellow bile humor.
2. The spleen secreted the earth element through the black bile humor.
3. The heart secreted air through the blood humor.
4. The brain secreted phlegm through the water humor.

The perspective that the cause of disease was a result of living out of harmony with the universe was passed on from ancient Egypt to ancient Greece—a continuation of the idea that health comes from the unfettered flow of energy in the body.

Ancient Europe

The discovery in the Swiss Alps of the frozen mummy dating back 5,300 years to the Copper Age, Ötzi the Iceman, suggests that the idea of treating a person's energy extends even to Europe and dates further back than many acknowledge. Ötzi was found with tattoos that corresponded to certain acupuncture points. Upon autopsy, he was found to have had ailments that corresponded to these points, which led many researchers to believe he was part of a society that practiced a well-developed form of acupuncture. From Asia to Africa to Europe, the idea of treating the energy flow of the body is evident across the globe.

The Maya

The importance of the energetic body is evident in the Americas as well. Ancient Mayan medicine was also intimately intertwined with the idea of energy flow throughout the body. The concept of hot versus cold is common in Mayan medicine. Like the polarity of yin and yang, the idea of hot and cold is applied to all sorts of objects such as animals, plants, food, air, and water. It is an energetic description that reflects the duality of the Mayas' cosmovision. This reflection pervades the universe and thus our health.

There are two variations of Mayan acupuncture: jup and tok. The Ritual of the Bacabs, written in the late-eighteenth century, mentions *ix hun pudzub kik*, the needle that bleeds, and *ix hun pudzub olom*, the needle that frees the blood. Mayan acupuncture is practiced with the spines and thorns of plants, bushes, and animals as well as the fang of a rattlesnake, beak of a carpenter bird, and porcupine quills. Jup and tok are the most common techniques for expelling evil winds of supernatural origin. Similar to Chinese acupuncture with many corresponding points, Mayan acupuncture demonstrates the same reverence for the healthy flow of energy in the body.

India

In ancient Ayurvedic medicine, there was also an appreciation of the impacts of the flow of energy in our body. Ayurvedic medicine used the term *nadi* to describe the flow of energy in the body. The nadis are subtle energy channels that flow throughout the body. These channels accompany the pulse as they deliver and disperse prana, the life force, to various parts of the body. This prana life force is dispersed through the chakras. Similar to Chinese meridians of energy flow, nadis can be used to diagnose and treat illness within our physiology. The pulse, bioelectrical signals of emotions, thoughts, energy, and information carried within make up the vast network of nadis, which is a subject of continued research today.

A UNIFIED FUTURE OF QUANTUM BIOLOGY

All of these cultures discussed have a practice of assessing, diagnosing, and treating the energetic flow throughout the body. Quantum biology holds a similar respect and practice in regard to light, sound, electrical charge in cells, electromagnetic communication, redox potential of electrons in the mitochondria, and the flow of protons in the fascia.

We are at a time in history when we can join the advances that come from the Newtonian model with the expanded perspective of quantum biology and the respect needed for ancient wisdom. One doesn't negate the others. We can actively hold all three as we reach a higher level of health and longevity.

Quantum biology speaks to the invisible order of life. We now have the ability to reveal some of this order. The role of light, sound, fields of electricity and magnetism, vibration, electromagnetic resonance, and water are gaining acceptance for their vital role in health and healing. The body has a language of resonant frequency that initiates recognition, interaction, and action in biomolecules. The liquid crystalline water and structures within the body can capture, store, and transmit information and energy. The biological six-sided ring plays a special role in this ability to transfer data and power action in the body. We should utilize what is known about the impacts of quantum biology on health and actively research what we still don't know.

Electromagnetic Fields and Health

Weak magnetic fields influence genetic expression and damage, cancer progression, immune system function, blood flow, pain, metabolism, and even our circadian rhythms. Quantum biology brings evidence of electromagnetic fields guiding cell behavior, movement, and differentiation. The Resonant Recognition Model shows how electromagnetics of biomolecules can be used to recognize, communicate, and initiate action in the body. Cells have been found to use their own electromagnetic fields to guide movement, behavior, and differentiation. We can no longer ignore the importance of electromagnetic fields on health.

Electricity and Health

The role of electricity in biology is becoming clearer. Pi electrons in the six-sided biomolecules and biological lattices can also serve the purpose of nonchemical information and energy transfer.

The cell's electrical field is critical for health and longevity. Specific frequencies of electricity can direct wound and bone healing. The cell's electrical voltage plays a vital part in cell function and health as evidenced in its role in directing cancer, infection, and autoimmunity. There is a perspective in health that views health as ample electrical charge and pain, inflammation and disease as a loss of vital electrical charge. Tending to our negative electrical charge is foundational to health and longevity. Devices that utilize electrical currents to treat cardiac conditions, vagal nerve health, and pain broaden options for a longer, healthier life.

Light and Health

There is emerging evidence of the overarching role light plays in biological action throughout the body. Natural light entrains almost every cell in the body. Natural light received through our eyes stimulates the release of hormones, neurotransmitters, and proteins that help mitigate pain and burn fat. Our metabolism, hormonal balance, sex hormones, stress resilience, neurological function, and mood are all regulated by the light in our environment. Light is now being used to improve aging eyesight, Alzheimer's disease, blood sugar, wound healing, pain, mitochondrial function, and more.

Light on the skin also contributes to hormonal and metabolic balance. It increases melanin, which has the capacity to create a flow of energy from the production of free electrons and the splitting of water that surrounds melanin. Melanin also has a role in sequestering toxins and heavy metals. Light offers an incredible avenue toward achieving improved health and longevity.

Our body has an internal network of light communication. The internal biophoton emission plays a role in a mode of communication that is not chemical. Our cells are constantly emitting ultralow-level light. Our body has light-sensitive proteins in internal organs, the lining of the gastrointestinal tract, and in the brain. This brings photonic communication internal. The microbiome also communicates via light, electricity, and electromagnetic fields. Combined with the light and electrical-sensitive proteins that are part of the gastrointestinal tract, this has implications for a messaging network between the microbiome and our own body via the gut.

Water and Health

A quantum biological understanding of the water within the body as a backdrop and amplifier of the unseen frequency information continues to grow. Water can receive, store, harness, amplify, and transmit vibratory information and energy. We see the association between the liquid crystalline water that lines our tissues, cells, and DNA and robust health. Dehydration is associated with aging whereas true hydration is associated with healthy functioning cells. There is a potential link between a loss in electrical charge and diminished negatively charged liquid crystalline water in cancer, infection severity, and immune dysregulation. The water within us has the potential to create a water battery, contributes to our vital negative electrical charge, and could be a source of valuable free electrons while acting as a vital receiver, transmitter, and amplifier of frequency information in the body. Water seems to be the backdrop on which quantum biology occurs in the body, making it vital to our health and longevity.

Sound and Health

Sound is gaining evidence for its role in health and medicine. New research on low-frequency sound and blood cells shows sound's potential to repair, preserve life span, and increase oxygen binding in cells. The relationship between the vagus nerve and sound offers tools for decreasing pain, inflammation, and nervous system support that aren't dependent on chemicals. The vibrations of sound have the power to influence and organize matter. Sound offers a noninvasive intervention that expands our options for health.

A NEW PERSPECTIVE ON HEALTH AND LONGEVITY

Quantum biology also offers a new perspective on the body. Fascia is no longer just the body's scaffolding. It is a piezoelectric structure that could be shuttling energy and information throughout the body. Mitochondria aren't just the cells' powerhouses. They form an intricate messaging system that guides action throughout the body. The immune system is no longer just a defensive line. It is an interconnected web of communication throughout the body. Our cells, proteins, and biomolecules can receive, store, and transmit the energy and information held in vibrations. Molecules within the biological structures, such as the benzene ring found in our DNA, fascia, neurotransmitters, and neurons, are not only able to capture, store, harness, and transmit vibrational energy and information, but frequencies of the quantum field seem to be an intimate part of their structure, total energy, and unique vibrational signature. Vibrations of light, sound, and fields of energy guide life, and it's time to acknowledge and tend to that. We are receivers and transmitters of energy in a universal field of information.

Our current perspective on disease has brought us this far and now quantum biology could take us even farther. By marrying the two, the Newtonian model and the quantum biology perspective, while respecting the ancient wisdom that came before, we can elevate our approach to wellness and longevity. With simple daily practices of earthing, drinking quality water, exposure to soothing sounds and silence, managing stress, cultivating a practice of coherence, utilizing breathwork, eating a diet rich in quality fats, colorful fruits and vegetables, and protein, exposure to natural light in the morning and throughout the day while lowering the lights at night we support our quantum terrain.

Quantum biology offers a new view of interconnection, where our life is entwined with the world around us, leading to a deeper relationship that has us tending to ourselves, each other, and the planet we live on.

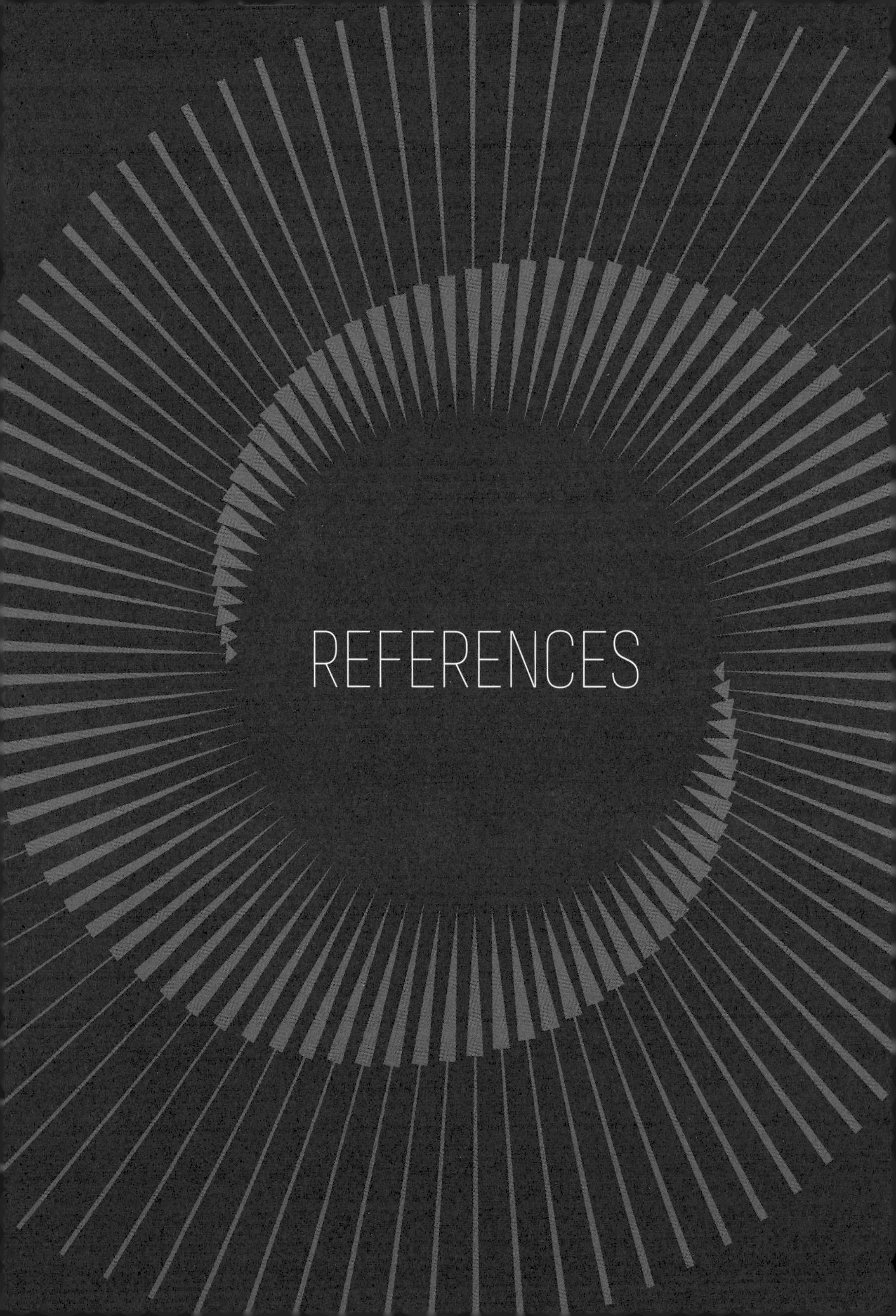

REFERENCES

CHAPTER ONE

Barrett, Terence W., and Herbert A. Pohl. *Energy Transfer Dynamics: Studies and Essays in Honor of Herbert Frohlich on His Eightieth Birthday*. Springer-Verlag, 1987.

Bartell, L. S. "Complementarity in the Double-Slit Experiment: On Simple Realizable Systems for Observing Intermediate Particle-Wave Behavior." *Physical Review D* 21 (1980). https://doi.org/10.1103/PhysRevD.21.1698.

Bennett, James. P. "Medical Hypothesis: Neurodegenerative Diseases Arise from Oxidative Damage to Electron Tunneling Proteins in Mitochondria." *Medical Hypotheses* 127 (2019): 1–4. https://doi.org/10.1016/j.mehy.2019.03.034.

Bennett, James P. Jr., and Isaac G. Onyango. "Energy, Entropy and Quantum Tunneling of Protons and Electrons in Brain Mitochondria: Relation to Mitochondrial Impairment in Aging-Related Human Brain Diseases and Therapeutic Measures." *Biomedicines* 9, no. 2 (2021): 225. https://doi.org/10.3390/biomedicines9020225.

Binhi, Vladimir N. "Statistical Amplification of the Effects of Weak Magnetic Fields in Cellular Translation." *Cells* 12 (2023). https://doi.org/10.3390/cells12050724.

Buchachenko, A. L. "Does Biological Longevity Depend on the Magnetic Fields?" *Russian Journal of Physical Chemistry B* 17 (2023): 128–134. https://doi.org/10.1134/S1990793123010037.

Cha, Yuan, Christopher J. Murray, and Judith P. Klinman. "Hydrogen Tunneling in Enzyme Reactions." *Science* 243, no. 4896 (1989): 1325–4896. https://doi.org/10.1126/science.2646716.

Chae, Kwon-Seok, Soo-Chan Kim, Hye-Jin Kwon, and Yongkuk Kim. 2022. "Human Magnetic Sense Is Mediated by a Light and Magnetic Field Resonance-Dependent Mechanism." *Scientific Reports* 12, no. 8997. https://doi.org/10.1038/s41598-022-12460-6.

Davisson, C. J. "The Diffraction of Electrons by a Crystal of Nickel." *The Bell System Technical Journal* 7, no. 1 (1928): 90–105. https://doi.org/10.1002/j.1538-7305.1928.tb00342.x.

de Arriba, M. M. Carretero, Nuria Illera, A. Holguin, Blanca Duarte, Sara Llames, et al. "169 Olfactory Receptors in Skin. Localization, Specific Expression Pattern and Their Potential Role in Wound Healing." *Journal of Investigative Dermatology* 137, no. 10 (2017). https:doi.org/10.1016/j.jid.2017.07.479.

DeVault, Don D., and Britton Chance. "Studies of Photosynthesis Using a Pulsed Laser. I. Temperature Dependence of Cytochrome Oxidation Rate in Chromatium. Evidence for Tunneling." *Biophysical Journal* 6, no. 6 (1966): 825–847. https://doi.org/10.1016/s0006-3495(66)86698-5.

Dirac, Paul. *The Principles of Quantum Mechanics*, 4th ed. Oxford University Press, 1967.

Einstein, Albert. "Concerning an Heuristic Point of View Toward the Emission and Transformation of Light." 1965 Translation into English *American Journal of Physics* 33, no. 5 (1905). https://inters.org/files/einstein1905_photoeff.pdf.

Editors of Encyclopedia Britannica, The. "Schrodinger Equation | Explanation & Facts." *Encyclopedia Britannica*, 2025. www.britannica.com/science/Schrodinger-equation.

Engel, Gregory. "Quantum Coherence in Photosynthesis." *Procedia Chemistry* 3 (2011): 222–231. https://doi.org/10.1016/j.proche.2011.08.029.

Engel, Gregory. S., Tessa R. Calhoun, Elizabeth L. Read, Tae-Kyu Ahn, Tomáš Mančal, Yuan-Chung Cheng, et al. "Evidence for Wavelike Energy Transfer Through Quantum Coherence in Photosynthetic Systems. *Nature* 446 (2007): 782–786. https://doi.org/10.1038/nature05678. https://pitpas1.phas.ubc.ca/varchive/qbio2014/2014_06_galiano_fleming.pdf.

Godbeer, A.D., J. S. Al-Khalili, and P. D. Stevenson. 2015 "Modelling Proton Tunnelling in the Adenine-Thymine Base Pair." *Physical Chemistry Chemical Physics* 17 (2015): 13034–13044. https://doi.org/10.1039/C5CP00472A.

Griffin, Christine A., Kimberly A. Kafadar, and Grace K. Pavlath. "MOR23 Promotes Muscle Regeneration and Regulates Cell Adhesion and Migration." *Developmental Cell* 17, no. 5 (2009): 649–61. https:// doi.org/10.1016/j.devcel.2009.09.004.

Gu Xiaoling, Philip H. Karp, Stephen L. Brody, Richard A. Pierce, Michael J. Welsh, Michael J. Holtzman, et al. "Chemosensory Functions for Pulmonary Neuroendocrine Cells." *American Journal of Respiratory Cell and Molecular Biology* 50, no. 3 (2014): 637–46. https://doi.org/10.1165/rcmb.2013-0199OC.

Huang Nengwen, Hianghe Qiao, Longjiang Li, Zhonghua Kou, Qiang Yi, and Xue Za Zhi. "Research Progress in Mitochondrial Transfer Mediated by Tunneling Nanotube in the Field of Tumor." *PubMD* 56, no. 10 (2021): 1045–1049. https://doi.org/10.3760/cma.j.cn112144-20210320-00131.

Ikeya, Noboru, and Jonathan R. Woodward. "Cellular Autofluorescence Is Magnetic Field Sensitive." *Proceedings of the National Academy of Sciences of the United States of America* 118, no. 3 (2021). https://doi.org/10.1073/pnas.2018043118.

Kim, Soochan, Baek Soonbong, and Quan Xiaoyuan. "Electromagnetic Fields Mediate Efficient Cell Reprogramming into a Pluripotent State." *ACS Nano* 8, no. 10 (2014): 10125–10138. https://doi.org/10.1021/nn502923s.

Kohen, Amnon, Raffaele Cannio, Simonetta Bartolucci, and Judith P. Klinman. "Enzyme Dynamics and Hydrogen Tunnelling in a Thermophilic Alcohol Dehydrogenase." *Nature* 399 (1999): 496–499. https://doi.org/10.1038/20981.

Liu, Shu, Rao Fu, and Guangwu Li. "Exploring the Mechanism of Olfactory Recognition in the Initial Stage by Modeling the Emission Spectrum of Electron Transfer." *PLOS One* 15 (1) (2020): e0217665. https://doi.org/10.1371/journal.pone.0217665.

Masgrau, Laura, Anna Roujeinikova, Linus O. Johannissen, Parvinder Hothi, Jaswir Basran, Kara E. Ranaghan, et al. "Atomic Description of an Enzyme Reaction Dominated by Proton Tunneling." *Science* 312 (2006): 237–241. https://doi.org/10.1126/science.1126002.

McFadden J., Al-Khalili J. "A Quantum Mechanical Model of Adaptive Mutation." *Biosystems* 50 (1999): 203–211. https://doi.org/10.1016/s0303-2647(99)00004-0.

Mohseni, Masoud, Patrick Rebentrost, Seth Lloyd, and Alán Aspuru-Guzik. "Environment-Assisted Quantum Walks in Photosynthetic Energy Transfer." *The Journal of Chemical Physics* 129, no. 174106 (2008). https://doi.org/10.1063/1.3002335.

Mo Wei-chuan, Zi-jian Zhang, Ying Liu, Perry F. Bartlett, and Rong-qiao He. "Magnetic Shielding Accelerates the Proliferation of Human Neuroblastoma Cell by Promoting G1-Phase Progression." *PLOS One* 8 (1) (2013): e54775. https://doi.org/10.1371/journal.pone.0054775.

Neuhaus Eva M., Weiyi Zhang, Lian Gelis, Ying Deng, Joachim Noldus, and Hanns Hatt. "Activation of an Olfactory Receptor Inhibits Proliferation of Prostate Cancer Cells." *Journal of Biological Chemistry* 284, no. 24 (2009): 16218–16225. https://doi.org/10.1074/jbc.M109.012096.

Nishattasnim Liza, and Enrique P. Blair. "An Explicit Electron-Vibron Model for Olfactory Inelastic Electron Transfer Spectroscopy." *Journal of Applied Physics* 125, no. 144701 (2019). https://doi.org/10.1063/1.5086053.

NobelPrize.org. "The Nobel Prize in Physics 1921." *NobelPrize.org* (2019). www.nobelprize.org/prizes/physics/1921/summary/.

Page, Christopher C., Christopher C. Moser, Xiaoxi Chen, and P. Leslie Dutton. "Natural Engineering Principles of Electron Tunnelling in Biological Oxidation–Reduction." *Nature* 402 (1999): 47–52. https://doi.org/10.1038/46972.

Pandey Nidhi, Debasattam Pal, Dipankar Saha, and Swaroop Ganguly. "Vibration-Based Biomimetic Odor Classification." *Scientific Reports* 11, no. 11389 (2021): 11389. https://doi.org/10.1038/s41598-021-90592-x.

Pluznick, Jennifer L., Dong-Jing Zou, Xiaohong Zhang, Qingshang Yan, Diego J. Rodriguez-Gil, Christopher Eisner, et. al. "Functional Expression of the Olfactory Signaling System in the Kidney." *Proceedings of the National Academy of Sciences of the United States of America* 106, no. 6 (2009): 2059–2064. https://doi.org/10.1073/pnas.0812859106.

Rodríguez-Santana, Elizabeth, and Luis Santana-Blank. "Emerging Evidence on the Crystalline Water-Light Interface in Ophthalmology and Therapeutic Implications in Photobiomodulation: First Communication." *Photomedicine and Laser Surgery* 32 (2014). https://doi.org/10.1089/pho.2013.3682.

Schrodinger, Erwin. *What Is Life: The Physical Aspect of a Living Cell*. Cambridge University Press, 1944.

Solov'yov Ilia A., Po-Yao Chang, and Schulten K. "Vibrationally Assisted Electron Transfer Mechanism of Olfaction: Myth or Reality?" *Physical Chemistry Chemical Physics* 14 (40) (2012): 13861–13871. https://doi.org/10.1039/C2CP41436H.

Solov'yov, Ilia A., Peter J. Hore, Thorsten Ritz, and Klaus Schulten, Klaus. "10. A Chemical Compass for Bird Navigation In *Quantum Effects in Biology*." Masoud Mohseni, Yasser Omar, Gregory S. Engel, and Martin B. Plenio (eds.) Cambridge University Press. (2013): 218–236. ISBN 978-1107010802.

Spehr, Marc, Gunter Gisselmann, Alexandra Poplawski, Jeffrey A. Riffell, Christian H. Wetzel, Richard K. Zimmer, et al. "Identification of a Testicular Odorant Receptor Mediating Human Sperm Chemotaxis." *Science* 299, no. 5615 (2003): 2054–2058. https://doi.org/10.1126/science.1080376.

Stovbun, Sergey V., Dmitry V. Zlenko, Alexander A. Bukhvostov, Alexander S. Vedenkin, Alexeyy A. Skoblin, Dmitry A. Kuznetsove, et al. "Magnetic Field and Nuclear Spin Influence on the DNA Synthesis Rate." *Scientific Reports* 13, no. 465 (2023). https://doi.org/10.1038/s41598-022-26744-4.

Usselman, Robert J., Cristina Chavarriage, Pablo R. Castello, Maria Procopio, Thorsten Ritz, Edward Dratz, et al. "The Quantum Biology of Reactive Oxygen Species Partitioning Impacts Cellular Bioenergetics." *Scientific Reports* 6, no. 38543 (2016). https://doi.org/10.1038/srep38543.

van Grondelle, Rienk, and Vladimir I. Novoderezhkin. "Quantum Effects in Photosynthesis." *Procedia Chemistry* 3 (2011): 198–210. https://doi.org/10.1016/j.proche.2011.08.027.

van Huizen, Alanna V., Jacob M. Morton, Luke J. Kinsey, Donald G. Von Kannon, Marwa A. Saad, Taylor R. Birkholz, et al. "Weak Magnetic Fields Alter Stem Cell–Mediated Growth." *Science Advances* 5, no. 1 (2019). https://doi.org/10.1126/sciadv.aau7201.

Xin, Hongbao, Wen Jing Sim, Bumseok Namgung, Yeonho Choi, Baojun Li, and Luke P. Lee. "Quantum Biological Tunnel Junction for Electron Transfer Imaging in Live Cells." *Nature Communications* 10, 3245 (2019). https://doi.org/ 10.1126/sciadv.aau7201.

Young, Thomas. "The Bakerian Lecture: On the Theory of Light and Colours." *Philosophical Transactions of the Royal Society* 92 (1802): 12–48. https://doi.org/10.1098/rstl.1802.0004.

Zadeh-Haghighi, Hadi, and Christoph Simon. "Magnetic Field Effects in Biology from the Perspective of the Radical Pair Mechanism." *Journal of the Royal Society Interface* 19 (2022). https://doi.org/10.1098/rsif.2022.0325.

Zadeh-Haghighi, Hadi, and Christoph Simon. "Magnetic Isotope Effects: A Potential Testing Ground for Quantum Biology." *Frontiers in Physiology* (2023). https://doi.org/10.3389/fphys.2023.1338479.

CHAPTER TWO

Alberola, Juan, and Francisco Coll. "Marine Therapy and its Healing Properties." *Current Aging Science* 6, no. 1 (2013): 63–75. https://doi.org/10.2174/18746098113060l0009.

Ańalemma. "Effects on Gut Microbiome 2022 Double-Blind Placebo-Blind Study." *Ańalemma* (2023). https://analemma-water.com/wp-content/uploads/2024/01/Analemma-Microbiome-Study-Report-2022.pdf.

Raffaella, Arani, Ivan Bono, Emilio Del Giudice, and Giuliano Preparata. "QED Coherence and the Thermodynamics of Water." *International Journal of Modern Physics B* 9 (1995): 1813–1842. https://doi.org/10.1142/S0217979295000744.

Armstrong, Lawrence E., and Evan C. Johnson. "Water Intake, Water Balance, and the Elusive Daily Water Requirement." *Nutrients* 10, no. 12 (2018): 1928. https://doi.org/10.3390/nu10121928.

Barancik, Miroslav, Branislav Kura, Tyler W. LeBaron, Roberto Bolli, Jozef Buday, and Jan Slezak. "Molecular and Cellular Mechanisms Associated with Effects of Molecular Hydrogen in Cardiovascular and Central Nervous Systems." *Antioxidants* 9, no. 12 (2020): 1281. https://doi.org/10.3390/antiox9121281.

Batmanghelidj, F. "Pain: A Need for Paradigm Change." *Anticancer Research* 7, no. 5B (1987): 971–989. PMID: 2829704.

Bellissent-Funel, Marie-Claire, Ali Hassanali, Martine Havenith, Richard Henchman, Peter Pohl, Fabio Sterpone, et al. "Water Determines the Structure and Dynamics of Proteins." *Chemical Reviews*, 116, no. 13 (2016): 7673–7697. https://doi.org/10.1021/acs.chemrev.5b00664.

Bono, Ivan, Emilio Del Giudice, Luca Gamberale, and Marc Henry. "Emergence of the Coherent Structure of Liquid Water." *Water* 4, no. 3 (2012): 510–532. https://doi.org/10.3390/w4030510.

Cusack, Carole. "Scotland's Sacred Waters: Holy Wells and Healing Springs." *Sydney Society for Scottish History Journal* 16 (2016): 67–83.

Davenas, E., F. Beauvais, J. Amara, M. Oberbaum, B. Robinzon, A. Miadonna, et al. "Human Basophil Degranulation Triggered by Very Dilute Antiserum Against IgE." *Nature* 333, no. 6176 (1988): 816–818. https://doi.org/10.1038/333816a0.

Davidson, Robert M., Ann Lauritzen, and Stephanie Seneff. "Biological Water Dynamics and Entropy: A Biophysical Origin of Cancer and Other Diseases." *Entropy* 15, no. 9 (2013): 3822–3876. https://doi.org/10.3390/e15093822.

De Ninno, A., A. C. Castellano, and E. Del Giudice. "The Supramolecular Structure of Liquid Water and Quantum Coherent Processes in Biology." *Journal of Physics: Conference Series* 442, no. 012031 (2013). https://doi.org/10.1088/1742-6596/442/1/012031.

De Ninno, Antonella. "Dynamics of Formation of the Exclusion Zone Near Hydrophilic Surfaces." *Chemical Physics Letters* 667 (2017): 322–326. https://doi.org/10.1016/j.cplett.2016.11.015.

Ebrahim, Shaban, and Azab Azab. "Biological Effects of Magnetic Water on Human and Animals." *Biomedical Sciences* 3 (2017): 78–85. https://doi.org/10.11648/j.bs.20170304.12.

Emoto, Masura. *The Hidden Messages in Water.* Beyond Words Pub, 2004. ISBN 97815827011412.

Geesink, Hans J. H., and Dirk K. F. Meijer. "Quantum Wave Information of Life Revealed: An Algorithm for Electromagnetic Frequencies that Create Stability of Biological Order, With Implications for Brain Function and Consciousness." *NeuroQuantology* 14, no. 1 (2016): 106–125. http://dx.doi.org/10.14704/nq.2016.14.1.911.

Geesink, Hans J. H., and Dirk K. F. Meijer. "Bio-Soliton Model that Predicts Non-Thermal Electromagnetic Frequency Bands, That Either Stabilize or Destabilize Living Cells." *Electromagnetic Biology and Medicine* 36 (2017): 357–378. https://doi.org/10.1080/15368378.2017.1389752.

Geesink, Hans J. H., and Dirk K. F. Meijer. "Electromagnetic Frequency Patterns That Are Crucial for Health and Disease Reveal a Generalized Biophysical Principle: The GM Scale." *Quantum Biosystems* 8 (2017): 1–16. ISSN 1970-223X.

GlycanAge. *GlycanAge Study*. Analemma: The Architect of Life. https://analemma-water.com/wp-content/uploads/2024/01/glycanage-study.pdf.

Ho, Mae-Wan. "Illuminating Water and Life: Emilio Del Giudice." *Electromagnetic Biology and Medicine* 34, no. 2 (2015): 113–22. https://doi.org/10.3109/15368378.2015.1036079.

Hwang, Seong Gu, Ho-Sung Lee, Byung-Cheon Lee, and GunWoong Bahng. "Effect of Antioxidant Water on the Bioactivities of Cells." *International Journal of Cell Biology* 2017, no. 1917239 (2017). https://doi.org/10.1155/2017/1917239.

Kang, Ki-Mun, Young-Nam Jang, Ihil-Bong Choi, Yeunhwa Gu, Tomohiro Kawamura, Yoshiya Toyoda, et al. "Effects of Drinking Hydrogen-Rich Water on the Quality of Life of Patients Treated with Radiotherapy for Liver Tumors." *Medical Gas Research* 1, no. 1 (2011): 11. https://doi.org/10.1186/2045-9912-1-11.

Karnib, Mona, Ahmad Kabbani, Hanafy Holail, and Zakia Olama. "Heavy Metals Removal Using Activated Carbon, Silica and Silica Activated Carbon Composite." *Energy Procedia* 50 (2014): 113–120. https://doi.org/10.1016/j.egypro.2014.06.014.

Kerch, Garry. "Role of Changes in State of Bound Water and Tissue Stiffness in Development of Age-Related Diseases." *Polymers* 12, no. 6 (2020): 1362. https://doi.org/10.3390/polym12061362.

Korotkov, K. G., O. A. Churganov, E. A. Gavrilova, M. A. Belodedova, and A. K. Korotkova. "Influence of Drinking Structured Water to Human Psychophysiology." *Journal of Applied Biotechnology & Bioengineering* 6 (2019): 171–177. https://doi.org/10.15406/jabb.2019.06.00190.

LeBaron, Tyler W., Randy Sharpe, and Kinji Ohno. "Electrolyzed-Reduced Water: Review I. Molecular Hydrogen Is the Exclusive Agent Responsible for the Therapeutic Effects." *International Journal of Molecular Sciences* 23, no. 23 (2022): 14750. https://doi.org/10.3390/ijms232314750.

Li, Tian-Ren, Fabian Huck, GiovanniMaria Piccini, and Konrad Tiefenbacher. "Mimicry of the Proton Wire Mechanism of Enzymes Inside a Supramolecular Capsule Enables -Selective O-Glycosylations." *Nature Chemistry* 14 (2022): 985–994. https://doi.org/10.1038/s41557-022-00981-6.

Li, Zheng, and Gerald H. Pollack. "On the Driver of Blood Circulation Beyond the Heart." *PLOS One* 18, no. 10 (2023): e0289652. https://doi.org/10.1371/journal.pone.0289652.

Lindinger, Michae l. "Structured Water: Effects on Animals." *Journal of Animal Science* 99, no. 5 (2021). https://doi.org/10.1093/jas/skab063.

Ling, Gilbert. "Nano-Protoplasm: The Ultimate Unit of Life" *Physiological Chemistry and Physics and Medical NMR* 39, no. 2 (2007): 111–234.

Ling, Gilbert N., and Margaret M. Ochsenfeld. "A Historically Significant Study That at Once Disproves the Membrane (Pump) Theory and Confirms That Nano-Protoplasm Is the Ultimate Physical Basis of Life-Yet so Simple and Low-Cost That It Could Easily be Repeated in Many High School Biology Classrooms Worldwide." *Physiological Chemistry and Physics and Medical NMR* 40 (2008): 89–113.

Ling, Gilbert. "An Ultra Simple Model of Protoplasm to Test the Theory of Its Long-Range Coherence and Control So Far Tested (and Affirmed) Mostly on Intact Cell(s)." *Physiological Chemistry and Physics and Medical NMR* 38, no. 2 (2206): 105–145.

Ling, Gilbert N. "A Physical Theory of the Living State: Application to Water and Solute Distribution." *Scanning Microscopy* 2, no. 2 (1988): 899–913.

Lorenzo, Isabel, Mateu Serra-Prat, and Juan Carlos Yébenes. "The Role of Water Homeostasis in Muscle Function and Frailty: A Review." *Nutrients* 11, no. 8 (2019): 1857. https://doi.org/10.3390/nu11081857

Maestro L. M., M. I. Marqués, E. Camarillo, D. Jaque, J. García Solé, J. A. Gonzalo, et al. "On the Existence of Two States in Liquid Water: Impact on Biological and Nanoscopic Systems." *International Journal of Nanotechnology* 13 (2016): 8-9, 667–677. https://doi.org/10.1504/IJNT.2016.079670.

Manil, Christian, and Laurent Lichtenstein; Daniel Leconte, prod. *Water Memory: 2014 Documentary about Nobel Prize Laureate Luc Montagnier*, (2014). https://www.youtube.com/watch?v=R8VyUsVOico.

Mitchell, H. H., T. S. Hamilton, F. R. Steggerda, and H. W. Bean. "The Chemical Composition of the Adult Human Body and Its Bearing on the Biochemistry of Growth." *Journal of Biological Chemistry* 158, no. 3 (1945): 625–637. https://doi.org/10.1016/S0021-9258(19)51339-4.

Mojica, Karina Torres, Jorge R. Miranda-Massari, Jose R. Rodriguez, Jose Olalde, Miguel Berdiel, and Michael J. Gonzalez. "Structured Water and Cancer: Orthomolecular Hydration Therapy." *Journal of Cancer Research Updates* 12 (2023): 5–9. https://doi.org/10.30683/1929-2279.2023.12.2.

Montagnier, L., J. Aissa, E. Del Giudice, C. Lavallee, A. Tedeschi, and G. Vitiello. "DNA Waves and Water." *In Journal of Physics: Conference Series* 306, no. 012007 (2011).https://doi.org/10.1088/1742-6596/306/1/012007.

Perakis, Fivos, Katrin Amann-Winkel, Felix Lehmkühler, Michael Sprung, Daniel Mariedahl, Jonas A. Sellberg, et al. "Diffusive Dynamics During the High-to-Low Density Transition in Amorphous Ice." *Proceedings of the National Academy of Sciences of the United States of America* 14, no. 31 (2017): 8193–8198. https://doi.org/10.1073/pnas.1705303114.

Pollack, G. H. "Cancer: An Unexpectedly Critical Role of Cell Water?" *Advances in Preventive Medicine and Health Care* 7 (2024): 1060. https://doi.org/10.29011/2688-996X.001060.

Pollack, Gerald. *The Fourth Phase of Water.* Ebner & Sons, 2013.

Pomès, R., and B. Roux. "Structure and Dynamics of a Proton Wire: A Theoretical Study of H+ Translocation Along the Single-File Water Chain in the Gramicidin A Channel." *Biophysical Journal* 71, no. 1 (1996): 19–39. https://doi.org/10.1016/S0006-3495(96)79211-1.

Popielska-Grzybowska, Joanna. "Contexts of Appearance of Water in the Pyramid Texts an Introduction." *Études et Travaux* 29 (2016): 157–167. https://www.researchgate.net/publication/328543262_Contexts_of_Appearance_of_Water_in_the_Pyramid_Texts_An_Introduction.

Quinton, Rene. "L'eau de Mer Milieu Organique: Constance du Milieu Marin Originel, Comme Milieu Vital des Cellules." *Hachette Bibliothèque Nationale de France* (in French), 1904.

Rabia, A. R., Abdul Haqi Ibrahim, and Nik Noriman Zulkepli. "Activated Alumina Preparation and Characterization: The Review on Recent Advancement." *E3S Web of Conferences* 34, no. 02049 (2018). https://doi.org/10.1051/e3sconf/20183402049.

Ramsey, Craig L. "Case Study: Long-Term Monitoring of Health Biomarkers after Drinking Structured Water Over 43 Months." *Journal of Basic & Applied Sciences* 20 (2024): 151–181. https://doi.org/10.29169/1927-5129.2024.20.16.

Ramsey, Craig. L. "Biologically Structured Water—A Review (Part 2): Redox Biology, Plant Resilience, SW Drinking Water Types, BSW Water and Aging, BSW Water and Immunity." *Journal of Basic & Applied Sciences* 19 (2023): 207–229. https://doi.org/10.29169/1927-5129.2023.19.17.

Ramsey, C. L. "Biologically Structured Water (BSW)—A Review (Part 3): Structured Water (SW) Generation, BSW Water, Bioenergetics, Consciousness and Coherence." *Journal of Basic & Applied Sciences* 19 (2023): 230–248. https://doi.org/10.29169/1927–5129.2023.19.18.

Ramsey, Craig. "Biologically Structured Water (BSW)—A Review (Part 1): Structured Water (SW) Properties, BSW and Redox Biology, BSW and Bioenergetics." *Journal of Basic & Applied Sciences* 19 (2023): 174–201. https://doi.org/10.29169/1927-5129.2023.19.15.

Raptim Research Pvt. Ltd. "The Effects of Analemma Water on Human ATP Levels: Research Report." (2022). https://analemma-water.com/wp-content/uploads/2024/01/ATP-STUDY-2022.pdf.

Rohani, Mina, and Pollack, Gerald. "Flow through Horizontal Tubes Submerged in Water in the Absence of a Pressure Gradient: Mechanistic Considerations." *Langmuir: The ACS Journal of Surfaces and Colloids* 29, no. 22 (2013). https://doi.org/10.1021/la4001945.

Shen, Yuchen, Alexis Theodorou, Zheng Li, and Gerald H. Pollack. "Ultraviolet (UV) Light Effect on the Electrical Potential of Interfacial Water." *Colloids and Surfaces A: Physicochemical and Engineering Aspects* 691, no. 133816 (2024). https://doi.org/10.1016/j.colsurfa.2024.133816.

Ebrahim, Shaban Ali, and Azab Elsayed Azab. "Biological Effects of Magnetic Water on Human and Animals." *Biomedical Sciences* 3, no. 4 (2017): 78–85. https://doi.org/10.11648/j.bs.20170304.12.

Singh, Rana P. B. "Sacrality and Waterfront Sacred Places in India." In *Sacred Waters: A Cross-cultural Compendium of Hallowed Springs and Holy Wells*, Celeste Ray (ed.), 80–94. Routledge, 2020. https://doi.org/10.1007/978-100-30-1014-2_6.

Szent-Györgyi, A. *Introduction to a Submolecular Biology*. Academic Press, 1960.

Szent-Györgyi, A. "Introductory Comments." In *Light and Life,* W.D. McElroy and B. Glass (eds.), 7–10. John Hopkins Press, Baltimore, 1961.

Tankersley, Kenneth Barnett, Nicholas P. Dunning, Christopher Carr, David L. Lentz, and Vernon L. Scarborough. "Zeolite Water Purification at Tikal, An Ancient Maya City in Guatemala." *Scientific Reports* 10, no. 18021 (2020). https://doi.org/10.1038/s41598-020-75023-7.

Vidal-Lorenzo, Cristina, and Patricia Horcajada-Campos. "Water Rituals and Offerings to the Mayan Rain Divinities." *European Journal of Science and Theology* 16, no. 2 (2020): 111–123.

Wu, Jishan, Miao Cao, Draco Tong, Zach Finkelstein, and Eric M. V. Hoek. "A Critical Review of Point-of-Use Drinking Water Treatment in the United States." *Clean Water* 4, no. 40 (2021). https://doi.org/10.1038/s41545-021-00128-z.

Yang, Yi, Yong Sik Ok, Ki-Hyun Kim, Eilhann E. Kwon, and Y. F. Tsang. "Occurrences and Removal of Pharmaceuticals and Personal Care Products (PPCPs) in Drinking Water and Water/Sewage Treatment Plants: A Review." *Science of the Total Environment* 596 (2017): 303–320. https://doi.org/10.1016/j.scitotenv.2017.04.102.

Ye, Tao, and Gerald H. Pollack. "Which Waters Hydrate Best? A Study Using Brine-Shrimp Cysts (*Artemia franciscana*)." *bioRxiv* (2020). https://doi.org/10.1101/2020.09.23.310326.

Yıldız, Fatmanur, Tyler W. LeBaron, and Duried Alwazeer. "A Comprehensive Review of Molecular Hydrogen as a Novel Nutrition Therapy in Relieving Oxidative Stress and Diseases: Mechanisms and Perspectives." *Biochemistry and Biophysics Reports* 41, no. 101933 (2025). https://doi.org/10.1016/j.bbrep.2025.101933.

Yu, Arthur, Peter Carlson, and Gerald Pollack. "Unexpected Axial Flow Through Hydrophilic Tubes: Implications for Energetics of Water." *The European Physical Journal Special Topics* 223 (2013). https://doi.org/10.1140/epjst/e2013-01837-8.

Zheng, Jian-Ming, Wei-Chun Chin, Eugene Khijniak, Eugene Khijniak Jr., and Gerald H. Pollack. "Surfaces and Interfacial Water: Evidence That Hydrophilic Surfaces Have Long-Range Impact." *Advances in Colloid and Interface Science* 127 (2006): 19–2. https://doi.org/10.1016/j.cis.2006.07.002.

Zheng, Yijun, and Duming Zhu. "Molecular Hydrogen Therapy Ameliorates Organ Damage Induced by Sepsis." *Oxidative Medicine and Cellular Longevity* 2016, no. 5806057 (2016): https://doi.org/10.1155/2016/5806057.

Zuo, Guanghong, Jun Hu, and Haiping Fang. "Effect of the Ordered Water on Protein Folding: An Off-Lattice Gō-Like Model Study." *Physical Review E* 79, no. 031925 (2009). https://doi.org/10.1103/PhysRevE.79.031925.

CHAPTER THREE

Ahn, Andrew C., and Ørjan G. Martinsen. "Electrical Characterization of Acupuncture Points: Technical Issues and Challenges." *Journal of Alternative and Complementary Medicine* 13, no. 8 (2007): 817–24. https://doi.org/10.1089/acm.2007.7193.

Andrews, John, and Saeed Seif Mohammadi. "Towards a Proton Flow Battery: Investigation of a Reversible PEM Fuel Cell with Integrated Metal-Hydride Hydrogen Storage." *International Journal of Hydrogen Energy* 39, no. 4 (2014): 1740–1751. https://doi.org/10.1016/j.ijhydene.2013.11.010.

Barry, C. M., G. Kestell, M. Gillan, R. V. Haberberger, and I. L. Gibbins. "Sensory Nerve Fibers Containing Calcitonin Gene-Related Peptide in Gastrocnemius, Latissimus Dorsi and Erector Spinae Muscles and Thoracolumbar Fascia in Mice." *Neuroscience* 2015 Apr 16, no. 291 (2015): 106–17. https://doi.org/10.1016/j.neuroscience.2015.01.062.

Berlin, Yuri A., Alexander L. Burin, and Mark A. Ratner. "DNA as a Molecular Wire." *Superlattices and Microstructures* 28, no. 4 (2000): 241–252. https://doi.org/10.1006/spmi.2000.0915.

Berrueta, L., J. Bergholz, D. Munoz, I. Muskaj, G. J. Badger, A. Shukla, et al. "Stretching Reduces Tumor Growth in a Mouse Breast Cancer Model." *Scientific Reports* 8, no. 7864 (2018). https://doi.org/10.1038/s41598-018-26198-7.

Berrueta, Lisbeth, Igla Muskaj, Sara Olenich, Taylor Butler, Gary J. Badger, Romain A. Colas, et al. "Stretching Impacts Inflammation Resolution in Connective Tissue." *Journal of Cellular Physiology* 231, no. 7 (2015): 1621–1627. https://doi.org/10.1002/jcp.25263.

Bordoni, Bruno, Fabiola Marelli, Bruno Morabito, and Beatrice Sacconi. "Emission of Biophotons and Adjustable Sounds by the Fascial System: Review and Reflections for Manual Therapy." *Journal of Evidence-Based Integrative Medicine* 23 (2018). https://doi.org/10.1177/2515690X17750750.

Bordoni, Bruno, and Fabiola Marelli. "Emotions in Motion: Myofascial Interoception." *Complement Medicine Research* 24, no. 2 (2017): 110–113. https://doi.org/10.1159/000464149.

Chevalier, Gaétan, Stephen T. Sinatra, James L. Oschman, Karol Sokal, and Pawel Sokal. "Earthing: Health Implications of Reconnecting the Human Body to the Earth's Surface Electrons." *Journal of Environmental and Public Health* (2012). doi:10.1155/2012/291541.

Chevalier, Gaétan, Stephen T. Sinatra, James L. Oschman, and Richard M. Delany. "Earthing (Grounding) the Human Body Reduces Blood Viscosity-A Major Factor in Cardiovascular Disease." *Journal of Alternative and Complementary Medicine* 19, no. 2 (2013): 102–10. https://doi.org/10.1089/acm.2011.0820.

Comeaux, Zachary. "Dynamic Fascial Release and the Role of Mechanical/Vibrational Assist Devices in Manual Therapies." *Journal of Bodywork and Movement Therapies* 15, no. 1 (2011): 35–41. https://doi.org/10.1016/j.jbmt.2010.02.006.

Cooper, Geoffrey M., *The Cell: A Molecular Approach*, 2nd edition. Sinauer Associates, 2000. ISBN-10: 0-87893-106-6.

Cosic, Irena, and Drasko Cosic. "DNA-Protein Interactions at Distance Explained by the Resonant Recognition Model." *International Journal of Sciences* 13 (2024): 1–5. https://doi.org/10.18483/ijSci.2805.

Cosic, Irena, Hodder A. N., Aguilar M. I., and Hearn M. T. "Resonant Recognition Model and Protein Topography. Model Studies with Myoglobin, Hemoglobin and Lysozyme." *European Journal of Biochemistry* 198, no. 1 (1991): 113–9. https://doi.org/10.1111/j.1432-1033.1991.tb15993.x.

Cosic, Irena. "The Resonant Recognition Model of Bio-Molecular Interactions: Possibility of Electromagnetic Resonance." *Polish Journal of Medical Physics and Engineering* 7, no. 1 (2001): 73–87.

Cosic, Irena, Drasko Cosic, and Katarina Lazar. "Environmental Light and Its Relationship with Electromagnetic Resonances of Biomolecular Interactions, as Predicted by the Resonant Recognition Model." *International Journal of Environmental Research and Public Health* 13, no. 7 (2016): 647. https://doi.org/10.3390/ijerph13070647.

Cosic, Irena, and Drasko Cosic. "DNA-Protein Interactions at Distance Explained by the Resonant Recognition Model." *International Journal of Sciences* 13, no. 11 (2024): 1–5. https://doi.org/10.18483/ijSci.2805.

Cosic, Irena, and Elena Pirogova. "Bioactive Peptide Design Using the Resonant Recognition Model." *Nonlinear Biomedical Physics* 1, no. 7 (2007). https://doi.org/10.1186/1753-4631-1-7.

Cosic, Irena, Vasilis Paspaliaris, and Drasko Cosic. "Analysis of Protein–Receptor Interactions on an Example of Leptin–Leptin Receptor Interaction Using the Resonant Recognition Model." *Applied Sciences* 2019, 9, no. 23 (2019): 5169. https://doi.org/10.3390/app9235169.

Dedic, J., H. I. Okur, and S. Roke. "Hyaluronan Orders Water Molecules in its Nanoscale Extended Hydration Shells." *Science Advances* 7, no. 10 (2021). https://doi.org/10.1126/sciadv.abf2558.

Elango, Jeevithan, Chunyu Hou, Bin Bao, Shujun Wang, José Eduardo Maté Sánchez de Val, and Wu Wenhui. "The Molecular Interaction of Collagen with Cell Receptors for Biological Function." *Polymers* 14, no. 5 (2022): 876. https://doi.org/10.3390/polym14050876.

Fischer, Michael J., Gergo Horvath, Martin Krismer, Erich Gnaiger, Georg Goebel, and Dominik H. Pesta. "Evaluation of Mitochondrial Function in Chronic Myofascial Trigger Points - A Prospective Cohort Pilot Study Using High-Resolution Respirometry." *BMC Musculoskeletal Disorders* 19, no. 388 (2018). https://doi.org/10.1186/s12891-018-2307-0.

Ghannam, Jack Y., Jason Wang, and Arif Jan. *Biochemistry, Structure.* StatPearls, 2025. https://www.ncbi.nlm.nih.gov/books/NBK538241/.

González-Jiménez, Mario, Gopakumar Ramakrishnan, Thomas Harwood, Adrian J. Lapthorn, Sharon M. Kelly, Elizabeth M. Ellis, et al. "Observation of Coherent Delocalized Phonon-Like Modes in DNA Under Physiological Conditions." *Nature Communications* 7, no. 11799 (2016). https://doi.org/10.1038/ncomms11799.

Gozalo-Pascual, Rodrigo, Héctor González-Ordi, María Ángeles Atín-Arratibel, Javier Llames-Sánchez, and Ángela C. Álvarez-Melcón. "Efficacy of the Myofascial Approach as a Manual Therapy Technique in Patients with Clinical Anxiety: A Randomized Controlled Clinical Trial." *Complementary Therapies in Clinical Practice* 51, no. 101753 (2023). https://doi.org/10.1016/j.ctcp.2023.101753.

Guimberteau, Jean-Claude, and Colin Armstrong. *Architecture of Human Living Fascia.* Handspring Publishing Ltd., 2015.

Gutiérrez, R., S. Mandal, and G. Cuniberti. "Quantum Transport Through a DNA Wire in a Dissipative Environment." *Nano Letters* 5, no. 6 (2005): 1093–1097. https://doi.org/10.1021/nl050623g.

Khesbak, Hassan, Olesya Savchuk, Satoru Tsushima, and Karim Fahmy. "The Role of Water H-Bond Imbalances in B-DNA Substate Transitions and Peptide Recognition Revealed by Time-Resolved FTIR Spectroscopy." *Journal of the American Chemical Society* 133, no. 15 (2011): 5834. https://doi.org/10.1021/ja108863v.

Ho, Mae-Wan, Julian Haffegee, Richard Newton, Yu-ming Zhou, John S. Bolton, and Stephen Ross. "Organisms as Polyphasic Liquid Crystals." *Bioelectrochemistry and Bioenergetics* 41 (1996): 81–91. https://doi.org/10.1016/0302-4598(96)05075-1.

Ho, Mae-Wan. "Super-Conducting Liquid Crystalline Water Aligned with Collagen Fibres in the Fascia as Acupuncture Meridians of Traditional Chinese Medicine." *Forum on Immunopathological Diseases and Therapeutics* 3, no. 3–4 (2012): 221–236. https://doi.org/10.1615/ForumImmunDisTher.2013007869.

Hoyle, Nathaniel P., Estere Seinkmane, Marrit Putker, Kevin A. Feeny, Toke P. Krogager, Johanna E. Chesham, et al. "Circadian Actin Dynamics Drive Rhythmic Fibroblast Mobilization During Wound Healing." *Science Translational Medicine* 9, no. 415 (2017). https://doi.org/10.1126/scitranslmed.aal2774

Humphrey, Kristen M., Sumali Pandey, Jeffery Martin, Tamara Hagoel, Anne Grand Mison, and Joyce E. Ohm. "Establishing a Role for Environmental Toxicant Exposure Induced Epigenetic Remodeling in Malignant Transformation." *Seminars in Cancer Biology* 57 (2019): 86–94. https://doi.org/10.1016/j.semcancer.2018.11.002.

Hunt, Tam. "The Rainbow and the Worm: Establishing a New Physics of Life." *Communicative & Integrative Biology* 6, no. 2 (2013). https://doi.org/10.4161/cib.23149.

Ibbotson, James Norman, and Sushant Shekhar. "Electromagnetic Field-Induced Amplification of Proton Tunneling and Tautomeric Shifts in DNA: A Quantum Mechanism for Accelerated Genetic Mutations." *Cambridge Open Engage* (2024). https://doi.org/10.33774/coe-2024-8qvz7.

Kolay, Jayeeta, Sudipta Bera, and Rupa Mukhopadhyay. "Electron Transport in Muscle Protein Collagen." *Langmuir* 35, no. 36 (2019): 11950–11957. https://doi.oeg/10.1021/acs.langmuir.9b01685/.

Lowles, Katherine, Marie F. A. Cutiongco, Joshua J. Hughes, Shiyang Li, John Knox, Madeleine Coy, Wei-Hsiang Lin, et al. "Macrophages Promote Collagen Deposition Through Circadian Regulation of Fibroblasts." *bioRxiv* (2025). https://doi.org/10.1101/2025.02.25.640115.

Lynes, Matthew D., Farnaz Shamsi, Elahu Gosney Sustarsic, Luiz O. Leiria, Chih-Hao Wang, Shen-Chiang Su, et al. "Cold-Activated Lipid Dynamics in Adipose Tissue Highlights a Role for Cardiolipin in Thermogenic Metabolism." *Cell Reports* 24, no. 3 (2018): 781–790. https://doi.org/10.1016/j.celrep.2018.06.073.

Lyons, Carey E., Jean Pierre Pallais, Seth McGonigle, Rachel P. Mansk, Charles W. Collinge, Matthew J. Yousefzadeh, et al. "Chronic Social Stress Induces p16-Mediated Senescent Cell Accumulation in Mice." *Nature Aging* 5 (2025): 48–64. https://doi.org/10.1038/s43587-024-00743-8.

MacDonald, Donald Ian, Monessha Jayabalan, Jonathan T. Seaman, Rakshita Balaji, Alec R. Nickolls, and Alexander Chesler. "Pain Persists in Mice Lacking Both Substance P and CGRPα Signaling." *Elife* 13 (2025). https://doi.org/10.7554/eLife.93754.

Maki, Kevin C., Fulya Eren, Martha E. Cassens, Mary R. Dicklin, and Michael H. Davidson. "ω-6 Polyunsaturated Fatty Acids and Cardiometabolic Health: Current Evidence, Controversies, and Research Gaps, Advances in Nutrition." *Advances in Nutrition* 9, no. 6 (2018): 688–700. https://doi.org/0.1093/advances/nmy038.

Masic, Admir, Luca Bertinetti, Roman Schuetz, Shu-Wei Chang, Till Hartmut Metzger, Markus J. Buehler, et al. "Osmotic pressure induced tensile forces in tendon collagen." *Nature Communications* 6, no. 5942 (2015). https://doi.org/10.1038/ncomms6942.

Matsuno, Yusuke, Yuko Atsumi, Md. Alauddin, Md. Masud Rana, Harula Fujimori, Mai Hyodo, et al. "Resveratrol and Its Related Polyphenols Contribute to the Maintenance of Genome Stability." *Scientific Reports* 10, no. 5388 (2020). https://doi.org/10.1038/s41598-020-62292-5.

Mense, S., U. Hoheisel, and A. Reinert. "The Possible Role of Substance P in Eliciting and Modulating Deep Somatic Pain." *Progress in Brain Research* 110 (1996): 125–35. https://doi.org/10.1016/s0079-6123(08)62570-4. PMID: 9000721.

Michalak, Johannes, Lanre Aranmolate, Antonia Bonn, Karen Grandin, Robert Schleip, Jaqueline Schmiedtke, et al. "Myofascial Tissue and Depression." *Cognitive Therapy and Research* 46, no. 3 (2022): 560–572. https://doi.org/10.1007/s10608-021-10282-w.

Miroslav, Stefanov. "Primo Vascular System: Before the Past, Bizarre Present, and Peek After the Future." *Journal of Acupuncture and Meridian Studies* 15, no. 1 (2022): 61–73. https://doi.org/10.51507/j.jams.2022.15.1.61.

Ogłuszka, Magdalena, Paweł Lipiński, and Rafał R. Starzyński. "Effect of Omega-3 Fatty Acids on Telomeres—Are They the Elixir of Youth?" *Nutrients* 14, no. 18 (2022): 3723. https://doi.org/10.3390/nu14183723.

Ortega-Campos, Sara M., Eva M. Verdugo-Sivianes, Ana Amiama-Roig, Josa R. Blanco, and Amancio Carnero. "Interactions of Circadian Clock Genes with the Hallmarks of Cancer." *Biochimica et Biophysica Acta (BBA)—Reviews on Cancer* 1878, no. 3 (2023): 188900. https://doi.org/10.1016/j.bbcan.2023.188900.

Oschman, James L., Gaétan Chevalier, and Richard Brown. "The Effects of Grounding (Earthing) on Inflammation, the Immune Response, Wound Healing, and Prevention and Treatment of Chronic Inflammatory and Autoimmune Diseases." *Journal of Inflammation Research* 8 (2015): 83–96. https://doi.org/10.2147/JIR.S69656.

Rainer, Peter P. "The Pulse of Fibroblasts: Circadian Rhythm in Pulmonary Fibrosis Development." *Cardiovascular Research* 116, no. 11 (2020): e134–e135. https://doi.org/10.1093/cvr/cvaa236.

Riera Aroche, R., Y. M. Ortiz García, M. A. Martínez Arellano, and A. Riera Leal. "DNA as a Perfect Quantum Computer Based on the Quantum Physics Principles." *Scientific Reports* 14, no. 11636 (2024). https://doi.org/10.1038/s41598-024-62539-5.

Sancar, Aziz, Laura A., Lindsey-Boltz, Tae-hong Kang, Joyce T. Reardon, Jin Hyup Lee, and Nuri Ozturk. "Circadian Clock Control of the Cellular Response to DNA Damage." *FEBS Lettersers* 584, no. 12 (2010): 2618–2625. https://doi.org/10.1016/j.febslet.2010.03.017.

Schleip, Robert. "Fascial Plasticity–A New Neurobiological Explanation: Part 1." *Journal of Bodywork and Movement Therapies* 7, no. 1 (2003): 11–19. ISSN 1360-8592. https://doi.org/10.1016/S1360-8592(02)00067-0.

Schwartz, Martin Alexander. "Integrins and Extracellular Matrix in mechanotraMsduction." *Cold Spring Harbor Perspectives in Biology* 2, no. 12 (2010): a005066. https://doi.org10.1101/cshperspect.a005066.

Silva, Bruna Luísa, Lara Alves de Oliveira, Camila Medeiros Costa, Cristiano Queiroz Guimarães, Leonardo Sette Vieira, and Andrei Pereira Pernambuco. "A Pilot Study of the Effects of Suboccipital Fascial Release on Heart Rate Variability in Workers in the Clothing Industry: Randomized Clinical Trial." *Journal of Bodywork and Movement Therapies* 25 (2021): 223–229. https://doi.org10.1016/j.jbmt.2020.10.020.

Singh, Abhishek K., Chengyuan Wen, Shengfeng Cheng, and Nguyen Q. Vinh. "Long-Range DNA-Water Interactions." *Biophysical Journal* 120, no. 22 (2021): 4966–4979. https://doi.org/10.1016/j.bpj.2021.10.016.

Slater, Alison M., S. Jade Barclay, Rouha M. S. Granfar, and Rebecca L. Pratt. "Fascia as a Regulatory System in Health and Disease." *Frontiers in Neurology* 15 (2024). https://doi.org/10.3389/fneur.2024.1458385.

Slocombe, Louie, Marco Sacchi, and Jim Al-Khalili. "An Open Quantum Systems Approach to Proton Tunnelling in DNA." *Communications Physics* 5, no. 109 (2022). https://doi.org/10.1038/s42005-022-00881-8

Slocombe, Louie, Jim Al-Khalili, and Marco Sacchi. "Quantum and Classical Effects in DNA Point Mutations: Watson–Crick Tautomerism in AT and GC Base Pairs." *Physical Chemistry Chemical Physics* 23, no. 7 (2021). https://doi.org/10.1039/D0CP05781A.

Stecco, Carla, Caterina Fede, Veronica Macchi, Andrea Porzionato, Lucia Petrelli, Carlo Biz, et al. "The Fasciacytes: A New Cell Devoted to Fascial Gliding Regulation." *Clinical Anatomy* 31, no. 5 (2018): 667–676. https://doi.org/10.1002/ca.23072.

Sustarsic, Elahu G., Tao Ma, Matthew D. Lynes, Michael Larsen, Iuliia Karavaeva, Jesper F. Havelund, et al. "Cardiolipin Synthesis in Brown and Beige Fat Mitochondria Is Essential for Systemic Energy Homeostasis." *Cell Metaboolism* 28, no.1 (2018): 159–174. https://doi.org/10.1016/j.cmet.2018.05.003.

Svineng, Gunbjørg, Chandra Ravuri, Oddveig Rikardsen, Nils-Erik Huseby, and Jan-Olof Winberg. "The Role of Reactive Oxygen Species in Integrin and Matrix Metalloproteinase Expression and Function." *Connective Tissue Research* 49, no. 3 (2008): 197–202. https://doi.org/10.1080/03008200802143166.

Tozzi, Paolo. "Does Fascia Hold Memories?" *Journal of Bodywork and Movement Therapies* 18, no. 2 (2014): 259–265. https://doi.org/10.1016/j.jbmt.2013.11.010.

van der Veen, Jelske N., John P. Kennelly, Sereana Wan, Jean E. Vance, Dennis E. Vance, and René L. Jacobs. "The Critical Role of Phosphatidylcholine and Phosphatidylethanolamine Metabolism in Health and Disease." *Biochimica et Biophysica Acta* 1859, no. 9 Part B, (2017): 1558–1572. https://doi.org/10.1016/j.bbamem.2017.04.006.

Van Parys, Anthea, Therese Karlsson, Katherine J. Vinknes, Thomas Olsen, Jannike Øyen, Jutta Dierkes, et al. "Food Sources Contributing to Intake of Choline and Individual Choline Forms in a Norwegian Cohort of Patients with Stable Angina Pectoris." *Frontiers in Nutrition* 8 (2021). https://doi.org/10.3389/fnut.2021.676026.

Vodyanoy, Vitaly, Oleg Pustovyy, Ludmila Globa, and Iryna Sorokulova. "Primo-Vascular System as Presented by Bong Han Kim." *Evidence-Based Complementary and Alternative Medicine* 2015, no. 361974 (2015). https://doi.org/10.1155/2015/361974.

Wang, Likun, Na Li, Mengyao Cao, Yun Zhu, Xiewei Xiong, Li Li, et al. "Predicting DNA Reactions with a Quantum Chemistry-Based Deep Learning Model." *Advanced Science* 11, no. 2409880 (2024). https://doi.org/10.1002/advs.202409880.

Wong, Zhi Yi, Elosie Nee, Mark Coles, and Christopher D. Buckley. "Why Does Understanding the Biology of Fibroblasts in Immunity Really Matter?" *PLOS Biology* 21, no. 2 (2023). https://doi.org/10.1371/journal.pbio.3001954.

Xu, Tiezhu, Zhenming Xu, Tengyu Yao, Miaoran Zhang, Duo Chen, Xiaogang Zhang, et al. "Discovery of Fast and Stable Proton Storage in Bulk Hexagonal Molybdenum Oxide." *Nature Communications* 14, no. 8360 (2023). https://doi.org/10.1038/s41467-023-43603-6.

Zheng, Li, and Gerald H. Pollack. "Surface-Induced Flow: A Natural Microscopic Engine Using Infrared Energy as Fuel." *Science Advances* 6, no. 19 (2020). https://doi.org/10.1126/sciadv.aba0941.

Zullo, Alberto, Johannes Fleckenstein, Robert Schleip, Kerstin Hoppe, Scott Wearing, and Werner Klingler. "Structural and Functional Changes in the Coupling of Fascial Tissue, Skeletal Muscle, and Nerves During Aging." *Frontiers in Physiology* 11 (2020). https://doi.org/10.3389/fphys.2020.00592.

CHAPTER FOUR

Aguilar-López, Bruno A., María Maximina Moreno-Altamirano, Hazel M. Dockrell, Michael R. Duchen, and Francisco Javier Sánchez-García. "Mitochondria: An Integrative Hub Coordinating Circadian Rhythms, Metabolism, the Microbiome, and Immunity." *Frontiers in Cell and Developmental Biology* 8, no. 51 (2020). https://doi.org/10.3389/fcell.2020.00051.

Ahlbom, Anders, Adele Green, Leeka Kheifets, David Savitz, Anthony Swerdlow, and ICNIRP (International Commission for Non-Ionizing Radiation Protection) Standing Committee on Epidemiology. "Epidemiology of Health Effects of Radiofrequency Exposure." *Environmental Health Perspectives* 112, no. 17 (2004): 1741–1754. https://doi.org10.1289/ehp.7306.

Balasubramanian, Swarnalatha, David A. Weston, Michael Levin, and Devon Charles Cardoso Davidian. "Electroceuticals: Emerging Applications Beyond the Nervous System and Excitable Tissues." *Trends in Pharmacological Sciences* 45 no. 5 (2024): 391–394. https://10.1016/j.tips.2024.03.001.

Banerjee, Tatsat, Debojyoti Biswas, Dhiman Sankar Pal, Yuchuan Miao, Pablo A. Iglesias, and Peter N. Devreotes. "Spatiotemporal Dynamics of Membrane Surface Charge Regulates Cell Polarity and Migration." *Nature Cell Biology* 24, no. 10 (2022): 1499–1515. https://doi.org/10.1038/s41556-022-00997-7.

Becker, R. O., and J. A. Spadaro. "Electrical Stimulation of Partial Limb Regeneration in Mammals." *Bulletin of the New York Academy of Medicine* 48, no. 4 (1972): 627–641. https://doi.org/10.1038/235109a0.

Bittner, Stefan, and Sven G. Meuth. "Targeting Ion Channels for the Treatment of Autoimmune Neuroinflammation." *Therapeutic Advances in Neurological Disorders* 6, no. 5 (2013): 322–336. https://doi.org/10.1177/1756285613487782.

Cadenas, Susana. "Mitochondrial Uncoupling, ROS Generation and Cardioprotection." *Biochimica et Biophysica Acta - Bioenergetics* 1859, no. 9 (2018): 940–950. https://doi.org/10.1016/j.bbabio.2018.05.019.

Alvarez-Lorenzo, Carmen, Mariana Zarur, Alejandro Seijo-Rabina, Barbara Blanco-Fernandez, Isabel Rodríguez-Moldes, and Angel Concheiro. "Physical Stimuli-Emitting Scaffolds: The Role of Piezoelectricity in Tissue Regeneration." *Materials Today Bio* 22, no. 100740 (2023). ISSN 2590-0064. https://doi.org/10.1016/j.mtbio.2023.100740.

Cervera, Javier, José A. Manzanares, Michael Levin, and Salvador Mafe. "Transplantation of Fragments from Different Planaria: A Bioelectrical Model for Head Regeneration." *Journal of Theoretical Biology* 558, no. 111356 (2022). https://doi.org/10.1016/j.jtbi.2022.111356.

Chernet, Brook, and Michael Levin. "Endogenous Voltage Potentials and the Microenvironment: Bioelectric Signals that Reveal, Induce and Normalize Cancer." *Journal of Clinical & Experimental Oncology* 1 (2013): S1–002. https://doi.org10.4172/2324-9110.S1-002.

Chen, Ruijing, and Jun Chen. "Mitochondrial Transfer—A Novel Promising Approach for the Treatment of Metabolic Diseases." *Frontiers in Endocrinology (Lausanne)* 14, no. 1346441 (2024). https://doi.org10.3389/fendo.2023.1346441.

Cheng, Danyu, Jiangang Long, Lin Zhao, and Kiankang Liu. "Hydrogen: A Rising Star in Gas Medicine as a Mitochondria-Targeting Nutrient via Activating Keap1-Nrf2 Antioxidant System." *Antioxidants* 12, no. 12 (2023): 2062. https://doi.org/10.3390/antiox12122062.

Chevalier, G., S. T. Sinatra, J. L. Oschman, K. Sokal, and P. Sokal. "Earthing: Health Implications of Reconnecting the Human Body to the Earth's Surface Electrons." *Journal of Environmental and Public Health* 12, no. 12 (2023): 291541. https://doi.org/10.1155/2012/291541.

Chevalier, Gaétan, Gregory Melvin, and Tiffany Barsotti. "One-Hour Contact with the Earth's Surface (Grounding) Improves Inflammation and Blood Flow a Randomized, Doubled-Blind, Pilot Study." *Health* 7, no. 8 (2015). https://doi.org/10.4236/health.2015.78119.

Chevalier, Gaétan. "Grounding the Human Body Improves Facial Blood Flow Regulation: Results of a Randomized, Placebo Controlled Pilot Study." *Journal of Cosmetic Dermatology* 2014, no. 5 (2014). https://doi.org/10.4236/jcdsa.2014.45039.

Chevalier, Gaétan. "Changes in Pulse Rate, Respiratory Rate, Blood Oxygenation, Perfusion Index, Skin Aging Conductance, and their Variability Induced During and After Grounding Human Subjects for 40 Minutes." *Journal of Alternative and Complementary Medicine* 16, no. 1 (2010): 81–87. https://doi.org/10.1089/acm.2009.0278.

Chevalier, Gaétan, Stephen T. Sinatra, James L. Oschman, and Richard M. Delany. "Earthing (Grounding) the Human Body Reduces Blood Viscosity-A Major Factor in Cardiovascular Disease." *Journal of Alternative and Complementary Medicine* 19, no. 2 (2013): 102–10. https://doi.org/10.1089/acm.2011.0820.

Chevalier, Gaétan. "The Effect of Grounding the Human Body on Mood." *Psychological Reports* 116, no. 2 (2015): 534–542. https://doi.org/10.2466/06.PR0.116k21w5.

Chevalier Gaétan, Kazuhito Mori, and James L. Oschman. "The Effect of Earthing (Grounding) on Human Physiology." *European Biology and Bioelectromagnetics* 2, no. 1 (2006): 600–621.

Chung, Nate, Jonghoon Park, and Kiwon Lim. "The Effects of Exercise and Cold Exposure on Mitochondrial Biogenesis in Skeletal Muscle and White Adipose Tissue." *Journal of Exercise Nutrition & Biochemistry* 21, no. 2 (2017): 39–47. https://doi.org/10.20463/jenb.2017.0020.

Clemente-Suárez Vicente, Javier, Alexandra Martín-Rodríguez, Rodrigo Yáñez-Sepúlveda, and José Francisco Tornero-Aguilera. "Mitochondrial Transfer as a Novel Therapeutic Approach in Disease Diagnosis and Treatment." *International Journal of Molecular Sciences* 24, no. 10 (2023): 8848. https://doi.org/10.3390/ijms24108848.

Demine, Stéphane, Patricia Renard, and Thierry Arnould. "Mitochondrial Uncoupling: A Key Controller of Biological Processes in Physiology and Diseases." *Cells* 28, no. 8 (2019): 795. https://doi.org/10.3390/cells8080795.

Eil, Robert L., Rahul Roychoudhuri, David Clever, Shashank Patel, Madhu Sukumar, Jenny H. Pan, et al. "Elevated Potassium Levels Suppress T Cell Activation Within Tumors." *Journal for ImmunoTherapy of Cancer* 3, no. 2 (2015): P403. https://doi.org/10.1186/2051-1426-3-S2-P403.

Elkin, Howard K., and Angela Winter. "Grounding Patients with Hypertension Improves Blood Pressure: A Case History Series Study." *Alternative Therapies in Health and Medicine* 24 no. 6 (2018): 46–50. PMID: 30982019.

Chevalier, Gaétan, and Stephen T. Sinatra. "Emotional Stress, Heart Rate Variability, Grounding, and Improved Autonomic Tone: Clinical Applications." *Integrative Medicine* 10, no. 3 (2011).

Gergely, Peter Jr., Brian Niland, Nick Gonchoroff, Rudolf Pullmann Jr., Paul E. Phillips, and Andreas Perl. "Persistent Mitochondrial Hyperpolarization, Increased Reactive Oxygen Intermediate Production, and Cytoplasmic Alkalinization Characterize Altered IL-10 Signaling in Patients with Systemic Lupus Erythematosus." *Journal of Immunology* 169, no. 2 (2002): 1092–101. https://doi.org/10.4049/jimmunol.169.2.1092.

Gertz, S. David, Sonya Malekzadeh, Allen L. Dollar, Amy H. Kragel, and William C. Roberts. "Composition of Atherosclerotic Plaques in the Four Major Epicardial Coronary Arteries in Patients Greater Than or Equal to 90 Years of Age." *American Journal of Cardiology* 67, no. 15 (1991): 1228–33. https://doi.org/10.1016/0002-9149(91)90932-b.

Ghaly, Maurice, and Dale Teplitz. "The Biologic Effects of Grounding the Human Body During Sleep as Measured by Cortisol Levels and Subjective Reporting of Sleep, Pain, and Stress." *Journal of Alternative and Complementary Medicine* 10, no. 5 (2004): 767–776. https://doi.org/10.1089/acm.2004.10.767.

Godley, Bernard F., Farrukh A. Shamsi, Fong-Qi Liang, Stuart G. Jarrett, Sallyanne Davies, and Mike Boulton. "Blue Light Induces Mitochondrial DNA Damage and Free Radical Production in Epithelial Cells." *Journal of Biological Chemistry* 280, no. 22 (2005): 21061–21066. https://doi.org/10.1074/jbc.M502194200.

Grba, Daniel N., and Judy Hirst. "Mitochondrial Complex I Structure Reveals Ordered Water Molecules for Catalysis and Proton Translocation." *Nature Structural & Molecular Biology* 27, no. 10 (2020): 892–900. https://doi.org/10.1038/s41594-020-0473-x.

Guan, Shuting, Li Zhao, and Ruiyun Peng. "Mitochondrial Respiratory Chain Supercomplexes: From Structure to Function." *International Journal of Molecular Sciences* 23, no. 22 (2022): 13880. https://doi.org/10.3390/ijms232213880.

Gvozdjáková, Anna, Jarmila Kucharská, Zuzana Sumbalova, and Zuzana Rausova. "Molecular Hydrogen: A New Treatment Strategy of Mitochondrial Disorders." In *Molecular Hydrogen in Health and Disease*, eds. Jan Slezak, and Branislav Kura. Springer, Nature, 2024, 55–68. https://doi.org/10.1007/978-3-031-47375-3_4.

Hoitzing, Hanne, Iain G. Johnston, and Nick S. Jones. "What Is the Function of Mitochondrial Networks? A Theoretical Assessment of Hypotheses and Proposal for Future Research." *Bioessays* 37, no. 6 (2015): 687–700. https://doi.org/10.1002/bies.201400188.

Holden, Constance. "Albert Szent-Györgyi, Electrons, and Cancer." *Science* 203, no. 4380 (1979): 522–24. https://doi.org/10.1126/science.366748.

Huang, N. W., X. H. Qiao, and L. J. Li. "[Research Progress in Mitochondrial Transfer Mediated by Tunneling Nanotube in the Field of Tumor]." *Zhonghua Kou Qiang Yi Xue Za Zhi.* 56, no. 10 (2021): 1045–1049. Chinese. https://doi.org/10.3760/cma.j.cn112144-20210320-00131. PMID: 34619902.

International Commission on Non-Ionizing Radiation Protection (ICNIRP). "Guidelines for Limiting Exposure to Time-Varying Electric and Magnetic Fields (1 Hz to 100 kHz)." *Health Physics* 99, no. 6 (2010): 818–836. https://doi.org10.1097/HP.0b013e3181f06c86.

Jamieson, Isaac A. "Grounding (Earthing) as Related to Electromagnetic Hygiene: An Integrative Review." *Biomedical Journal* 46, no. 1 (2023): 30–40. https://doi.org/10.1016/j.bj.2022.11.005.

Jerath, Ravinder, and Connor Beveridge. "Respiratory Rhythm, Autonomic Modulation, and the Spectrum of Emotions: The Future of Emotion Recognition and Modulation." *Frontiers in Psychology* 11 (2020): 1980. https://doi.org/10.3389/fpsyg.2020.01980.

Kıvrak, Elfide Gizem, Kıymet Kübra Yurt, Arife Ahsen Kaplan, Işınsu Alkan, and Gamze Altun. "Effects of Electromagnetic Fields Exposure on the Antioxidant Defense System." *Journal of Microscopy and Ultrastructure* 5, no. 4 (2017): 167–176. https://doi.org/10.1016/j.jmau.2017.07.003.

Kohler, Andreas, Antoni Barrientos, Flavia Fontanesi, and Martin Ott. "The Functional Significance of Mitochondrial Respiratory Chain Supercomplexes." *EMBO Reports* 24 (2023). https://doi.org/10.15252/embr.202357092.

Lee, ChiaHuang, Douglas C. Wallace, and Peter J. Burke. "Super-Resolution Imaging of Voltages in the Interior of Individual, Vital Mitochondria." *ACS Nano* 18, no. 2 (2024): 1345–1356. https://doi.org/10.1021/acsnano.3c02768.

Lee, Ji Won, and Gerald Pollack. "Impact of Wi-Fi Energy on EZ Water." *ScienceOpen Preprints* (2021). https://doi.org10.14293/S2199-1006.1.SOR-.PPIQ9G6.v1.

Lin, Yiqi, Garett Cheung, Edith Porter, and Vassilios Papadopoulos. "The Neurosteroid Pregnenolone Is Synthesized by a Mitochondrial P450 Enzyme Other than CYP11A1 in Human Glial Cells." *Journal of Biological Chemistry* 298, no. 7 (2022): 102110. https://doi.org/10.1016/j.jbc.2022.102110.

Liu D, Y Gao, J Liu, Y Huang, J Yin, Y Feng, L Shi, BP Meloni, C Zheng, and J Gao. "Intercellular Mitochondrial Transfer as a Means of Tissue Revitalization." *Signal Transduction and Targeted Therapy* 6, no. 1 (2021): 65. https://doi.org10.1038/s41392-020-00440-z.

Manolios, Nicholas, John Papaemmanouil, and David J. Adams. "The Role of Ion Channels in T Cell Function and Disease." *Frontiers in Immunology* 14 (2023). doi=10.3389/fimmu.2023.1238171.

Marie, Mélanie, Karine Bigot, Claire Angebault, Coralie Barrau, Pauline Gondouin, Delphine Pagan, et al. "Light Action Spectrum on Oxidative Stress and Mitochondrial Damage in A2E-Loaded Retinal Pigment Epithelium Cells." *Cell Death & Disease.* 9, no. 3 (2018): 287. https://doi.org/10.1038/s41419-018-0331-5.

Marino, Andrew A., James M. Cullen, and R. O. Becker. "Fracture Healing in Rats Exposed to Extremely Low-Frequency Electric Fields." *Clinical Orthopaedics and Related Research* 149 (1979): 239–44. https://doi.org/10.1097/00003086-197911000-00039.

Martin, Daniel R., and Dmitry V. Matyushov. "Electron-Transfer Chain in Respiratory Complex I." *Scientific Reports* 7, no. 5495 (2017). https://doi.org/10.1038/s41598-017-05779-y.

Maassen, J. A., J. A. Romijn, and R. J. Heine. "Fatty Acid-Induced Mitochondrial Uncoupling in Adipocytes as a Key Protective Factor Against Insulin Resistance and Beta Cell Dysfunction: A New Concept in the Pathogenesis of Obesity-Associated Type 2 Diabetes Mellitus." *Diabetologia* 50, no. 10 (2007): 2036–2041. https://doi.org10.1007/s00125-007-0776-z.

Malhotra, Varun, Tanusha Pathak, Danish Javed, Francisco Jose Cidral-Filho, Chanchal Suryawanshi, and Mohit Agrawal. "Comparative Neurodynamic Analysis of Spinal Energy Enhancement in Experienced Yoga Practitioners Using Various Breathing Techniques." *Cureus* 16, no. 11 (2024): e73541. https://doi.org/10.7759/cureus.73541.

Melhuish Beaupre, Lindsay M., Gregory M. Brown, Vanessa F. Gonçalves, and James L. Kennedy. "Melatonin's Neuroprotective Role in Mitochondria and Its Potential as a Biomarker in Aging, Cognition and Psychiatric Disorders." *Translational Psychiatry* 11, no. 339 (2021). https://doi.org/10.1038/s41398-021-01464-x.

Menigoz, Wendy, Tracy T. Latz, Robin A. Ely, Cimone Kamei, Gregory Melvin, and Drew Sinatra. "Integrative and Lifestyle Medicine Strategies Should Include Earthing (Grounding): Review of Research Evidence and Clinical Observations." *Explore* 16, no. 3 (2020): 152–160. https://doi.org/10.1016/j.explore.2019.10.005.

Moser, Christopher C., Tammer A. Farid, Sarah E. Chobot, and P. Leslie Dutton. "Electron Tunneling Chains of Mitochondria." *Biochimica et Biophysica Acta (BBA) Bioenergetics* 1757, no. 9–10 (2006): 1096–1109. https://doi.org/10.1016/j.bbabio.2006.04.015.

Ober, Clinton A., Stephen T. Sinatra, and Martin Zucker. *Earthing: The Most Important Health Discovery Ever?* 2nd edition. Basic Health Publications, 2014.

Ober, C. "Grounding the Human Body to Neutralize Bioelectrical Stress from Static Electricity and EMFs." *ESD Journal* (2000).

Oschman, James L., Gaétan Chevalier, and Richard Brown. "The Effects of Grounding (Earthing) on Inflammation, the Immune Response, Wound Healing, and Prevention and Treatment of Chronic Inflammatory and Autoimmune Diseases." *Journal of Inflammation Research* 8 (2015): 83–96. https://doi.org/10.2147/JIR.S69656.

Park, Hyun-Jung, Woojin Jeong, Hyo Jeong Yu, Minsook Ye, Yunki Hong, Minji Kim, et al. "The Effect of Earthing Mat on Stress Induced Anxiety-like Behavior and Neuroendocrine Changes in the Rat." *Biomedicines* 11, no. 1 (2023): 57. https://doi.org/10.3390/biomedicines11010057.

Passi, Rohit, Kim K. Doheny, Yuri Gordin, Hans Hinssen, and Charles Palmer. "Electrical Grounding Improves Vagal Tone in Preterm Infants." *Neonatology* 112, no. 2 (2017): 187–192. https://doi.org/10.1159/000475744.

Picard, Martin, Bruce S. McEwen, Elissa S. Epel, and Carmen Sandi. "An Energetic View of Stress: Focus on Mitochondria." *Frontiers in Neuroendocrinology* 49, (2018): 72–85. https://doi.org/10.1016/j.yfrne.2018.01.001.

Picard Martin, Douglas C. Wallace, and Yan Burelle. "The Rise of Mitochondria in Medicine." *Mitochondrion* 30 (2016): 105–116, ISSN 1567-7249. https://doi.org/10.1016/j.mito.2016.07.003.

Picard, Martin. "Energy Transduction and the Mind–Mitochondria Connection." *Biochemest* 44, no. 4 (2022): 14–18. https://doi.org/10.1042/bio_2022_118.

Pio-Lopez, Léo, and Michael Levin. "Aging as a Loss of Morphostatic Information: A Developmental Bioelectricity Perspective." *Ageing Research Reviews* 97, no. 102310 (2024). https://doi.org/10.1016/j.arr.2024.102310.

Pizzorno, Joseph. "Mitochondria-Fundamental to Life and Health." *Journal of Integrative Medicine* 13, no. 2 (2014): 8–15. PMID: 26770084.

Pollack, Gerald H. "Is it Oxygen, or Electrons, That Our Respiratory System Delivers? *Medical Hypotheses* 192, no. 111467 (2024). https://doi.org/10.1016/j.mehy.2024.111467.

Powner, Michael B., and Glen Jeffery. "Light Stimulation of Mitochondria Reduces Blood Glucose Levels." *Journal of Biophotonics* 15, no. 5 (2024). https://doi.org/10.1002/jbio.202300521.

Rahnama, Majid, Jack A. Tuszynski, István Bókkon, Michael Cifra, Peyman Sardar, and Vahid Salari. "Emission of Mitochondrial Biophotons and Their Effect on Electrical Activity of Membrane via Microtubules." *Journal of Integrative Neuroscience* 10, no. 1 (2011): 65–88. https://doi.org/10.1142/S0219635211002622.

Rajput, Prabha, Dhanananajay Kumar, and Sairam Krishnamurthy. "Chronic Exposure to Dim Artificial Light Disrupts the Daily Rhythm in Mitochondrial Respiration in Mouse Suprachiasmatic Nucleus." *Chronobiology International* 40, no. 7 (2023): 938–951. https://doi.org/10.1080/07420528.2023.2236708.

Ramach, Ulrich, Rosmarie Schöfbeck, Jakob Andersson, and Markus Valtiner. "Self-Assembling Redox-Wires Form the 2D Power Grid of Energy Converting Cell Membranes." *Cornell University* (2021). https://doi.org/10.48550/arXiv.2104.07709.

Rascalou, Adeline, Jérôme Lamartine, Pauline Poydenot, Frédéric Demarne, and Nicolas Bechetoille. "Mitochondrial Damage and Cytoskeleton Reorganization in Human Dermal Fibroblasts Exposed to Artificial Visible Light Similar to Screen-Emitted Light." *J Dermatol Sci.* S0923–1811, no. 18 (2018): 30213–30215. https://doi.org/10.1016/j.jdermsci.2018.04.018.

Reiter, Russel J., Ramaswamy Sharma, Sergio Rosales-Corral, Walter Manucha, Luiz Gustavo de Almeida Chuffa, and Debora Aparecida Pires de Campos Zuccari. "Melatonin and Pathological Cell Interactions: Mitochondrial Glucose Processing in Cancer Cells." *International Journal of Molecular Sciences* 22, no. 22 (2021): 12494. https://doi.org/10.3390/ijms222212494.

Richtar, Jan, Patricie Heinrichova, Dogukan Hazar Apaydin, Veronika Schmiedova, Cigdem Yumusak, Aslexander Kovalenko, et al. "Novel Riboflavin-Inspired Conjugated Bio-Organic Semiconductors." *Molecules* 23, no. 9 (2018): 2271. https://doi.org/10.3390/molecules23092271.

Roland, Thar, and Michael Kühl. "Propagation of Electromagnetic Radiation in Mitochondria?" *Journal of Theoretical Biology* 230, no. 2 (2004): 261–270. https://doi.org/10.1016/j.jtbi.2004.05.021.

Rosenburg, Barnett. "Electrical Conductivity of Proteins." *Nature* 193, no. 364–365 (1962). https://doi.org/10.1038/193364a0

Sardon Puig, Laura, Miriam Valera-Alberni, Carles Cantó, and Nicolas J. Pillon. "Circadian Rhythms and Mitochondria: Connecting the Dots." *Front Genet.* 9 (2018): 452. https://doi.org/10.3389/fgene.2018.00452.

Schüz, J. "Exposure to Extremely Low-Frequency Magnetic Fields and the Risk of Childhood Cancer: Update`1e of the Epidemiological Evidence." *Progress in Biophysics and Molecular Biology* 107, no. 3 (2011): 339–342. https://doi.org/10.1016/j.pbiomolbio.2011.09.008.

Sepa-Kishi, Diane M., Shailee Jani, Daniel Da Eira, and Rolando B. Ceddia. "Cold Acclimation Enhances UCP1 Content, Lipolysis, and Triacylglycerol Resynthesis, but Not Mitochondrial Uncoupling and Fat Oxidation, in Rat White Adipocytes." *American Journal of Physiology-Cell Physiology* 2019 Mar 1;316, no. 3 (2019): C365–C376. https://doi.org/10.1152/ajpcell.00122.2018.

Seppälä, Emma M., Jack B. Nitschke, Dana L. Tudorascu, Andrea Hayes, Michael R. Goldstein, Dong T. H. Nguyen, et al. "Breathing-Based Meditation Decreases Posttraumatic Stress Disorder Symptoms in U.S. Military Veterans: A Randomized Controlled Longitudinal Study." *Journal of Traumatic Stress* 27, no. 4 (2014): 397–405. https://doi.org/10.1002/jts.21936.

Shinhmar, Harpreet, Manjot Grewal, Sobha Sivaprasad, Chris Hogg, Victor Chong, Magella Neveu, et al. "Optically Improved Mitochondrial Function Redeems Aged Human Visual Decline." *The Journals of Gerontology* 75, no. 9 (2020): e49–e52. https://doi.org/10.1093/gerona/glaa155.

Sinatra, Stephen T., Drew S. Sinatra, Stephen W. Sinatra, and Gaétan Chevalier. "Grounding—The Universal Anti-Inflammatory Remedy." *Biomedical Journal* 46, no. 1 (2023): 11–16. https://doi.org/10.1016/j.bj.2022.12.002

Stefano, Geroge B., Tobias Esch, and Richard M. Kream. "Augmentation of Whole-Body Metabolic Status by Mind-Body Training: Synchronous Integration of Tissue- and Organ-Specific Mitochondrial Function." *Medical Science Monitor Basic Research* 25 (2019): 8–14. https://doi.org/10.12659/MSMBR.913264.

Sullivan, Patrick G., Nancy A. Rippy, Kristina Dorenbos, Rachele C. Concepcion, Aakash K. Agarwal, and Jong M. Rho. "The Ketogenic Diet Increases Mitochondrial Uncoupling Protein Levels and Activity." *Annals of Neurology* 55 (2004): 576–580. https://doi.org/10.1002/ana.20062.

Sun, Guogui, Jiong Li, Wei Zhou, Rosalie G. Hoyle, and Yue Zhao. "Electromagnetic Interactions in Regulations of Cell Behaviors and Morphogenesis." *Frontiers in Cell and Developmental Biology* 10 (2022): 1014030. https://doi.org/10.3389/fcell.2022.1014030.

Tafur, Joseph, and Paul J. Mills. "Low-Intensity Light Therapy: Exploring the Role of Redox Mechanisms." *Photomedicine and Laser Surgery* 26, no. 4 (2008): 323–8. https://doi.org/10.1089/pho.2007.2184.

Li, Ting-Ting, Hong-Ying Wang, Hui Zhang, Ping-Ping Zhang, Ming-Chen Zhang, Hai-Yang Feng, et al. "Effect of Breathing Exercises on Oxidative Stress Biomarkers in Humans: A Systematic Review and Meta-Analysis." *Frontiers in Medicine* 10 (2023). https://doi.org/10.3389/fmed.2023.1121036.

Trainini, Jorge, Mario Beraudo, Mario Wernicke, Francesc Carreras Costa, Alejandro Trainini, Vicente Mora Llabata, et al. "Evidence That the Myocardium Is a Continuous Helical Muscle with One Insertion." *REC: CardioClinics* 57, no. 3 (2022): 194–202. https://doi.org/10.1016/j.rccl.2022.01.006.

Wallace, Douglas C. "A Mitochondrial Paradigm of Metabolic and Degenerative Diseases, Aging, and Cancer: A Dawn for Evolutionary Medicine." *Annual Review of Genetics* 39 (2005): 359–407. https://doi.org/10.1146/annurev.genet.39.110304.095751.

Wallace, Douglas C. "Mitochondria as Chi." *Genetics* 179, no. 2 (2008): 727–735. https://doi.org/10.1534/genetics.104.91769.

Waisberg, Ethan, Joshua Ong, Mouayad Masalkhi, and Andrew G. Lee. "Near Infrared/Red Light Therapy a Potential Countermeasure for Mitochondrial Dysfunction in Spaceflight Associated Neuro-Ocular Syndrome (SANS)." *Eye* 38 (2024): 2499–2501. https://doi.org/10.1038/s41433-024-03091-4.

Williams, E. R., and S. J. Heckman. "The Local Diurnal Variation of Cloud Electrification and the Global Diurnal Variation of Negative Charge on the Earth." *Journal of Geophysical Research* 98, no. 3 (1993): 5221–5234. https://doi.org/10.1029/92JD02642.

Wood Dos Santos, Tanila, Quélita Cristina Pereira, Lucimara Teixeira, Alessandra Gambero, Josep A. Villena, and Marcelo Lima Ribeiro. "Effects of Polyphenols on Thermogenesis and Mitochondrial Biogenesis." *International Journal of Molecular Sciences* 19, no. 9 (2018): 2757. https://doi.org/10.3390/ijms19092757.

Zhang, GuangJun, and Michael Levin. "Bioelectricity Is a Universal Multifacedsignaling Cue in Living Organisms." *Molecular Biology of the Cell* 36, no. 2 (2025). https://doi.org/10.1016/j.plrev.2025.01.008.

Zhang, L., J. R. Lu, and T. A. Waigh. "Electronics of Peptide- and Protein-Based Biomaterials." *Advances in Colloid and Interface Science* 287, no. 102319 (2021). https://doi.org/10.1016/j.cis.2020.102319.

Zhao, Linlin, Shuqing Wang, Qianli Zhu, Bin Wu, Zhijun Liu, Bo OuYang, et al. "Specific Interaction of the Human Mitochondrial Uncoupling Protein 1 with Free Long-Chain Fatty Acid." *Structure* 25, no. 9 (2017): 1371–1379. https://doi.org/10.1016/j.str.2017.07.005.

Zhang, Tiang, Qi Liu, Zhuo Li, Siqi Tang, Qimin An, Dongdong Fan, et al. "The Role of Ion Channels in Immune-Related Diseases." *Progress in Biophysics and Molecular Biology* 177 (2023): 129–140. https://doi.org10.1016/j.pbiomolbio.2022.11.003.

Zhang, Wenbo, Blanc Star, W. R. A. K. J. S. Rajapaksha, and Thomas E. Fisher. "Dehydration Increases L-Type Ca(2+) Current in Rat Supraoptic Neurons." *Journal of Physiology* 2580 (Pt 1) (2007): 181–93. https://doi.org/10.1113/jphysiol.2006.126680.

Zhang, Xiaoyue, Fei Xie, Shiwen Ma, Chen Ma, Xue Jiang, Yang Yi, et al. "Mitochondria: One of the Vital Hubs for Molecular Hydrogen's Biological Functions." *Frontiers in Cell and Developmental Biology* 11, no. 1283820 (2023). https://doi.org10.3389/fcell.2023.1283820.

Zhang, Yanjun, Ziliang Ye, Yuanyuan Zhang, Sisi Yang, Mengyi Liu, Qimeng Wu, et al. "Regular Mobile Phone Use and Incident Cardiovascular Diseases: Mediating Effects of Sleep Patterns, Psychological Distress, and Neuroticism." *Canadian Journal of Cardiology* 40, no. 11 (2024): 2156 – 2165. https://doi.org/10.1016/j.cjca.2024.06.006.

Zhao, Yipeng, Jie Huang, Xiaolu Yuan, Biwen Peng, Wanhong Liu, Song Han, et al. "Toxins Targeting the Kv1.3 Channel: Potential Immunomodulators for Autoimmune Diseases." *Toxins* 7, no. 5 (2015): 1749–64. https://doi.org/10.3390/toxins7051749.

CHAPTER FIVE

Aguida, Blance, Marie-Marthe Chabi, Soria Baouz, Rhys Mould, Jimmy D. Bell, Marootpong Pooam, et al. "Near-Infrared Light Exposure Triggers ROS to Downregulate Inflammatory Cytokines Induced by SARS-CoV-2 Spike Protein in Human Cell Culture." *Antioxidants* 12, no. 10 (2023): 1824.

Albrecht, Urs. "Timing to Perfection: The Biology of Central and Peripheral Circadian Clocks." *Neuron* 74, no. 2 (2012): 246–260. https://doi.org/10.1016/j.neuron.2012.04.006.

Allen, Mary J., and Sandeep Sharma. *Physiology, Adrenocorticotropic Hormone (ACTH).* StatPearls Publishing, 2024. https://www.ncbi.nlm.nih.gov/books/NBK500031/.

Azeemi, Samina T. Yousuf, and S. Mohsin Raza. "A Critical Analysis of Chromotherapy and Its Scientific Evolution." *Evidence-Based Complementary and Alternative Medicine* 2, no. 4 (2005): 481–488. https://doi.org10.1093/ecam/neh137.

Barolet, A. C, I. V. Litvinov, and D. Barolet. "Light-Induced Nitric Oxide Release in the Skin Beyond UVA and Blue Light: Red & Near-Infrared Wavelengths." *Nitric Oxide* 117 (2021): 16–25. https://doi.org/10.1016/j.niox.2021.09.003.

Bikle, Daniel D. "Vitamin D: An Ancient Hormone." *Experimental Dermatology* 20, no. 1 (2011): 7–13. https://doi.org/10.1111/j.1600-0625.2010.01202.x.

Brand, Martin D., and David G. Nicholls. "Assessing Mitochondrial Dysfunction in Cells." *The Biochemical Journal* 435, no. 2 (2011): 297–312. https://doi.org10.1042/BJ20110162.

Bulat, Vedrana, Mirna Situm, Iva Dediol, Ivana Ljubicić, and Lada Bradić. "The Mechanisms of Action of Phototherapy in the Treatment of the Most Common Dermatoses." *Collegium Antropologicum* 35, no. 2 (2011): 147–151. PMID: 22220423.

Cajochen, Christian, Mirjam Münch, Szymon Kobialka, Kurt Kräuchi, Rolan Steiner, Peter Oelhafen, et al. "High Sensitivity of Human Melatonin, Alertness, Thermoregulation, and Heart Rate to Short Wavelength Light." *Journal of Clinical Endocrinology & Metabolism* 90 (2005): 1311–1316. https://doi.org/10.1210/jc.2004-0957.

Callaway, Ewen, and Heidi Ledford. "Medicine Nobel Awarded for Work on Circadian Clocks." *Nature* 550, no. 18 (2017). https://doi.org/10.1038/nature.2017.22736.

Castrucci, Ana Maria de Lauro, Maurício S. Baptista, and Leonardo Vinicius Monteiro de Assis. "Opsins as Main Regulators of Skin Biology." *Journal of Photochemistry and Photobiology* 15, no. 100186 (2023). https://doi.org/10.1016/j.jpap.2023.100186.

Cheung, Ivy N., Phyllis C. Zee, Dov Shalman, Roneil G. Malkani, Joseph Kang, and Kathryn J. Reid. "Morning and Evening Blue-Enriched Light Exposure Alters Metabolic Function in Normal Weight Adults." *PLOS One* 11, no. 5 (2016): e0155601. https://doi.org/10.1371/journal.pone.0155601.

Coclivo, A. "Coloured Light Therapy: Overview of Its History, Theory, Recent Developments and Clinical Applications Combined With Acupuncture." *American Journal of Acupuncture* 27 (1999): 71–83. PMID: 10513100.

Daubner, S. Colette, Tiffany Le, and Shanzhi Wang. "Tyrosine Hydroxylase and Regulation of Dopamine Synthesis." *Archives of Biochemistry and Biophysics* 508, no. 1 (2011): 1–12. https://doi.org/10.1016/j.abb.2010.12.017.

Del Olmo-Aguado, Susana, Claudia Núñez-Álvarez, and Neville N. Osborne. "Blue Light Action on Mitochondria Leads to Cell Death by Necroptosis." *Neurochemical Research* 41, no. 9 (2016): 2324–2335. https://doi.org/10.1007/s11064-016-1946-5.

Dobson, Ruth, Ute C. Meier, Monic Marta, Sreeram Ramagopalan, and Gavin Giovannoni. "Vitamin D Deficiency—Do We Follow Our Own Advice?" *Clinical Medicine* 11, no. 6 (2011): 521–523. https://doi.org10.7861/clinmedicine.11-6-521.

Driller, Matthew William, Gregory Jacobson, and Liis Uiga. "Hunger Hormone and Sleep Responses to the Built-In Blue-Light Filter on an Electronic Device: A Pilot Study." *Sleep Science* 12, no. 3 (2019): 171–177. https://doi.org/10.5935/1984-0063.20190074.

Ebrahimzadeh, Mohammad Ali, Reza Enayatifard, Masoumeh Khalili, Mahdieh Ghaffarloo, Majid Saeedi, and Jamshid Yazdani Charati. "Correlation between Sun Protection Factor and Antioxidant Activity, Phenol and Flavonoid Contents of some Medicinal Plants." *Iranian Journal of Pharmaceutical Research* 13, no. 3 (2014): 1041–1047. PMID: 25276206.

Elrashid, Nesrein A. Abd, Doaa A. Sanad, Noha F. Mahmoud, Hamada A. Hamada, Alshaimaa M. Abdelmoety, and Ahmed M. Kenawy. "Effect of Orange Polarized Light on Post Burn Pediatric Scar: A Single Blind Randomized Clinical Trial." *Journal of Physical Therapy Science* 30, no. 10 (2018): 1227–1231. https://doi.org/10.1589/jpts.30.1227.

Foster, Russell G., Mark W. Hankins, and Stuart N. Peirson. "Light, Photoreceptors, and Circadian Clocks." *Methods in Molecular Biology* 362 (2007): 3–28. https://doi.org/10.1007/978-1-59745-257-1_1.

Ge, Li, Ming Yang, Na-Na Yang, Xin-Xin Yin, and Wen-Gang Song. "Molecular Hydrogen: A Preventive and Therapeutic Medical Gas for Various Diseases." *Oncotarget* 8, no. 60 (2017): 102653–102673. https://doi.org/10.18632/oncotarget.21130.

Ghazi, Sara. "Do the Polyphenolic Compounds from Natural Products Can Protect the Skin from Ultraviolet Rays?" *Results in Chemistry* 4, no. 100428 (2022). https://doi.org/10.1016/j.rechem.2022.100428.

Gold, Michael H., Anneke Andriessen, Julie Biron, and Hinke Andriessen. "Clinical Efficacy of Self-Applied Blue Light Therapy for Mild-to-Moderate Facial Acne." *Journal of Clinical and Aesthetic Dermatology* 2, no. 3 (2009): 44–50. PMID: 20729943.

Gómez-Vela, Paula, Margarita Pérez-Ruiz, María Fátima Hernández Martín, Javier Román, and Eneko Larumbe-Zabala. "Acute Effect of Orange Chromatic Environment on Perceived Health Status, Pain, and Vital Signs During Chemotherapy Treatment." *Support Care Cancer* 28, no. 5 (2020): 2321–2329. https://doi.org/10.1007/s00520-019-05064-w.

Gooley, Joshua J., Kyle Chamberlain, Kurt A. Smith, Sat Bir S. Khalsa, Shantha M. W. Rajaratnam, Eliza Van Reen, et al. "Exposure to Room Light Before Bedtime Suppresses Melatonin Onset and Shortens Melatonin Duration in Humans." *Journal of Clinical Endocrinology & Metabolism* 96, no. 3 (2011): E463–472. https://doi.org/10.1210/jc.2010-2098.

Gurwitsch, A. A. "A Historical Review of the Problem of Mitogenetic Radiation." *Experientia* 44, no. 7 (1998): 545–550. https://doi.org/10.1007/BF01953301.

Harno, Erika, Thanuja Gali Ramamoorthy, Anthony P. Coll, and Anne White. "POMC: The Physiological Power of Hormone Processing." *Physiological Reviews* 2018 Oct 1;98, no. 4 (2018): 2381–2430. https://doi.org/10.1152/physrev.00024.2017.

Herrera, Arturo Solís, María del Carmen Arias Esparza, Paola Eugenia Solís Arias, Marco Ávila-Rodriguez, George Emilio Barreto, et al. "Unsuspected Intrinsic Property of Melanin to Dissociate Water Can Be Used for the Treatment of CNS Diseases." *CNS & Neurological Disorders - Drug Targets* 15, no. 2 (2016): 135–140. https://doi.org/10.2174/1871527315666160202122943.

Holick, Michael F. "Biological Effects of Sunlight, Ultraviolet Radiation, Visible Light, Infrared Radiation and Vitamin D for Health." *Anticancer Research* 36, no. 3 (2016): 1345–1356. PMID: 26977036.

Hong, Ji Yeon, Hye Sung Han, Ji Hyun Youn, Hyun-Wook Kim, Hyun-Seung Ryu, and Kui Young Park. "Irradiation With 590-nm Yellow Light-Emitting Diode Light Attenuates Oxidative Stress and Modulates UVB-Induced Change of Dermal Fibroblasts." *Experimental Dermatology* 31, no. 6 (2022): 931–935. https://doi.org/10.1111/exd.14542.

Huang, Xiaodan, Qian Tao, and Chaoran Ren. "A Comprehensive Overview of the Neural Mechanisms of Light Therapy." *Neuroscience Bulletin* 40, no. 3 (2024): 350–362. https://doi.org/10.1007/s12264-023-01089-8.

Isaias, Ioannis U., Paula Trujillo, Paul Summers, Giorgio Marotta, Luca Mainardi, Gianni Pezzoli, et al. "Neuromelanin Imaging and Dopaminergic Loss in Parkinson's Disease." *Frontiers in Aging Neuroscience* 8, no. 196 (2016). https://doi.org/10.3389/fnagi.2016.00196.

Iuvone, Michael P., C. L. Galli, C. K. Garrison-Gund, and N. H. Neff. "Light Stimulates Tyrosine Hydroxylase Activity and Dopamine Synthesis in Retinal Amacrine Neurons." *Science* 202, no. 4370 (1978): 901–902. https://doi.org/10.1126/science.30997.

Jia, Chuanlong, Chengchen Gong, Yongzhou Lu, and Nan Xu. "Low-Energy Green Light Alleviates Senescence-Like Phenotypes in a Cell Model of Photoaging." *Journal of Cosmetic Dermatology* 22, no. 2 (2023): 505–511. https://doi.org/10.1111/jocd.15175.

Kemény, Lajos, and Andrea Koreck. "Ultraviolet Light Phototherapy for Allergic Rhinitis." *Journal of Photochemistry and Photobiology B: Biology* 87, no. 1 (2007): 58–65. https://doi.org/10.1016/j.jphotobiol.2007.01.001.

Kent, Jeremy B., Li Jin, and Zudong Joshua Li. "Quantifying Biofield Therapy Through Biophoton Emission in a Cellular Model." *Journal of Scientific Exploration* 34, no. 3 (2020): 434–454. https://doi.org/10.31275/20201691.

Kleszczyński, Konrad, Lena H. Hardkop, and Tobias W. Fischer. "Differential Effects of Melatonin as a Broad Range UV-Damage Preventive Dermato-Endocrine Regulator." *Dermato-Endocrinology* 3, no. 1 (2011): 27–31. https://doi.org/:10.4161/derm.3.1.14842.

Laakso, M. L., T. Hätönen, D. Stenberg, A. Alila, and S. Smith. "One-Hour Exposure to Moderate Illuminance (500 lux) Shifts the Human Melatonin Rhythm." *Journal of Pineal Research* 15, no. 1 (1993): 21–26. https://doi.org/10.1111/j.1600-079x.1993.tb00505.x.

Li, Yajia, Ziqin Cao, Jia Guo, Qiangxiang Li, Wu Zhu, Yehong Kuang, et al. "Assessment of Efficacy and Safety of UV-Based Therapy for Psoriasis: A Network Meta-Analysis of Randomized Controlled Trials." *Annals of Medicine* 54, no. 1 (2022): 159–169. https://doi.org/10.1080/07853890.2021.2022187.

Lister, Tom, Philip A. Wright, and Paul H. Chappell. "Optical Properties of Human Skin." *Journal of Biomedical Optics* 17, no. 9 (2012): 090901–1. https://doi.org/10.1117/1.JBO.17.9.090901.

Ma, Melina A., and Elizabeth H. Morrison. *Neuroanatomy, Nucleus Suprachiasmatic.* StatPearls Publishing, 2024.

Malthiery, Eve, Batoul Chouaib, Ana María Hernandez-Lopez, Marta Martin, Csilla Gergely, Jacques-Herni Torres, et al. "Effects of Green Light Photobiomodulation on Dental Pulp Stem Cells: Enhanced Proliferation and Improved Wound Healing by Cytoskeleton Reorganization and Cell Softening." *Lasers in Medical Science* 36, no. 2 (2021): 437–445. https://doi.org/10.1007/s10103-020-03092-1.

Marcos, José, José Marcos Teixeira de Alencar Filho, Pedrita Alves Sampaio, Emanuella Chiara, Emanuella Chiara Valença Pereira, Raimundo Gonçalves de Oliveira Junior, et al. "Flavonoids as Photoprotective Agents: A Systematic Review." *Journal of Medicinal Plant Research* 10, no. 47 (2017): 848–864. https://doi.org/10.5897/JMPR2016.6273.

Martin, Laurent F., Amol M. Patwardhan, Sejal V. Jain, Michella M. Salloum, Julia Freeman, Rajesh Khanna, et al. "Evaluation of Green Light Exposure on Headache Frequency and Quality of Life in Migraine Patients: A Preliminary One-Way Cross-Over Clinical Trial." *Cephalalgia* 41, no. 2 (2021): 135–147. https://doi.org/10.1177/0333102420956711.

Martin, Laurent, Frank Porreca, Elizabeth I. Mata, Michel Salloum, Vasudha Goel, Pooja Gunnala, et al. "Green Light Exposure Improves Pain and Quality of Life in Fibromyalgia Patients: A Preliminary One-Way Crossover Clinical Trial." *Pain Medicine* 22, no. 1 (2021): 118–130. https://doi.org/10.1093/pm/pnaa329.

Martin, Laurent F., Kevin Cheng, Stephanie M. Washington, Millie Denton, Vasudha Goel, Maithili Khandekar, et al. "Green Light Exposure Elicits Anti-inflammation, Endogenous Opioid Release and Dampens Synaptic Potentiation to Relieve Post-Surgical Pain." *Journal of Pain* 24, no. 3 (2023): 509–529. https://doi.org/10.1016/j.jpain.2022.10.011.

Mason, Ivy C., Daniela Grimaldi, Kathryn J. Reid, Chloe D. Warlick, Roneil G. Malkani, Sabra M. Abbott, et al. "Light Exposure During Sleep Impairs Cardiometabolic Function." *Proceedings of the National Academy of Sciences of the United States of America* 119, no. 12 (2022): e2113290119. https://doi.org/10.1073/pnas.2113290119.

Minich, Deanna M., Melanie Henning, Catherine Darley, Mona Fahoum, Cory B. Schuler, and James Frame. "Is Melatonin the "Next Vitamin D"?: A Review of Emerging Science, Clinical Uses, Safety, and Dietary Supplements." *Nutrients* 14, no. 19 (2022): 3934. https://doi.org/10.3390/nu14193934.

Mohawk, Jennifer A., Carla B. Green, and Joseph S. Takahashi. "Central and Peripheral Circadian Clocks in Mammal." *Annual Review of Neuroscience* 35 (2013): 445–462. https://doi.oeg/10.1146/annurev-neuro-060909-153128.

Monteiro de Assis, Leonardo Vinicius, Paulo Newton Tonolli, Maria Nathalia Moraes, Maurício S. Baptista, and Ana Maria de Lauro Castrucci. "How Does the Skin Sense Sun Light? An Integrative View of Light Sensing Molecules." *Journal of Photochemistry and Photobiology C: Photochemistry Reviews* 47, no. 100403 (2021). https://doi.org/10.1016/j.jphotochemrev.2021.100403.

Musters, Annelie H., Soudeh Mashayekhi, Jane Harvey, Emma Axon, Stephanie J. Lax, Carsten Flohr, et al. "Phototherapy for Atopic Eczema." *Cochrane Database of Systematic Reviews*; no. 10 (2021): CD013870. https://doi.org10.1002/14651858.CD013870.pub2.

Nguyen, Nhu T., and David E. Fisher. "MITF and UV Responses in Skin: From Pigmentation to Addiction." *Pigment Cell & Melanoma Research* 32, no. 2 (2019): 224–236. https://doi.org/10.1111/pcmr.12726.

Nguyen, Thuy Trang, Qui Thanh Hoai Ta, Thi Kim Oanh Nguyen, Thi Thuy Dung Nguyen, and Vo Van Giau. "Type 3 Diabetes and Its Role Implications in Alzheimer's Disease." *International Journal of Molecular Sciences* 21, no. 9 (2020): 3165. https://doi.org/10.3390/ijms21093165.

Niggli, Hugo J., Salvatore Tudisco, Giuseppe Privitera, Lee Ann Applegate, Agata Scordino, and Franco Musumeci. "Laser-Ultraviolet-A-Induced Ultraweak Photon Emission in Mammalian Cells." *Journal of Biomedical Optics* 10, no. 2 (2005): 024006. https://doi.org/10.1117/1.1899185.

Oren, D. A., G. C. Brainard, S. H. Johnston, J. R. Joseph-Vanderpool, E. Sorek, and N. E. Rosenthal. "Treatment of Seasonal Affective Disorder with Green Light and Red Light." *American Journal of Psychiatry* 148, no. 4 (1991): 509–511. https://doi.org10.1176/ajp.148.4.509.

Phan, Thieu X., Barbara Jaruga, Sandeep C. Pingle, Bidhan C. Bandyopadhyay, and Gerard P. Ahern. "Intrinsic Photosensitivity Enhances Motility of T Lymphocytes." *Scientific Reports* 6, no. 39479 (2016). https://doi.org/10.1038/srep39479.

Pilozzi, Alexander, Caitlin Carro, and Xudong Huang. "Roles of β-Endorphin in Stress, Behavior, Neuroinflammation, and Brain Energy Metabolism." *International Journal of Molecular Sciences* 22, no. 1 (2020): 338. https://doi.org/10.3390/ijms22010338.

Popp, F. A., W. Nagl, K. H. Li, W. Scholz, O. Weingärtner, and R. Wolf. "Biophoton Emission. New Evidence for Coherence and DNA as Source." *Biophysical Journal* 6, no. 1 (1984): 33–52. https://doi.org/10.1007/BF02788579.

Powner, Michael B., and Glen Jeffery. "Light Stimulation of Mitochondria Reduces Blood Glucose Levels." *Journal of Biophotonics* 17, no. 5 (2024). https://doi.org/10.1002/jbio.202300521.

Rastogi, Anshu, and Pavel Pospísil. "Spontaneous Ultraweak Photon Emission Imaging of Oxidative Metabolic Processes in Human Skin: Effect of Molecular Oxygen and Antioxidant Defense System." *Journal of Biomedical Optics* 16, no. 9 (2011): 096005. https://doi.org/10.1117/1.3616135.

Rees, Jonathan. "Industrialization and Urbanization in the United States 1880–1929." *Oxford Research Encyclopedia of American History* (2016). https://doi.org/10.1093/acrefore/9780199329175.013.327.

Reiter, Russel J., Qiang Ma, and Ramaswamy Sharma. "Melatonin in Mitochondria: Mitigating Clear and Present Dangers." *Physiology* 35, no. 2 (2020): 86–95.

Reyes, Marc G., Francesco Faraldi, Robert Rydman, and Charles Ce Wang. "Decreased Nigral Neuromelanin in Alzheimer's Disease." *Neurological Research* 25, no. 2 (2003): 179–82. https://doi.org/10.1179/016164103101201166.

Rhodes, L. E., S. O'Farrell, M. J. Jackson, and P. S. Friedmann. "Dietary Fish-Oil Supplementation in Humans Reduces UVB-Erythemal Sensitivity but Increases Epidermal Lipid Peroxidation." *Journal of Investigative Dermatology* 103, no. 2 (1994): 151–4. https://doi.org/10.1111/1523-1747.ep12392604.

Richards, Jacobs, and Michelle L. Gumz. "Advances in Understanding the Peripheral Circadian Clocks." *FASEB JOURNAL* 26, no. 9 (2012): 3602–3613. https://doi.org/10.1096/fj.12-203554.

Rodríguez-Cano, Ameyalli M., Claudia Caldaza-Mendoza, Guadalupe Estrada-Gutierrez, Jonatan A. Mendoza-Ortega, and Otilia Perichart-Perera. "Nutrients, Mitochondrial Function, and Perinatal Health." *Nutrients* 12 (2020): 2166. https://doi.org/10.3390/nu12072166.

Sadowska, Magdalena, Joanna Narbutt, and Aleksandra Lesiak. "Blue Light in Dermatology." *Life* 11, no. 7 (2021): 670. https://doi.org/10.3390/life11070670.

Schiller, Meinhard, Thomas Brzoska, Markus Böhm, Dieter Metze, Thomas E. Scholzen, André Rougier, et al. "Solar-Simulated Ultraviolet Radiation-Induced Upregulation of the Melanocortin-1 Receptor, Proopiomelanocortin, and α-Melanocyte-Stimulating Hormone in Human Epidermis In Vivo." *Journal of Investigative Dermatology* 122, no. 2 (2004): 468–476. https://doi.org/10.1046/j.0022-202X.2004.22239.x.

Shinhmar, Harpreet, Manjot Grewal, Sobha Sivaprasad, Chris Hogg, Victoria Chong, Magella Neveu, et al. "Optically Improved Mitochondrial Function Redeems Aged Human Visual Decline." *The Journals of Gerontology* 75, no. 9 (2020): e49–e52. https://doi.org/10.1093/gerona/glaa155.

Shinhmar, Harpreet, Chris Hogg, Magella Neveu, and Glen Jeffery. "Weeklong Improved Colour Contrasts Sensitivity After Single 670 nm Exposures Associated with Enhanced Mitochondrial Function. *Scientific Reports* 11, no. 1 (2021). https://doi.org/10.1038/s41598-021-02311-1.

Słominski, Andrzej, Gisela Moellmann, Elizabeth Kuklinska, Andrzej Bomirski, and John Pawelek. "Positive Regulation of Melanin Pigmentation by Two Key Substrates of the Melanogenic Pathway, L-Tyrosine and L-Dopa." *Journal of Cell Science* no. 3 (1988): 287–296. https://doi.org/10.1242/jcs.89.3.287.

Slominski, Andrzej T., Michal A. Zmijewski, Przemyslaw M. Plonka, Jerzy P. Szaflarski, and Ralf Paus. "How UV Light Touches the Brain and Endocrine System Through Skin, and Why."*Endocrinology* 159, no. 5 (2018): 1992–2007. https://doi.org/10.1210/en.2017-03230.

Solis, Arturo, Maria E. Lara, and Luis E. Rendon. "Photoelectrochemical Properties of Melanin." *Nature Precedings* (2007). https://doi.org/10.1038/npre.2007.1312.1.

Tafur, Joseph, and Paul J. Mills. "Low-Intensity Light Therapy: Exploring the Role of Redox Mechanisms." *Photomedicine and Laser Surgery* 26, no. 4 (2008): 323–8. https://doi.org/10.1089/pho.2007.2184.

Takahashi, Akiyoshi, and Kanta Mizusawa. "Posttranslational Modifications of Proopiomelanocortin in Vertebrates and Their Biological Significance." *Frontiers in Endocrinology* 4, no. 143 (2013). https://doi.org/10.3389/fendo.2013.00143.

Takahashi, Joseph S. "Transcriptional Architecture of the Mammalian Circadian Clock." *Nature Reviews Genetics* 18 (2017): 164–179.

Tan, Dun-Xian, Lucien C. Manchester, Lilan Qin, and Russel J. Reiter. "Melatonin: A Mitochondrial Targeting Molecule Involving Mitochondrial Protection and Dynamics." *International Journal of Molecular Sciences* 17, no. 12 (2016): 2124. https://doi.org/10.3390/ijms17122124.

Tao, Jin-Xin, Wen-Chuan Zhou, and Xin-Gen XG. "Mitochondria as Potential Targets and Initiators of the Blue Light Hazard to the Retina." *Oxidative Medicine and Cellular Longevity* 2019, no. 6435364 (2019). https://doi.org/10.1155/2019/6435364.

Thau, Lauren, Jayashree Gandhi, and Sandeep Sharma. *Physiology, Cortisol.* StatPearls Publishing, 2024.

Torii, Hidemasa, Toshihide Kurihara, Yuko Seko, Kazuno Negishi, Kazuhiko Ohnuma, Takaaki Inaba, et al. "Violet Light Exposure Can Be a Preventive Strategy Against Myopia Progression." *eBioMedicine* 15 (2017): 210–219. https://doi.org/10.1016/j.ebiom.2016.12.007.

Tsai, Shang-Ru, and Michael R. Hamblin. "Biological Effects and Medical Applications of Infrared Radiation." *Journal of Photochemistry and Photobiology B: Biology* 170 (2017): 197–207. https://doi.org/10.1016/j.jphotobiol.2017.04.014.

Uzunbajakava, Natalia E., Desmond J. Tobin, Natalia V. Botchkareva, Christine Dierickx, Peter Bjerring, and Godfrey Town. "Highlighting Nuances of Blue Light Phototherapy: Mechanisms and Safety Considerations." *Journal of Biophotonics* 16, no. 2 (2023): e202200257. https://doi.org/10.1002/jbio.202200257.

van Wijk, Eduard, Masaki Kobayashi M,Roeland van Wijk, and Jan van der Greef. "Imaging of Ultra-Weak Photon Emission in a Rheumatoid Arthritis Mouse Model." *PLOS One* 8, no. 12 (2013): e84579. https://doi.org/10.1371/journal.pone.0084579.

van Wijk Roeland, Eduard PA van Wijk, Jingxiang Pang, Meina Yang, Yu Yan, and Jinxiang Han. "Integrating Ultra-Weak Photon Emission Analysis in Mitochondrial Research." *Frontiers in Physiology* 11, no. 717 (2020). https://doi:10.3389/fphys.2020.00717.

Vandersee, Staffan, Marc Beyer, Juergen Lademann, and Maxim E. Darvin. "Blue-Violet Light Irradiation Dose Dependently Decreases Carotenoids in Human Skin, Which Indicates the Generation of Free Radicals." *Oxidative Medicine and Cellular Longevity* 2015, no. 579675 (2015). https://doi.org/10.1155/2015/579675.

Vila, Miguel. "Neuromelanin, Aging, and Neuronal Vulnerability in Parkinson's Disease." *Movement Disorders* 34, no. 10 (2019): 1440–1451. https://doi.org/10.1002/mds.27776.

Vinck, Elke M., Cagnie Barbara, Ria Cornelissen, Heidi Declercq, and Dirk Cambier. "Green Light Emitting Diode Irradiation Enhances Fibroblast Growth Impaired by High Glucose Level." *Photomedicine and Laser Surgery* 23, no. 2 (2005): 167–171. https://doi.org/10.1089/pho.2005.23.167.

Wahl, Siegfried, Moritz Engelhardt, Patrick Schaupp, Christian Lappe, and Iliya V. Ivanov. "The Inner Clock-Blue Light Sets the Human Rhythm." *Journal of Biophotonics* 12, no. 12 (2019): e201900102. https://doi.org/10.1002/jbio.201900102.

Wang, Liyin, Xin Yu, Dongyan Zhang, Yingying Wen, Liyue Zhang, Yutong Xia, et al. "Long-Term Blue Light Exposure Impairs Mitochondrial Dynamics in the Retina in Light-Induced Retinal Degeneration in Vivo and in Vitro." *Journal of Photochemistry and Photobiology B: Biology* 240, no. 112654 (2023). https://doi.org/10.1016/j.jphotobiol.2023.112654.

Weller RB, Wang Y, He J, et al. "Does Incident Solar Ultraviolet Radiation Lower Blood Pressure?" *Journal of the American Heart Association* 9, no. 5 (2020): e013837. https://doi.org10.1161/JAHA.119.013837.

Wilson, James M. "Henry Ford vs. Assembly Line Balancing." *International Journal of Production Research* 52, no. 3 (2014): 757–765. https://doi.org/10.1080/00207543.2013.836616.

Wu, Fan, Shuo Wu, Qiuqi Gui, Kaixin Tang, Qiqi Xu, Yue Tao, et al. "Blue Light Insertion at Night Is Involved in Sleep and Arousal-Promoting Response Delays and Depressive-Like Emotion in Mice." *Bioscience Reports* 41, no. 3 (2021): BSR20204033. https://doi.org/10.1042/BSR20204033.

Wunsch, Alexander, and Karsten Matuschka. "A Controlled Trial to Determine the Efficacy of Red and Near-Infrared Light Treatment in Patient Satisfaction, Reduction of Fine Lines, Wrinkles, Skin Roughness, and Intradermal Collagen Density Increase." *Photomedicine and Laser Surgery* 32, no. 2 (2014): 93–100. https://doi.org/10.1089/pho.2013.3616.

Young, A. R. "Chromophores in Human Skin." *Physics in Medicine & Biology* 42, no. 5 (1997): 789–802. https://doi.org10.1088/0031-9155/42/5/004.

Zeitzer, Jamie M., Derk-Jan Dijk, Richard E. Kronauer, Emery N. Brown, and Charles A. Czeisler. "Sensitivity of the Human Circadian Pacemaker to Nocturnal Light: Melatonin Phase Resetting and Suppression." *Journal of Physiology* 526 Pt 3 (2000): 695–702. https://doi.org/10.1111/j.1469-7793.2000.00695.x.

Zapata, Félix, Victoria Pastor-Ruiz, Fernando Ortega-Ojeda, Gemma Montalvo, Ana Victoria Ruiz-Zolle, and Carmen García-Ruiz C. "Human Ultra-Weak Photon Emission as Non-Invasive Spectroscopic Tool for Diagnosis of Internal States—A Review." *Journal of Photochemistry and Photobiology B: Biology* 216, no. 112141 (2021). https://doi.org/10.1016/j.jphotobiol.2021.112141.

CHAPTER SIX

Antonelli, Michele, Grazia Barbieri, and Davide Donelli. "Effects of Forest Bathing (Shinrin-Yoku) on Levels of Cortisol as a Stress Biomarker: A Systematic Review and Meta-Analysis." *International Journal of Biometeorology* 63, no. 8 (2019): 1117–1134. https://doi.org/10.1007/s00484-019-01717-x.

Aubrecht, L., Z. Stanek, and J. Koller. "Corona Discharge on Coniferous Trees—Spruce and Pine." *Europhysics Letters* 53 (2001): 304–390. https://doi.org/10.1209/epl/i2001-00153-2.

Bachman, C. H., and D. G. Hademenos. "Ozone and Air Ions Accompanying Biological Applications of Electric Fields." *Journal of Atmospheric and Solar-Terrestrial Physics* 33 (1971): 497–505. https://doi.org/10.1016/0021-9169(71)90153-X.

Barnes, Christopher, and Holli-Anne Passmore. "Development and Testing of the Night Sky Connectedness Index (NSCI)." *Journal of Environmental Psychology* 93, no. 102198 (2024). https://doi.org/10.1016/j.jenvp.2023.102198.

Besser, B. P. "Synopsis of the Historical Development of Schumann Resonances." *Radio Science* 42 (2007). https://doi.org/10.1029/2006RS003495.

Borra, J.P., R. A. Roos, D. Renard, H. Lazar, A. Goldman, and M. Goldman. "Electrical and Chemical Consequences of Point Discharges in a Forest During a Mist and a Thunderstorm." *Journal of Physics D: Applied Physics* 30 (1997): 84–93. https://doi.org/10.1088/0022-3727/30/1/011.

Bouchama, Abderrezak, Mohammad Azhar Aziz, Saeed Al Mahri, Musa Nur Gabere, Meshan Al Dlamy, Sameer Mohammad, et al. "A Model of Exposure to Extreme Environmental Heat Uncovers the Human Transcriptome to Heat Stress." *Scientific Reports* 7, no. 9429 (2017). https://doi.org/10.1038/s41598-017-09819-5.

Bowers, Bonnie, Randall Flory, Joseph Ametepe, Lauren Staley, Anne Patrick, and Heather Carrington. "Controlled Trial Evaluation of Exposure Duration to Negative Air Ions for the Treatment of Seasonal Affective Disorder." *Psychiatry Research* 259 (2018): 7–14. https://doi.org/10.1016/j.psychres.2017.08.040.

Buxton, Rachel T., Amber L. Pearson, Claudia Allou, and George Wittemyer. "A Synthesis of Health Benefits of Natural Sounds and Their Distribution in National Parks." *Proceedings of the National Academy of Sciences of the United States of America* 118, no. 14 (2021). https://doi.org/10.1073/pnas.2013097118.

Chen, Wenyao, Ziye Xu, Wenjing You, Yanbing Zhou, Liyi Wang, Yuquin Huang, and Tizhong Shan. "Cold Exposure Alters Lipid Metabolism of Skeletal Muscle Through HIF-1α-Induced Mitophagy." *BMC Biology* 21, no. 27 (2023). https://doi.org/10.1186/s12915-023-01514-4.

Chung, Nana, Jonghoon Park, and Kiwon Lim. "The Effects of Exercise and Cold Exposure on Mitochondrial Biogenesis in Skeletal Muscle and White Adipose Tissue." *Journal of Exercise Nutrition & Biochemistry* 21, no. 2 (2017): 39–47. https://doi.org/10.20463/jenb.2017.0020.

Della Vecchia, Alessandra, Federico Mucci, Andrea Pozza, and Donatella Marazziti. "Negative Air Ions in Neuropsychiatric Disorders." *Current Medical Chemistry* 28, no. 13 (2013): 2521–2539. https://doi.org/10.2174/0929867327666200630104550.

Donelli, Davide, Francesco Meneguzzo, Michele Antonelli, Diago Ardissino, Giampaolo Niccoli, Giorgio Gronchi, et al. "Effects of Plant-Emitted Monoterpenes on Anxiety Symptoms: A Propensity-Matched Observational Cohort Study." *International Journal of Environmental Research and Public Health* 20, no. 4 (2023): 2773. https://doi.org/10.3390/ijerph20042773.

Gangwisch, James E. "Seasonal Variation in Metabolism: Evidence for the Role of Circannual Rhythms in Metabolism?" *Hypertension Research* 36 (2013): 392–393. https://doi.org/10.1038/hr.2012.229.

Goel, Namni, Michael Terman, Jiuan Su Terman, Mariana M. Macchi, and Jonathan W. Stewart. "Controlled Trial of Bright Light and Negative Air Ions for Chronic Depression." *Psychological Medicine* 35, no. 7 (2005): 945–955. https://doi.org/10.1017/S0033291705005027.

Gould van Praag, Cassandra D., Sarah N. Garfinkel, Oliver Sparasci, Alex Mees, Andrew O. Philippides, Mark Ware, et al. "Mind-Wandering and Alterations to Default Mode Network Connectivity When Listening to Naturalistic Versus Artificial Sounds." *Scientific Reports* 7, no. 45273 (2017). https://doi.org/10.1038/srep45273.

Hafen, Paul S., Coray N. Preece, Jacob R. Sorensen, Chad R. Hancock, and Robert D. Hyldahl. "Repeated Exposure to Heat Stress Induces Mitochondrial Adaptation in Human Skeletal Muscle." *Journal of Applied Physiology* 125, no. 5 (2018): 1447–1455. https://doi.org/10.1152/japplphysiol.00383.2018.

Hahad, Omar, Marin Kuntic, Sadeer Al-Kindi, Ivana Kuntic, Donya Gilan, Katja Petrowski, et al. "Noise and Mental Health: Evidence, Mechanisms, and Consequences." *Journal of Exposure Science & Environmental Epidemiology* 35 (2025): 16–23. https://doi.org/10.1038/s41370-024-00642-5.

Harrison, R.G., and K. S. Carslaw. "Ion-Aerosol-Cloud Processes in the Lower Atmosphere." *Reviews of Geophysics* 41, no. 3 (2003). https://doi.org/10.1029/2002RG000114.

Hawkins, L. H., and T. Barker. "Air Ions and Human Performance." *Ergonomics* 21, no. 4 (1978): 273–278. https://doi.org/10.1080/00140137808931724.

Hirvonen, Jorma, Sari Lindeman, Joukamaa Matti, and Pirkko Huttunen. "Plasma Catecholamines, Serotonin and Their Metabolites and Beta-Endorphin of Winter Swimmers During One Winter. Possible Correlations to Psychological Traits." *International Journal of Circumpolar Health* 61, no. 4 (2002): 363–372.

Hong-Viet V., Ngo, Thomas Martinetz, Jan Born, and Matthias Mölle. "Auditory Closed-Loop Stimulation of the Sleep Slow Oscillation Enhances Memory." *Neuron* 78, no. 3 (2013): 545–553. https://doi.org/10.1016/j.neuron.2013.03.006.

Hoppel, W.A., R. V. Anderson, and J. C. Willet. "Atmospheric Electricity in the Planetary Boundary Layer." In *The Earth's Electrical Environment.* NAS Press, 1986, 195–205.

Hotho, Gerard, Dietrich von Bonin, Daniel Krerke, Ursula Wolf, and Dirk Cysarz. "Unexpected Cardiovascular Oscillations at 0.1Â Hz During Slow Speech Guided Breathing (OM Chanting) at 0.05Â Hz." *Frontiers in Physiology* 13 (2022). https://doi.org/10.3389/fphys.2022.875583.

Imbeault, Pascal, Isabelle Dépault, and François Haman. "Cold Exposure Increases Adiponectin Levels in Men." *Metabolism* 58, no. 4 (2009): 552–559. https://doi.org/10.1016/j.metabol.2008.11.017.

Iwama, H. "Negative Air Ions Created by Water Shearing Improve Erythrocyte Deformability and Aerobic Metabolism." *Indoor Air* 14, no. 4 (2004): 293–297. https://doi.org/10.1111/j.1600-0668.2004.00254.x.

Jaruševičius, Gediminas, Tautvydas Rugelis, Rollin McCraty, Mantas Landauskas, Kristina Berškienė, and Alfonsas Vainoras. "Correlation between Changes in Local Earth's Magnetic Field and Cases of Acute Myocardial Infarction." *International Journal of Environmental Research and Public Health* 15, no. 3 (2018): 399. https://doi.org/10.3390/ijerph15030399.

Jo, Hyunju, Chorong Song, and Yoshifumi Miyazaki. "Physiological Benefits of Viewing Nature: A Systematic Review of Indoor Experiments." *International Journal of Environmental Research and Public Health* 16, no. 23 (2019): 4739. https://doi.org/10.3390/ijerph16234739.

Ju, K., and Kubo T. "Power Spectral Analysis of Autonomic Nervous Activity in Spontaneously Hypertensive Rats." *Biomedical Sciences Instrumentation* 33, no. 23 (1997): 338–343. PMID: 9731382.

Kobayashi, Hiromitsu, Chorong Song, Harumi Ikei, Bum-Jin Park, Juyoung Lee, Takahide Kagawa, et al. "Forest Walking Affects Autonomic Nervous Activity: A Population-Based Study." *Frontiers in Public Health* 6, no. 278 (2018). https://doi.org/10.3389/fpubh.2018.00278.

Kondrashove, M. N., E. V. Grigorenko, A. V. Tikhonov, T. V. Sirota, A. V. Temnov, I. G. Stavrovskaja, et al. "The Primary Physico-Chemical Mechanism for the Beneficial Biological/Medical Effects of Negative Air Ions." *IEEE Transactions on Plasma Science* 28, no. 1 (2000): 230–237. https://doi.org/10.1109/27.842910.

König, Herbert L., Albert P. Krueger, Siegnot Lang, and Walter Sönning. *Biologic Effects of Environmental Electromagnetism.* Springer, 2012.

Kühn, Simone, Anna Mascherek, Elisa Filevich, Nina Lisofsky, Maxi Becker, Oisin Butler, et al. "Spend Time Outdoors for Your Brain—An In-Depth Longitudinal MRI Study." *The World Journal of Biological Psychiatry* 23, no. 3 (2021): 201–207. https://doi.org/10.1080/15622975.2021.1938670.

Laukkanen, Tanjaniina, Hassan Khan, Francesco Zaccardi, and Jari A. Laukkanen. "Association Between Sauna Bathing and Fatal Cardiovascular and All-Cause Mortality Events." *JAMA Internal Medicine* 175, no. 4 (2015): 542–548. https://doi.org/10.1001/jamainternmed.2014.8187.

Lazzerini, Fabio, M. T. Orlando, and W. De Prá. "Progress of Negative Air Ions in Health Tourism Environments Applications." *Boletín de la Sociedad Española de Hidrología Médica* 33, no. 1 (2018): 27–46. https://doi.org/10.23853/bsehm.2018.0450.

Lee, Paul, Sheila Smith, Joyce Linderman, Amber B. Courville, Robert J. Brychta, William Dieckmann, et al. "Temperature-Acclimated Brown Adipose Tissue Modulates Insulin Sensitivity in Humans." *Diabetes* 63, no. 11 (2014): 3686–3698. https://doi.org/10.2337/db14-0513.

Li, Fuzhong, K. John Fisher, and Peter Harmer. "Improving Physical Function and Blood Pressure in Older Adults Through Cobblestone Mat Walking: A Randomized Trial." *Journal of the American Geriatrics Society* 53, no. 8 (2005): 1305–1312. https://doi.org/10.1111/j.1532-5415.2005.53407.x.

Li, G. F., Q. Y. Li, L. H. Yan, and J. Y. Liao. "Study on the Concentration Characteristics of Air Negative Oxygen Ions in Urban Forest." *Hunan Foresty Science & Technology* 46, no. 02 (2019): 52–56.

Li, Qing. "Effects of Forest Environment (Shinrin-yoku/Forest Bathing) on Health Promotion and DiseasePprevention—the Establishment of 'Forest Medicine.'" *Environmental Health and Preventive Medicine* 27, no. 43 (2022). https://doi.org10.1265/ehpm.22-00160.

Li, Q., M. Kobayashi, Y. Wakayama Y, H. Inagaki, M. Katsumata, Y. Hirata, et al. "Effect of Phytoncide from Trees on Human Natural Killer Cell Function." *International Journal of Immunopathology and Pharmacology* 22, no. 4 (2022): 951–959. https://doi.org/10.1177/039463200902200410.

Liu, Shan, Chen Li, Mengtian Chu, Wenlou Zhang, Wanzhou Wang, Yazheng Wang, et al. "Associations of Forest Negative Air Ions Exposure with Cardiac Autonomic Nervous Function and the Related Metabolic Linkages: A Repeated-Measure Panel Study." *Science of the Total Environment* 850, no. 158019 (2022). https://doi.org/10.1016/j.scitotenv.2022.158019.

Marazita, Elizabeth, and Michael Spano. *The Dao of Foot Reflexology Paths: A Global Self-Care Tradition.* Wanderer's Press, 2012.

Meuwese, Daphne, Karin Dijkstra, Jolanda Maas, and Sander Koole. "Beating the Blues by Viewing Green: Depressive Symptoms Predict Greater Restoration from Stress and Negative Affect After Viewing a Nature Video." *Journal of Environmental Psychology* 75, no. 101594. (2021). https://doi.org/10.1016/j.jenvp.2021.101594.

McCraty, Rollin, Mike Atkinson, Viktor Stolc, Abdullah A. Alabdulgader, Alfonsas Vainoras, and Minvydas Ragulskis. "Synchronization of Human Autonomic Nervous System Rhythms with Geomagnetic Activity in Human Subjects." *International Journal of Environmental Research and Public Health* 14, no. 7 (2017): 770. https:doi.org/10.3390/ijerph14070770.

McCraty, Rollin, and Doc Childre. “Coherence: Bridging Personal, Social, and Global Health.” *Alternative Therapies in Health and Medicine* 16, no. 4 (2010): 10–24. PMID: 20653292.

McCraty, Rollin, Annette Deyhle, and Doc Childre. “The Global Coherence Initiative: Creating a Coherent Planetary Standing Wave.” *Global Advances in Integrative Medicine and Health* 1, no. 1 (2012): 64–77. https://doi.org/10.7453/gahmj.2012.1.1.013.

Mohan, Mithra S., S. S. Aswani, N. S. Aparna, P. T. Boban, P. R. Sudhakaran, and K. Saja. “Effect of Acute Cold Exposure on Cardiac Mitochondrial Function: Role of Sirtuins.” *Molecular and Cellular Biochemistry* 478 (2023): 2257–2270. https://doi.org/10.1007/s11010-022-04656-1.

Morris, K. F., S. C. Nuding, L. S. Segers, D. M. Baekey, R. Shannon, B. G. Lindsey, and T. E. Dick. “Respiratory and Mayer Wave-Related Discharge Patterns of Raphé and Pontine Neurons Change with Vagotomy.” *Journal of Applied Physiology* 109, no. 1 (1985): 189–202. https://doi.org/10.1152/japplphysiol.01324.2009.

Murr, L. E. “Biophysics of Plant Growth in an Electrostatic Field.” *Nature* 206 (1965): 467–470. https://doi.org/10.1038/206467a0.

Nemeryuk, G. E. “Migration of Salts Into the Atmosphere During Transpiration.” *Russian Journal of Plant Physiology* (Engl. Transl.) 17 (1970): 560–566. Accession: 093321560.

Nichols, Wallace J., *Blue Mind: The Surprising Science That Shows How Being Near, In, On, or Under Water Can Make You Happier, Healthier, More Connected, and Better at What You Do* Reprint Edition. Back Bay Books/Little, Brown, and Company, 2015. ISBN: 978-0-316-25211-9.

Ong, Ju Lynn, June C. Lo, Nicholas I. Y. N. Chee, Giovanni Santostasi, Ken A. Paller, Phyllis C. Zee, et al. “Effects of Phase-Locked Acoustic Stimulation During a Nap on EEG Spectra and Declarative Memory Consolidation.” *Sleep Medicine* 20 (2016): 88–97. https://doi.org/10.1016/j.sleep.2015.10.016.

Papalambros, Nelly A., Sandra Weintraub, Tammy Chen, Daniela Grimaldi, Giovanni Santostasi, Ken. A. Paller, et al. “Acoustic Enhancement of Sleep Slow Oscillations in Mild Cognitive Impairment.” *Annals of Clinical and Translational Neurology* 6, no. 7 (2019): 1191–1201. https://doi.org/10.1002/acn3.796.

Peng, Cheng, Marco Sanchez-Guerra, Ander Wilson, Amar J. Mehta, Jia Zhong, Antonella Zanobetti, et al. “Short-Term Effects of Air Temperature and Mitochondrial DNA Lesions Within an Older Population.” *Environment International* 103 (2017): 23–29. https://doi.org/10.1016/j.envint.2017.03.017.

Peterfalvi, Agnes, Matyas Meggyes, Lilla Makszin, Nelli Farkas, Eva Miko, Attila Miseta, et al. “Forest Bathing Always Makes Sense: Blood Pressure-Lowering and Immune System-Balancing Effects in Late Spring and Winter in Central Europe.” *International Journal of Environmental Research and Public Health* 18, no. 4 (2021): 2067. https://doi.org/10.3390/ijerph18042067.

Persinger, Michael, and Kevin S. Saroka. “Human Quantitative Electroencephalographic and Schumann Resonance Exhibit Real-Time Coherence of Spectral Power Densities: Implications for Interactive Information Processing.” *Journal of Signal and Information Processing* 6, no. 2 (2015): 153. https://doi.org/10.4236/jsip.2015.62015.

Pino, Olimpia, and Frencesco La Ragione. "There's Something in the Air: Empirical Evidence for the Effects of Negative Air Ions (NAI) on Psychophysiological State and Performance." *Research in Psychology and Behavioral Sciences* 1, no. (2013): 48–53. https://doi.org/10.12691/rpbs-1-4-1.

Pobachenko, S. V., A. G. Kolesnik, A. S. Borodin, and V. V. Kalyuzhin. "The Contigency of Parameters of Human Encephalograms and Schumann Resonance Electromagnetic Fields Revealed in Monitoring Studies." *Complex Systems Biophysics* 51 (2006): 480–483.

Poggiogalle, Eleonora, Humaira Jamshed, and Courtney M. Peterson. "Circadian Regulation of Glucose, Lipid, and Energy Metabolism in Humans." *Metabolism: Clinical and Experimental* 84 (2018): 11–27. https://doi.org/10.1016/j.metabol.2017.11.017.

Price, Colin, Earle Williams, Gal Elhalel, and Dave Sentman. "Natural ELF Fields in the Atmosphere and in Living Organisms." *International Journal of Biometeorology* 65, no. 1 (2021): 85–92. https://doi.org/10.1007/s00484-020-01864-6.

Ratcliffe, Eleanor, Birgitta Gatersleben, and Paul T. Sowden. "Predicting the Perceived Restorative Potential of Bird Sounds Through Acoustics and Aesthetics." *Environment and Behavior* 52, no. 4 (2018). https://doi.org/10.1177/0013916518806952.

Ryushi, T., I. Kita, T. Sakurai, M. Yasumatsu, M. Isokawa, Y. Aihara, et al. "The Effect of Exposure to NegativeAair Ions on the Recovery of Physiological Responses After Moderate Endurance Exercise." *International Journal of Biometeorology* 41, no. 3 (1998): 132–136. https://doi.org/10.1007/s004840050066.

Scott, Mandy A., and Michael A. Persinger, "Quantitative Convergence for Cerebral Processing of Information Within the Geomagnetic Environment." *Journal of Signal and Information Processing* 4, no. 3 (2013): 282–287. https://doi.org/10.4236/jsip.2013.43036.

Smith, David G., Roberta Martinelli, Gurdyal S. Besra, Petr A. Illarionov, Istvan Szatmari, Peter Brazda, et al. "Identification and Characterization of a Novel Anti-Inflammatory Lipid Isolated from Mycobacterium Vaccae, a Soil-Derived Bacterium with Immunoregulatory and Stress Resilience Properties." *Psychopharmacology* 236, no. 5 (2019): 1653–1670. https://doi.org/10.1007/s00213-019-05253-9.

Šrámek, P., M. Šimečková, L. Janský, J. Šavlíková, and S. Vybiral. "Human Physiological Responses to Immersion Into Water of Different Temperatures." *European Journal of Applied Physiology* 81, no. 5 (2000): 436–442. https://doi.oeg/10.1007/s004210050065.

Sugasawa, T., N. Mukai, K. Tamura, T. Tamba, S. Mori, Y. Miyashiro, et al. "Effects of Cold Stimulation on Mitochondrial Activity and VEGF Expression in Vitro." *International Journal of Sports Medicine* 37, no. 10 (2016): 766–778. https://doi.org/10.1055/s-0042-102659.

Suzuki, Koji, Kenji Maekawa, Hajime Minakuchi, Hirofumi Yatani, Glenn T. Clark, Yoshizo Matsuka, et al. "Responses of the Hypothalamic–Pituitary–Adrenal Axis and Pain Threshold Changes in the Orofacial Region Upon Cold Pressor Stimulation in Normal Volunteers." *Archives of Oral Biology* 52, no. 8 (2007): 797–802.

Tang, Haosu, Congyi Zheng, Xue Cao, Su Wang, Linfeng Zhang, Xin Wang, et al. "Blue Sky as a Protective Factor for Cardiovascular Disease." *Frontiers in Public Health* 10, no. 1016853 (2022). https://doi.org/10.3389/fpubh.2022.1016853.

Timofejeva, Inga, Rollin McCraty, Mike Atkinson, Abdullah A. Alabdulgader, Alfonsas Vainoras, Mantas Landauskas, et al. "Global Study of Human Heart Rhythm Synchronization with the Earth's Time Varying Magnetic Field." *Applied Sciences* 11, no. 7 (2021): 2935. https://doi.org/10.3390/app11072935

Timofejeva, Inga, Rollin McCraty, Mike Atkinson, Roza Joffe, Alfonsas Vainoras, Abdullah A. Alabdulgader, et al. "Identification of a Group's Physiological Synchronization with Earth's Magnetic Field." *International Journal of Environmental Research and Public Health.* 14, no. 9 (2017): 998. https://doi.org/10.3390/ijerph14090998.

Ulrich, R. S. "View Through a Window May Influence Recovery from Surgery." *Science* 224, no. 4647 (1984): 420–421. https://doi.org/10.1126/science.6143402.

Varma, Vijay R., Yi-Fang Chuang, Gregory C. Harris, Erwin J. Tan, and Michelle C. Carlson. "Low-Intensity Daily Walking Activity is Associated with Hippocampal Volume in Older Adults." *Hippocampus* 25, no. 5 (2015): 605–615. https://doi.org/10.1002/hipo.22397.

Vickrey, Beverly, and Itamar Lerner. "Overnight Exposure to Pink Noise Could Jeopardize Sleep-Dependent Insight and Pattern Detection." *Frontiers in Human Neuroscience* 17, no. 1302836 (2023). https://doi.org/10.3389/fnhum.2023.1302836.

Voloshina, Alexandra S., Arthur D. Kuo, Monica A. Daley, and Daniel P. Ferris. "Biomechanics and Energetics of Walking on Uneven Terrain." *J Exp Biol.* 216 (Pt 21) (2013): 3963–70. https://doi.org/10.1242/jeb.081711.

Von Schulze, Alex T., and Paige C. Geiger. "Heat and Mitochondrial Bioenergetics." *Current Opinion in Physiology* 27, no. 100553 (2022). https://doi.org/10.1016/j.cophys.2022.100553.

Wang, Connie X., Isaac A. Hilburn, Daw-An Wu, Yuki Mizuhara, Christopher P. Cousté, Jacob N. H. Abrahams, et al. "Transduction of the Geomagnetic Field as Evidenced from Alpha-Band Activity in the Human Brain." *eNeuro* 6, no. 2 (2019). https://doi.org/10.1523/ENEURO.0483-18.2019.

Wang, Jun, and Shu-hua Li. "Changes in Negative Air Ions Concentration Under Different Light Intensities and Development of a Model to Relate Light Intensity to Directional Change." *Journal of Environmental Management* 90, no. 8 (2009): 2746–2754. https://doi.org/10.1016/j.jenvman.2009.03.003.

White, Matthew P., Ian Alcock, James Grellier, Benedict W. Wheeler, Terry Hartig, Sara L. Warber, et al. "Spending at Least 120Minutes a Week in Nature Is Associated with Good Health and Wellbeing." *Scientific Reports* 9, no. 7730 (2019). https://doi.org/10.1038/s41598-019-44097-3.

Wiszniewski Andrzej, Andrzej Suchanowski, and Bartosz Wielgomas. "Effects of Air-Ions on Human Circulatory Indicators." *Polish Journal of Environmental Studies* 23, no. 2 (2014): 521–531.

Yamada, Roppei, Syunsuke Yanoma, Makoto Akaike, Akira Tsuburaya, Yukio Sugimasa, Shoji, et al. "Water-Generated Negative Air Ions Activate NK Cell and Inhibit Carcinogenesis in Mice." *Cancer Lett.* 239 (2006): 190–197. https://doi.org/10.1016/j.canlet.2005.08.002.

Yau, Winifred W., Kiraely Adam Wong, Jin Zhou, Nivetha Kanakaram Thimmukonda, Yajun Wu, Boon-Huat Bay, Brijesh Kumar Singh, et al. "Chronic Cold Exposure Induces Autophagy to Promote Fatty Acid Oxidation, Mitochondrial Turnover, and Thermogenesis in Brown Adipose Tissue." *iScience* 24, no. 5 (2021): 102434. https://doi.org/10.1016/j.isci.2021.102434.

Xiao, Sha, Tianjing Wei, Jindong Ding Petersen, Jing Zhou, and Xiaobo Lu. "Biological Effects of Negative Air Ions on Human Health and Integrated Multiomics to Identify Biomarkers: A Literature Review." *Environmental Science and Pollution Research* 30, no. 27 (2023): 1–13. https://doi.org/10.1007/s11356-023-27133-8.

CHAPTER SEVEN

Anderson, Joel G., and Ann Gill Taylor. "Biofield Therapies in Cardiovascular Disease Management: A Brief Review." *Holistic Nursing Practice* 25, no. 4 (2011): 199–204. https://doi.org/10.1097/HNP.0b013e3182227185.

Andersen, Søren S. L., Andrew D. Jackson, and Thomas Heimburg. "Towards a Thermodynamic Theory of Nerve Pulse Propagation." *Progress in Neurobiology* 88, no. 2 (2009): 104–13. https://doi.org/10.1016/j.pneurobio.2009.03.002.

Aureli, Tiziana, Fabio Presaghi, and Maria Concetta Garito. "Mother-Infant Co-Regulation During Infancy: Developmental Changes and Influencing Factors." *Infant Behavior and Development* 202269, no. 101768 (2022). https://doi.org10.1016/j.infbeh.2022.101768.

Babcock, N. S., G. Montes-Cabrera, K. E. Oberhofer, M. Chergui, G. L. Celardo, and P. Kurian. "Ultraviolet Superradiance from Mega-Networks of Tryptophan in Biological Architectures." *Journal of Physical Chemistry B* 128, no. 17 (2024): 4035–4046. https://doi.org/10.1021/acs.jpcb.3c07936.

Balaji, Sai, Nachum Plonka, Mike Atkinson, Malathy Muthu, Minvydas Ragulskis, Alfonsas Vainoras, et al. "Heart Rate Variability Biofeedback in a Global Study of the Most Common Coherence Frequencies and the Impact of Emotional States." *Scientific Reports* 15, no. 3241 (2025). https://doi.org/10.1038/s41598-025-87729-7.

Bartel, Lee, and Abdullah Mosabbir. "Possible Mechanisms for the Effects of Sound Vibration on Human Health." *Healthcare* 9, no. 5 (2021): 597. https://doi.org/10.3390/healthcare9050597.

Bastuji, Hélène, Maud Frot, Caroline Perchet, Koichi Hagiwara, and Luis Garcia-Larrea. "Convergence of Sensory and Limbic Noxious Input into the Anterior Insula and the Emergence of Pain from Nociception." *Scientific Reports* 8, no. 1 (2018): 13360. https://doi.org/10.1038/s41598-018-31781-z.

Behzadmehr Razieh, Neda Dastyar, Mahdieh Poodineh Moghadam, Mahnaz Abavisani, and Mandana Moradi. "Effect of Complementary and Alternative Medicine Interventions on Cancer Related Pain Among Breast Cancer Patients: A Systematic Review." *Complimentary Therapies in Medicine* 49, no. 102318 (2020). https://doi.org/10.1016/j.ctim.2020.102318.

Bengston, William, Paul Cizdziel, Akane Tanaka, and Hiroshi Matsuda. "Differential In Vivo Effects on Cancer Models by Recorded Magnetic Signals Derived from a Healing Technique." *Dose-Response* 21, no. 2 (2023). https://doi.org/10.1177/15593258231179903.

Beseme, Sarah, William Bengston, Dean Radin, Michael Turner, and John McMichael. "Transcriptional Changes in Cancer Cells Induced by Exposure to a Healing Method." *Dose-Response* 16, no. 3 (2018). https://doi.org/10.1177/1559325818782843.

Bilal, Saad Ahmed, Alfredo Obieta, Tamsin Santos, Saara Ahmad, and Joseph Elliot Ibrahim. "Effects of Nonpharmacological Interventions on Disruptive Vocalisation in Nursing Home Patients With Dementia—A Systematic Review." *Frontiers in Rehabilitation Sciences* 2 (2022). https://doi.org/10.3389/fresc.2021.718302.

Bohm, David. *Quantum Theory*. Phys Today, 1952. https://doi.org/10.1063/1.3067480.

Bonilla, Ernesto. "La Causalidad Formativa" [The Formative Causation]." *Instituto de Investigaciones Clínicas* 53, no. 4 (2012): 325–329. PMID: 23513483.

Bower, Julienne E., Arielle Radin, and Kate R. Kuhlman. "Psychoneuroimmunology in the Time of COVID-19: Why Neuro-Immune Interactions Matter for Mental and Physical Health." *Behaviour Research and Therapy* 154, no. 104104 (2022). https://doi.org/10.1016/j.brat.2022.104104.

Bruntrup, Godehard, and Ludwig Jaskolla, *Panpsychism: Contemporary Perspectives*. Oxford University Press, 2017. ISBN 978-0-19-935994-3.

Burroughs, Stephanie, and Denise French. "Depression and Anxiety: Role of Mitochondria." *Current Anaesthesia & Critical Care* 18, no. 1 (2007): 34–41. https://doi.org/10.1016/j.cacc.2007.01.007.

Butler, Emily A., and Ashley K. Randall. "Emotional Coregulation in Close Relationships." *Emotion Review* 5, no. 2 (2012): 202–210. https://doi.org/10.1177/1754073912451630.

Cakmak, Ayse S., Erick A. Perez Alday, Guilia Da Poian, Ali Bahrami Rad, Thomas J. Metzler, Thomas C. Neylan, et al. "Classification and Prediction of Post-Trauma Outcomes Related to PTSD Using Circadian Rhythm Changes Measured via Wrist-Worn Research Watch in a Large Longitudinal Cohort." *IEEE Journal of Biomedical and Health Informatics* 25, no. 8 (2021): 2866–2876. https://doi.org/10.1109/JBHI.2021.3053909.

Carrico, Adam W., Emily M. Cherenack, Leah H. Rubin, Roger McIntosh, Delaram Ghanooni, Jennifer V. Chavez, et al. "Through the Looking-Glass: Psychoneuroimmunology and the Microbiome-Gut-Brain Axis in the Modern Antiretroviral Therapy Era." *Biopsychosocial Science and Medicine* 84, no. 8 (2022): 984–994. https://doi.org/10.1097/PSY.0000000000001133.

Casuso-Holgado, María Jesús, Alberto Marcos Heredia-Rizo, Paula Gonzalez-Garcia, María Jesús Muñoz-Fernández, and Javier Martinez-Calderon. "Mind-Body Practices for Cancer-Related Symptoms Management: An Overview of Systematic Reviews Including One Hundred Twenty-Nine Meta-Analyses." *Support Care Cancer* 30, no. 12 (2022): 10335–10357. https://doi.org/10.1007/s00520-022-07426-3.

Coviello, Lorenzo, Yunkyu Sohn, Adam D. I. Kramer, Cameron Marlow, Massimo Franceschetti, Nicholas A. Christakis, et al. "Detecting Emotional Contagion in Massive Social Networks." *PLOS One* 9, no. 3 (2014): e90315. https://doi.org/10.1371/journal.pone.0090315.

Crawford, M. A., M. Thabet, Y. Wang, C. L. Broadhurst, and W. F. Schmidt. "A Theory on the Role of π-Electrons of Docosahexaenoic Acid in Brain Function: The Six Methylene-Interrupted Double Bonds and the Precision of Neural Signaling." *OCL* 25, no. 4 (2018). https://doi.org/10.1051/ocl/2018011.

Crawford, Michael A., C. Leigh Broadhurst, Martin Guest, Atulya Nagar, Yiqun Wang, Kebreab Ghebremeskel, et al. "A Quantum Theory for the Irreplaceable Role of Docosahexaenoic Acid in Neural Cell Signaling Throughout Evolution." *Prostaglandins, Leukotrienes and Essential Fatty Acids* 88, no. 1 (2013) 5–13. https://doi.org/10.1016/j.plefa.2012.08.005.

Crawford, Stephen E., V. Wayne Leaver, and Sanda D. Mahoney. "Using Reiki to Decrease Memory and Behavior Problems in Mild Cognitive Impairment and Mild Alzheimer's Disease." *Journal of Alternative and Complementary Medicine* 12, no. 9 (2006): 911–913. https://doi.org/10.1089/acm.2006.12.911.

D'Agata Amy, L., Jing Wu, Manushi K. V. Welandawe, Samia V. O. Dutra, Bradley Kane, and Maureen W. Groer. "Effects of Early Life NICU Stress on the Developing Gut Microbiome." *Developmental Psychobiology* 61, no. 5 (2019): 650–660.

Deleemans, Julie M., Haley Mather, Athina Spiropoulos, Kirsti Toivonen, Mohamad Baydoun, and Linda E. Carlson. "Recent Progress in Mind-Body Therapies in Cancer Care." *Current Oncology Reports* 25, no. 4 (2023): 293–307. https://doi.org/10.1007/s11912-023-01373-w.

Dinan, Timothy G., and John F. Cryan. "Microbes, Immunity, and Behavior: Psychoneuroimmunology Meets the Microbiome." *Neuropsychopharmacology* 42, no. 1 (2017): 178–192. https://doi.org/10.1038/npp.2016.103.

Dyer, Natlie L., Ann L. Baldwin, and William L. Rand. "A Large-Scale Effectiveness Trial of Reiki for Physical and Psychological Health." *Journal of Alternative and Complementary Medicine* 25, no. 12 (2019): 1156–1162. https://doi.org/10.1089/acm.2019.0022.

Evans, Courtney A., and Christin L. Porter. "The Emergence of Mother-Infant Co-Regulation During the First Year: Links to Infants' Developmental Status and Attachment." *Infant Behavior and Development* 32, no. 2 (2009): 147–158. https://doi.org/10.1016/j.infbeh.2008.12.005.

Fedele, Laura, and Thomas Brand. "The Intrinsic Cardiac Nervous System and Its Role in Cardiac Pacemaking and Conduction." *Journal of Cardiovascular Development and Disease* 7, no. 4 (2020): 54. https://doi.org/10.3390/jcdd7040054.

Ferrari, Pier Francesco, and Rizzolatti Giacomo. "Mirror Neuron Research: The Past and the Future." *Philosophical Transactions of the Royal Society* 369, no. 1644 (2014). https://doi.org/10.1098/rstb.2013.0169.

Ferrer, Emilio, and Jonathan L. Helm. "Dynamical Systems Modeling of Physiological Coregulation in Dyadic Interactions." *International Journal of Psychophysiology* 88, no. 3 (2012). https://doi.org/10.1016/j.ijpsycho.2012.10.013.

Fishburn, Frank A., Vishnu P. Murty, Christina O. Hlutkowsky, Caroline E. MacGillivray, Lisa M. Bemis, Meghan E. Murphy, et al. "Putting Our Heads Together: Interpersonal Neural Synchronization as a Biological Mechanism for Shared Intentionality." *Social Cognitive and Affective Neuroscience* 13, no. 8 (2018): 841–849. https://doi.org/10.1093/scan/nsy060.

FitzHenry, Fern, Nancy Wells, Victoria Slater, Mary S. Dietric, Panarut Wisawatapnimit, and A. Bapsi Chakravarthy. "A Randomized Placebo-Controlled Pilot Study of the Impact of Healing Touch on Fatigue in Breast Cancer Patients Undergoing Radiation Therapy." *Integrative Cancer Therapies* 13, no. 2 (2014): 105–13. https://doi.org/10.1177/1534735413503545.

Flux, M. C., and Christopher A. Lowry, "Inflammation as a Mediator of Stress-Related Psychiatric Disorders." In *Neurobiology of Brain Disorders.* 2nd edition. Academic Press, 2023, 885–911. ISBN 9780323856546. https://doi.org/10.1016/B978-0-323-85654-6.00052-6.

Friedman, Rachel S. C., Matthew M. Burg, Pamela Miles, Forrester Lee, and Rachel Lampert. "Effects of Reiki on Autonomic Activity Early After Acute Coronary Syndrome." *Journal of the American College of Cardiology* 56, no. 12 (2010): 995–996.

Goggins, Eibhlin, Shuhei Mitani, and Shinji Tanaka. "Clinical Perspectives on Vagus Nerve Stimulation: Present and Future." *Clinical Science* 136, no. 9 (2022): 695–709. doi:10.1042/CS20210507.

Goldman, Jonathan, and Andi Goldman. *The Humming Effect: Sound Healing for Health and Happiness*. Healing Arts Press, 2017.

Goldstein, Pavel, Irit Weissman-Fogel, Guillaume Dumas, and Simone G. Shamay-Tsoory. "Brain-to-Brain Coupling During Handholding Is Associated with Pain Reduction." *Proceedings of the National Academy of Sciences of the United States of America* 115, no. 11 (2018): E2528–E2537. https://doi.org/10.1073/pnas.1703643115 .

Gonzalez-Perez, Alfredo, Rima Budvytyte, Lars D. Mosgaard, Søren Nissen, and Thomas Heimburg. "Penetration of Action Potentials During Collision in the Median and Lateral Giant Axons of Invertebrates." *Physical Review X* 4, no. 3 (2014). https://doi.org/10.1103/PhysRevX.4.031047.

Gulsrud, Amanda C., Laudan B. Jahromi, and Connie Kasari. "The Co-Regulation of Emotions Between Mothers and Their Children with Autism." *Journal of Autism and Developmental Disorders* 40, no. 2 (2010): 227–237. https://doi.org/10.1007/s10803-009-0861-x.

Grof, Stanislav. "Ervin Laszlo's Akashic Field and The Dilemmas of Modern Consciousness Research." *World Futures* 62 (2006): 86–102. https://doi.org/10.1080/02604020500412717.

Hagelin, John S., Maxwell V. Rainforth, Kenneth L. C. Cavanaugh, Charles N. Alexander, Susan F. Shatkin, John L. Davies, et al. "Effects of Group Practice of the Transcendental Meditation Program on Preventing Violent Crime in Washington, D.C.: Results of the National Demonstration Project." *Social Indicators Research* 47 (1999): 153–201. https://doi.org/10.1023/A:1006978911496.

Hameroff, Stuart, and Roger Penrose. "Consciousness in the Universe: A Review of the 'Orch OR' Theory." *Physics of Life Reviews* 11, no. 1 (2014): 39–78. https://doi.org/10.1016/j.plrev.2013.08.002.

Hammerschlag, Richard, Michael Levin, Rollin McCraty, Namuun Bat, John A. Ives, Susan K. Lutgendorf, et al. "Biofield Physiology: A Framework for an Emerging Discipline." *Global Advances in Integrative Medicine and Health* 4 (2015): 35–41. https://doi.org/10.7453/gahmj.2015.015.suppl.

Hasson, Uri, Asif A. Ghazanfar, Bruno Galantucci, Simon Garrod, and Christian Keysers. "Brain-to-Brain Coupling: A Mechanism for Creating and Sharing a Social World." *Trends in Cognitive Sciences* 16, no. 2 (2012): 114–21. https://doi.org/10.1016/j.tics.2011.12.007.

He, Saike, Xiaolong Zheng, Daniel Zeng, Chuan Luo, and Zhu Zhang. "Exploring Entrainment Patterns of Human Emotion in Social Media." *PLOS One* 11, no. 3 (2016): e0150630. https://doi.org/10.1371/journal.pone.0150630.

Helm, Jonathan L., David Sbarra, and Emilio Ferrer. "Assessing Cross-Partner Associations in Physiological Responses via Coupled Oscillator Models." *Emotion* 12, no. 4 (2012): 748. https://doi.org/10.1037/a0025036.

Hertenstein Matthew J., Dacher Keltner, Betsy App, Brittany A. Bulleit, and Ariane R. Jaskolka. "Touch Communicates Distinct Emotions." *Emotion* 6, no. 3 (2006): 528–533. https://doi.org/10.1037/1528-3542.6.3.528.

Hertenstein, Matthew J., Rachel Holmes, Margaret McCullough, and Dacher Keltner. "The Communication of Emotion via Touch." *Emotion* 9, no. 4 (2009): 566–573. https://doi.org/10.1037/a0016108.

Heyes, Cecilia, and Caroline Catmur. "What Happened to Mirror Neurons?" *Perspectives on Psychological Science* 17, no. 1 (2021): 153–168. https://doi:10.1177/1745691621990638.

Holland, Anthony. "Digital Electronic Signal Synthesis Method For Synthesizing a Destructive Cancer Resonant Frequency Formant (DCRFF) And Preliminary Experimental Results of the Method Showing Inhibition of Cancer Cell Proliferation." (2023). https://doi.org/10.13140/RG.2.2.25528.11525.

Holland, Anthony. "Cell Fragmentation and Inhibition of Proliferation of Human Leukemia Cells in Vitro by Frenquency Specific Amplitude Modulated RF Pulsed Plasmas." Presented at BIOEM2015, Monterey, California, June 2015. https://www.researchgate.net/publication/304596455_cell_fragmentation_and_inhibition_of_proliferation_of_human_leukemia_cells_in_vitro_by_frequency_specific_amplitude_modulated_rf_pulsed_plasmas.

Jain, Shamini, Richard Hammerschlag, Paul Mills, Lorenzo Cohen, Richard Krieger, Cassandra Vieten, et al. "Clinical Studies of Biofield Therapies: Summary, Methodological Challenges, and Recommendations." *Global Advances in Integrative Medicine and Health* 4 (2015): 58–66. https://doi.org/10.7453/gahmj.2015.034.suppl.

Jain, Shamini, and Paul J Mills. "Biofield Therapies: Helpful or Full of Hype? A Best Evidence Synthesis." *International Journal of Behavioral Medicine* 17, no. 1 (2010): 1–16. https://doi.org/10.1007/s12529-009-9062-4.

Jain, Shamini, Desiree Pavlik, Janet Distefan, Rosalyn L. Bruyere, Julia Acer, Rosalie Garcia, et al. "Complementary Medicine for Fatigue and Cortisol Variability in Breast Cancer Survivors." *Cancer* 118, no. 3 (2012): 777–787.

Jerman, I., R. T. Leskovar, and R. Krašovec, *Evidence for Biofield: Philosophical Insights About Modern Science.* Nova Science Publishers, 2009, 199–216.

Keeler, Jason R., Edward A. Roth, Brittany L. Neuser, John M. Spitsbergen, Daiel J. Waters, and John-Mary Vianney. "The Neurochemistry and Social Flow of Singing: Bonding and Oxytocin." *Frontiers in Human Neuroscience* 9 (2015): 518. https://doi.org/10.3389/fnhum.2015.00518.

Kent, Jeremy B., Li Jin, and Xudong Joshua Li. "Quantifying Biofield Therapy Through Biophoton Emission in a Cellular Model." *Journal of Scientific Exploration* 34, no. 3 (2020): 434–454. https://doi.org/10.31275/20201691.

Kerna, Nicholas A., Sudeep Chawla, Victor Carsrud, Hilary M. Holets, Stephen M. Brown, John Flores, et al. "Sound Therapy: Vibratory Frequencies of Cells in Healthy and Disease States." *EC Clinical and Medical Case Reports* 5 (2022): 112–123. https://doi.org/10.31080/eccmc.2022.05.00532.

Khalid, Shehzad, and R. Shane Tubbs. "Neuroanatomy and Neuropsychology of Pain." *Cureus* 9, no. 10 (2017): e1754. https://doi.org/10.7759/cureus.1754.

Konvalinka, Ivana, Natalie Sebanz, and Günther Knoblich. "The Role of Reciprocity in Dynamic Interpersonal Coordination of Physiological Rhythms." *Cognition* 230 (2023): 105307. https://doi.org/10.1016/j.cognition.2022.105307.

Kozell, Anna, Aleksei Solomonov, and Ulyana Shimanovich. "Effects of Sound Energy on Proteins and Their Complexes." *FEBS Letters* 597 (2023): 3013–3037. https://doi.org/10.1002/1873-3468.14755.

Laszlo, Ervin. "Cosmic Connectivity: Toward a Scientific Foundation for Transpersonal Consciousness." *International Journal of Transpersonal Studies* 23, (2004): 21–31. https://doi.org/10.24972/ijts.2004.23.1.21.

Laszlo, Ervin, and Ralph A. Abraham, *The Connectivity Hypothesis: Foundations of an Integral Science of Quantum, Cosmos, Life, and Consciousness.* State University New York Press, 2003, 1–147.

Livingston, Gil, Lynsey Kelly, Elanor Lewis-Holmes, Gianluca Baio, Stephen Morris, Nishma Pate, et al. "A Systematic Review of the Clinical Effectiveness and Cost-Effectiveness of Sensory, Psychological and Behavioural Interventions for Managing Agitation in Older Adults with Dementia." *Health Technology Assessment* 18, no. 39 (2014): 1–vi. https://doi.org/10.3310/hta18390.

Lopez, Richard B., Bryan T. Denny, and Christopher P. Fagundes. "Neural Mechanisms of Emotion Regulation and Their Role in Endocrine and Immune Functioning: A Review with Implications for Treatment of Affective Disorders." *Neuroscience & Biobehavioral Reviews* 95 (2018): 508–514. https://doi.org/10.1016/j.neubiorev.2018.10.019.

Lucas, Alexander R., Heidi D. Klepin, Stephen W. Porges, and W. Jack. "Mindfulness-Based Movement: A Polyvagal Perspective." *Integrative Cancer Therapies* 17, no. 1 (2018): 5–15. https://doi.org/10.1177/1534735416682087.

Lutgendorf, Susan K., Elizabeth Mullen-Houser, Daniel Russell, Koen Degeest, Geraldine Jacobson, Laura Hart, et al. "Preservation of Immune Function in Cervical Cancer Patients During Chemoradiation Using a Novel Integrative Approach." *Brain, Behavior, and Immunity* 24, no. 8 (2010): 1231–40. https://doi.org/10.1016/j.bbi.2010.06.014.

Magal, Noa, Ophir Netzer, Eden Eldar, Noga Mandelblit, Michal Oren, Roy Salomon, et al. "Circadian Instability Predicts PTSD Symptom Severity Following Mass Trauma." *medRxiv* (2025). https://doi.org/10.1101/2025.03.19.25324240.

Maman, F., and T. Unsoeld. *The Tao of Sound: Acoustic Sound Healing for the 21st Century*. Tama-Do, the Academy of Sound, Color and Movement, 2008, 1–295. ISBN 0979552559/9780979552557.

Maruani, Jean, Roland Lefebvre, and Marja Rantanen. "Science and Music: From the Music of the Depths to the Music of the Spheres." In *Advanced Topics in Theoretical Chemical Physics*. Springer Science+Business Media, 2002, 479–514. ISBN 978-90-481-6401-1.

Matos, Luís Carlos, Jorge Pereira Machado, Fernando Jorge Monteiro, and Henry Johannes Greten. "Perspectives, Measurability and Effects of Non-Contact Biofield-Based Practices: A Narrative Review of Quantitative Research." *International Journal of Environmental Research and Public Health* 18, no. 12 (2021): 6397. https://doi.org/10.3390/ijerph18126397.

McCraty, R., M. Atkinson, W. A. Tiller, G. Rein, and A. D. Watkins. "The Effects of Emotions on Short-Term Power Spectrum Analysis of Heart Rate Variability." *American Journal of Cardiology* 76, no. 14 (1995): 1089–1093. https://doi.org/10.1016/S0002-9149(99)80309-9.

McCraty, Rollin. "New Frontiers in Heart Rate Variability and Social Coherence Research: Techniques, Technologies, and Implications for Improving Group Dynamics and Outcomes." *Frontiers in Public Health* 5, no. 267 (2017). https://doi.org/10.3389/fpubh.2017.00267.

McCraty, Rollin. "The Energetic Heart: Bioelectromagnetic Interactions Within and Between People." In *Clinical Applications of Bioelectromagnetic Medicine*. P. J. Rosch and M. S. Markov (eds.). Marcel Dekker, 2004, 541–562.

McCraty, Rollin, and Maria A. Zayas. "Cardiac Coherence, Self-Regulation, Autonomic Stability, and Psychosocial Well-Being." *Frontiers in Psychology* 5 (2014): 1090. https://doi.org/10.3389/fpsyg.2014.01090.

Mehra, Jagdish., and Helmut Rechenberg. "Planck's Half-Quanta: A History of the Concept of Zero-Point Energy." *Foundations of Physics* 29 (1999): 91–132. https://doi.org/10.1023/A:1018869221019.

Melzack R., and P.D. Wall. "Pain Mechanisms: A New Theory." *Science* 150, no. 3699 (1965): 971–979. https://doi.org/10.1126/science.150.3699.971.

Moraes, Lucam J., Márcia B. Miranda, Liliany F. Loures, Alessandra G. Mainieri, and Cláudia Helena C. Mármora. "A Systematic Review of Psychoneuroimmunology-Based Interventions." *Psychology, Health & Medicine.* 23, no. 6 (2018): 635–652. https://doi.org/10.1080/13548506.2017.1417607.

Müller, Viktor. "Neural Synchrony and Network Dynamics in Social Interaction: A Hyper-Brain Cell Assembly Hypothesis." *Frontiers in Human Neuroscience* 16 (2022): 848026. https://doi.org/10.3389/fnhum.2022.848026.

Müller, Viktor, Kira-Rahel P. Ohström, and Ulman Lindenberger. "Interactive Brains, Social Minds: Neural and Physiological Mechanisms of Interpersonal Action Coordination." *Neuroscience & Biobehavioral Reviews* 128 (2021): 661–677. https://doi.org/10.1016/j.neubiorev.2021.07.017.

Nassau, Jack H., Karen Tien, and Gregory K. Fritz. "Review of the Literature: Integrating Psychoneuroimmunology Into Pediatric Chronic Illness Interventions." *Journal of Pediatric Psychology* 33, no. 2 (2008): 195–207. https://doi.org/10.1093/jpepsy/jsm076.

Niu, Jian-Feir, Xiao-Feng Zhao, Han-Tong Hu, Jia-Jie Wang, Yan-Ling Liu, and De-Hua Lu. "Should Acupuncture, Biofeedback, Massage, Qi Gong, Relaxation Therapy, Device-Guided Breathing, Yoga and Tai Chi Be Used to Reduce Blood Pressure?: Recommendations Based on High-Quality Systematic Reviews." *Complimentary Therapies in Medicine* 42 (2019): 322–331. https://doi.org/10.1016/j.ctim.2018.10.017.

Ogolsky, Brian G., Shannon T. Mejia, Alexandra Chronopoulou, Kiersten Dobson, Christopher R. Maniotes, TeKisha M. Rice, et al. "Spatial Proximity as a Behavioral Marker of Relationship Dynamics in Older Adult Couples." *Journal of Social and Personal Relationships* 39, no. 10 (2021). https://doi.org/10.1177/02654075211050073.

Orme-Johnson, David W., Charles N. Alexander, John L. Davies, Howard M. Chandler, and Wallace E. Larimore. "International Peace Project in the Middle East: The Effects of the Maharishi Technology of the Unified Field." *The Journal of Conflict Resolution* 32, no. 4 (1988): 776–812. http://www.jstor.org/stable/174032.

Oschman, James L., Gaétan Chevalier, and Richard Brown. "The Effects of Grounding (Earthing) on Inflammation, the Immune Response, Wound Healing, and Prevention and Treatment of Chronic Inflammatory and Autoimmune Diseases." *Journal of Inflammation Research* 8 (2015): 83–96. https://doi.org/10.2147/JIR.S69656.

Paley, Blair, and Nastassia Hajal. "Conceptualizing Emotion Regulation and Coregulation as Family-Level Phenomena." *Clinical Child and Family Psychology Review* 25 (2022): 19–43. https://doi.org/10.1007/s10567-022-00378-4.

Pelling, Andrew E., Sadaf Sehati, Edith B. Gralla, Joan S. Valentine, and James K. Gimzewski. "Local Nanomechanical Motion of the Cell Wall of Saccharomyces Cerevisiae." *Science* 305, no. 5687 (2004): 1147–1150. https://doi.org/10.1126/science.1097640.

Perry, Gemma, Vince Polito, and William Forde Thompson. "Rhythmic Chanting and Mystical States Across Traditions." *Brain Sciences* 11, no. 1 (2021): 101. https://doi.org/10.3390/brainsci11010101.

Pinna, Thomas, and Darren J. Edwards. "A Systematic Review of Associations Between Interoception, Vagal Tone, and Emotional Regulation: Potential Applications for Mental Health, Wellbeing, Psychological Flexibility, and Chronic Conditions." *Frontiers in Psychology* 11 (2020): 1792. https://doi.org/10.3389/fpsyg.2020.01792.

Porges, S. W. "Orienting in a Defensive World: Mammalian Modifications of Our Evolutionary Heritage: A Polyvagal Theory." *Psychophysiology* 32, no. 4 (1995): 301–318. https://doi.org/10.1111/j.1469-8986.1995.tb01213.x.

Porges, Stephen W. "The Polyvagal Theory: New Insights Into Adaptive Reactions of the Autonomic Nervous System." *Cleveland Clinic Journal of Medicine* 76 (2009): S86–90. https://doi.org/10.3949/ccjm.76.s2.17.

Porges, Stephen W. "The Polyvagal Perspective." *Biological Psychology* 74, no. 2 (2007): 116–143. https://doi.org/10.1016/j.biopsycho.2006.06.009.

Porges, Stephen W. "Polyvagal Theory: A Science of Safety." *Frontiers in Integrative Neuroscience* 16 (2022): 871227. https://doi.org/10.3389/fnint.2022.871227.

Prakash, Shreya, Anindita Roy Chowdhury, and Anshu Gupta. "Monitoring the Human Health by Measuring the Biofield "Aura": An Overview." *International Journal of Applied Engineering Research* 10, no. 35 (2015). https://www.researchgate.net/publication/277575681_monitoring_the_human_health_by_measuring_the_biofield_aura_an_overview.

Pribram, Karl H. *Brain and Perception: Holonomy and Structure in Figural Processing.* Lawrence Erlbaum Associates, Inc., 1991. ISBN 0-89859-995-4.

Pusceddu, Matteo M., Sahar El Aidy, Fiona Crispie, Orla O'Sullivan, Paul Cotter, Catherine Stanton, et al. "N-3 Polyunsaturated Fatty Acids (PUFAs) Reverse the Impact of Early-Life Stress on the Gut Microbiota." *PLOS One* 10, no. 10 (2015): e0139721. https://doi.org/10.1371/journal.pone.0142228.

Radin, Dean, Peter A. Bancel, and Arnaud Delorme. "Psychophysical Interactions with Entangled Photons: Five Exploratory Experiments." *Journal of Anomalous Experience and Cognition* 1, no. 1–2 (2021): 9–54. https://doi.org/10.31156/23392.

Radin, Dean, Leena Michel, Karla Galdamez, Paul Wendland, Robert Rickenbach, and Arnaud Delorme. "Consciousness and the Double-Slit Interference Pattern: Six Experiments." *Physics Essays* 25, no. 2 (2021): 157–171. https://doi.org/10.4006/0836-1398-25.2.157.

Radin, Dean, Nancy Lund, Masaru Emoto, and Takashige Kizu. "Effects of Distant Intention on Water Crystal Formation: A Triple-Blind Replication." *Journal of Scientific Exploration* 22, no. 4 (2008). https://www.researchgate.net/publication/255669110_effects_of_distant_intention_on_water_crystal_formation_a_triple-blind_replication.

Radin, Dean, Gail Hayssen, Masaru Emoto, and Takashige Kizu. "Double-Blind Test of the Effects of Distant Intention on Water Crystal Formation." *Explore* 2, no. 5 (2006): 408–11. https://10.org/1016/j.explore.2006.06.004.

Reid, John Stuart. "Testing a 2,500 Year-Old Hypothesis: If Music Breathes New Life Into Old Blood Cells, Play On!" *Cymascope Institute* (2007). www.CymaScope.com. https://cymascope.com/testing-a-2500-year-old-hypothesis-%E2%80%8B/.

Reid, John Stuart, Beum Jun, and Sungchul Ji. "Imaging Cancer and Healthy Cell Sounds in Water by CymaScope, Followed by Quantitative Analysis by Planck-Shannon Classifier." *Water Journal* (2019). https://doi.org/10.14294/water.2019.6.

Ricciardi, L. M., and H. Umezawa. "Brain and Physics of Many-Body Problems." *Kybernetik* 4 (1967): 44–48. https:doi.org/10.1007/BF00292170.

Roy, Sisir, and Menas Kafatos. "Quantum Processes and Functional Geometry: New Perspectives in Brain Dynamics." *Forma* 19 (2004): 69–84. https://www.researchgate.net/profile/Sisir-Roy-2/publication/228382306_Quantum_processes_and_functional_geometry_new_perspectives_in_brain_dynamics/links/0fcfd50f6835ac3185000000/Quantum-processes-and-functional-geometry-new-perspectives-in-brain-dynamics.pdf.

Rubik, B., R. Pavek, E. Greene, D. Laurence, R. Ward, and E. Al. "Manual Healing Methods." In *Alternative Medicine: Expanding Medical Horizons: A Report to the National Institutes of Health on Alternative Medical Systems and Practices in the United States. Rubik B, et al., (eds.).* US Government Printing Office, 1995, 113–57.

Rubik, Beverly, and Harry Jabs. "Effects of Intention, Energy Healing, and Mind-Body States on Biophoton Emission." *Cosmos and History* 13, no. 2 (2017): 227–247. https://cosmosandhistory.org/index.php/journal/article/view/608.

Scaletti, Carla, Premila P. Samuel Russell, Kurt J. Hebel, Meredith M. Rickard, Mayank Boob, Franz Danksagmüller, et al. "Hydrogen Bonding Heterogeneity Correlates with Protein Folding Transition State Passage Time as Revealed by Data Sonification." *Proceedings of the National Academy of Sciences of the United States of America* 121, no. 22 (2024): e2319094121. https://doi.org/10.1073/pnas.2319094121.

Sheldrake, Rupert. "Morphic Fields." *World Futures, The Journal of New Paradigm Research* 62, no. 1–2 (2006): 31–41. https://doi.org/10.1080/02604020500406248.

Sheldrake, Rupert. "An Experimental Test of the Hypothesis of Formative Causation." *Rivista Di Biologia* 85, no. 3–4 (1992): 431–443. PMID: 1341836.

Sheldrake, Rupert, *A New Science of Life: The Hypothesis of Formative Causation*. Blond & Briggs, 1981. ISBN 978-0856341151.

Stuart, C., Y. Takahashi, and H. Umezawa. "Mixed-System Brain Dynamics: Neural Memory as a Macroscopic Ordered State." *Foundations of Physics* 9 (1979): 301–27. https://doi.org/10.1007/BF00715185.

Shiraishi, Masahiro, and Sotaro Shimada. "Inter-Brain Synchronization During a Cooperative Task Reflects the Sense of Joint Agency." *Neuropsychologia* 154, no. 16 (2021): 107770. https://doi.org/10.1016/j.neuropsychologia.2021.107770.

Soares, Sara, Vânia Rocha, Michelle Kelly-Irving, Silvia Stringhini, and Sílvia Fraga. "Adverse Childhood Events and Health Biomarkers: A Systematic Review." *Frontiers in Public Health* 9, no. (649825) (2021). https://doi.org/10.3389/fpubh.2021.649825.

Soma, Christina S., Brian R. W. Baucom, Bo Xiao, Jonathan E. Butner, Peter Hilpert, Shrikanth Narayanan, et al. "Coregulation of Therapist and Client Emotion During Psychotherapy." *Psychotherapy Research* 30, no. 5 (2020): 591–603. https://doi.org/10.1080/10503307.2019.1661541.

Song, Gdnqing, Claudio Fiocchi, and Jean-Paul Achkar. "Acupuncture in Inflammatory Bowel Disease." *Inflammatory Bowel Diseases* 25, no. 7 (2019): 1129–1139. https://doi.org/10.1093/ibd/izy371.

Song, Yu, Huan Cao, Chengchao Zuo, Zhongya Gu, Yaqi Huang, Jinfeng Miao, et al. "Mitochondrial Dysfunction: A Fatal Blow in Depression." *Biomedicine & Pharmacotherapy* 167 (2023): 115652. https://doi.org/10.1016/j.biopha.2023.115652.

Sternheimer, Joel. "Musique des Particules Élémentaires." *Comptes rendus de l'Académie des Sciences* 297, no. 829 (1983). https://www.researchgate.net/profile/Joel-Sternheimer/publication/261931616_Musique_des_particules_elementaires/links/55903fa008ae1e1f9bae15a9/Musique-des-particules-elementaires.pdf.

Straub, Rainer H., and Maurizio Cutolo. "Psychoneuroimmunology-Developments in Stress Research." *Wiener Medizinische Wochenschrift* 168, no. 3–4 (2018): 76–84. https://doi.org/10.1007/s10354-017-0574-2.

Stuart, C. I. J. M., Y. Takahashi, and H. Umezawa. "On the Stability and Non-Local Properties of Memory." *Journal of Theoretical Biology* 71, no. 4 (1978): 605–18. https://doi.org/10.1016/0022-5193(78)90327-2.

Subnis, Utkarsh B., Angela R. Starkweather, Nancy L. McCain, and Richard F. Brown. "Psychosocial Therapies for Patients with Cancer: A Current Review of Interventions Using Psychoneuroimmunology Based Outcome Measures." *Integrative Cancer Therapies* 13, no. 2 (2014): 85–104. https://doi.org/10.1177/1534735413503548.

Tabatabaee, Amir, Mansoureh Zagheri Tafresh, Maryam Rassouli, Seyed Amir Aledavood, Hamid AlaviMajd, and Seyed Kazem Farahmand. "Effect of Therapeutic Touch in Patients with Cancer: A Literature Review." *Medical Archives* 70, no. 2 (2016): 142–147. https://doi.org/10.5455/medarh.2016.70.142-147.

Thrane, Susan, and Susan M. Cohen. "Effect of Reiki Therapy on Pain and Anxiety in Adults: An In-Depth Literature Review of Randomized Trials with Effect Size Calculations." *Pain Management Nursing* 15, no. 4 (2014): 897–908. https://doi.org/10.1016/j.pmn.2013.07.008.

Timofejeva, Inga, Rollin McCraty, Mike Atkinson, Abdullah A. Alabdulgader, Alfonsas Vainoras, Mantas Landauskas, et al. "Global Study of Human Heart Rhythm Synchronization with the Earth's Time Varying Magnetic Field." *Applied Sciences* 11, no. 7 (2021): 2935. https://doi.org/10.3390/app11072935.

Tiller, W. A., R. McCraty, and M. Atkinson. "Cardiac Coherence: A New, Noninvasive Measure of Autonomic Nervous System Order." *Alternative Therapies in Health and Medicine* 2, no. 1 (1996): 52–65. PMID: 8795873.

Toppi, Jlenia, Gianluca Borghini, Manuela Petti, Eric J. He, Vittorio De Giusti, Bin He, Laura Astolfi, et al. "Investigating Cooperative Behavior in Ecological Settings: An EEG Hyperscanning Study." *PLOS One* 11, no. 4 (2016): e0154236. https://doi.org/10.1371/journal.pone.0154236.

Trivedi, Gunjan, Kamal Sharma, Banshi Saboo, Soundappan Kathirvel, Ashwati Konat, Vatsal Zapadia, et al. "Humming (Simple Bhramari Pranayama) as a Stress Buster: A Holter-Based Study to Analyze Heart Rate Variability (HRV) Parameters During Bhramari, Physical Activity, Emotional Stress, and Sleep." *Cureus* 15, no. 4 (2023): e37527. https://doi.org/10.7759/cureus.37527.

Urits, Ivan, Ruben H. Schwartz, Vwaire Orhurhu, Nishita V. Maganty, Brian T. Reilly, Parth M. Patel, et al. "A Comprehensive Review of Alternative Therapies for the Management of Chronic Pain Patients: Acupuncture, Tai Chi, Osteopathic Manipulative Medicine, and Chiropractic Care." *Advances in Therapy* 38, no. 1 (2021): 76–89. https://doi.org/10.1007/s12325-020-01554-0.

Valenti, Daniela, and Anna Atlante. "Sound Matrix Shaping of Living Matter: From Macrosystems to Cell Microenvironment, Where Mitochondria Act as Energy Portals in Detecting and Processing Sound Vibrations." *International Journal of Molecular Sciences* 25, no. 13 (2024): 6841. https://doi.org/10.3390/ijms25136841.

Valentovich, V., W. A. Goldberg, D. R. Garfin, and Y. Guo. "Emotion Coregulation Processes Between Parents and Their Children with ASD." In *Encyclopedia of Autism Spectrum Disorders.* F. R. Volkmar (ed.). Springer, 2021. https://doi.org/10.1007/978-3-319-91280-6_102422.

Valera-Calero, Juan Antonio, César Fernández-de-Las-Peñas, Marcos José Navarro-Santana, and Gustavo Plaza-Manzano. "Efficacy of Dry Needling and Acupuncture in Patients with Fibromyalgia: A Systematic Review and Meta-Analysis." *International Journal of Environmental Research and Public Health* 19, no. 16 (2022): 9904. https://doi.org/10.3390/ijerph19169904.

vanderVaart, Sondra, Violette M., G. J. Gijsen, Saskia N. de Wildt, and Gideon Koren. "A Systematic Review of the Therapeutic Effects of Reiki." *Journal of Alternative and Complementary Medicine* 15, no. 11 (2009): 1157–69. https://doi.org/10.1089/acm.2009.0036.

Weitzberg, Eddie, and Jon O. N. Lundberg. "Humming Greatly Increases Nasal Nitric Oxide." *American Journal of Respiratory and Critical Care Medicine* 166, no. 2 (2002): 144–5. https://doi.org/10.1164/rccm.200202-138BC.

Wikström, Valtteri, Katri Saarikivi, Mari Falcon, Tommi Makkonen, Silja Martikainen, Vesa Putkinen, et al. "Inter-Brain Synchronization Occurs Without Physical Co-Presence During Cooperative Online Gaming." *Neuropsychologia* 174 (2022): 108316. https://doi.org/10.1016/j.neuropsychologia.2022.108316.

Xu, Mingdi, Satoshi Morimoto, Eiichi Hoshino, Kenji Suzuki, and Yasuyo Minagawa. "Two-In-One System and Behavior-Specific Brain Synchrony During Goal-Free Cooperative Creation: An Analytical Approach Combining Automated Behavioral Classification and the Event-Related Generalized Linear Model." *Neurophotonics* 10, no. 1 (2023): 013511. https://doi.org/10.1117/1.NPh.10.1.013511.

Zadbood, A., J. Chen, Y. C. Leong, K. A. Norman, and U. Hasson. "How We Transmit Memories to Other Brains: Constructing Shared Neural Representations Via Communication." *Cerebral Cortex* 27, no. 10 (2017): 4988–5000. https://doi.org/10.1093/cercor/bhx202.

Zadro, Sonia, and Peta Stapleton. "Does Reiki Benefit Mental Health Symptoms Above Placebo?" *Frontiers in Psychology* 13 (2022): 897312. https://doi.org/10.3389/fpsyg.2022.897312.

CHAPTER EIGHT

Mohamed, Abdelrhman, Phuc T. Ha, Brent M. Peyton, Rebecca Mueller, Michelle Meagher, and Haluk Beyenal. "In Situ Enrichment of Microbial Communities on Polarized Electrodes Deployed in Alkaline Hot Springs." *Journal of Power Sources* 414, no. 28 (2019): 547–556. https://doi.org/10.1016/j.jpowsour.2019.01.027.

Agus, Allison, Julien Planchais, and Harry Sokol. "Gut Microbiota Regulation of Tryptophan Metabolism in Health and Disease." *Cell Host & Microbe* 23, no. 6 (2018): 716–724.

Akbar, Noor, Naveed Ahmed Khan, Jibran Sualeh Muhammad, and Ruqaiyyah Siddiqui. "The Role of Gut Microbiome in Cancer Genesis and Cancer Prevention." *Health Sciences Review* 2 (2022): 100010. https://doi.org/10.1016/j.hsr.2021.100010.

Altaha, Baraa, Marjolein Heddes, Violetta Pilorz, Yunhui Niu, Elizaveta Gorbunova, Michael Gigl, et al. "Genetic and Environmental Circadian Disruption Induce Weight Gain Through Changes in the Gut Microbiome." *Molecular Metabolism* 66 (2022). https://doi.org/10.1016/j.molmet.2022.101628.

Angajala, Anusha, Sangbin Lim, Joshua B. Phillips, Jin-Hwan Kim, Clayton Yates, and Zongbing You. "Diverse Roles of Mitochondria in Immune Responses: Novel Insights Into Immuno-Metabolism." *Frontiers in Immunology* 9 (2018): 1605. https://doi.org/10.3389/fimmu.2018.01605.

Arpaia, Nicholas, Clarissa Campbell, Xiying Fan, Stanislav Dikiy, Joris van der Veeken, Paul deRoos, et al. "Metabolites Produced by Commensal Bacteria Promote Peripheral Regulatory T-cell Generation." *Nature* 504 (2013): 451–455. https://doi.org/10.1038/nature12726.

Ballard, J. William O., and Samuel G. Towarnicki, "Mitochondria, the Gut Microbiome and ROS." *Cellular Signaling* 75 (2020): 109737. https://doi.org/10.1016/j.cellsig.2020.109737.

Bao, Li, Ying Zhang, Guoying Zhang, Dechun Jiang, and Dan Yan. "Abnormal Proliferation of Gut Mycobiota Contributes to the Aggravation of Type 2 Diabetes." *Communications Biology* 6, no. 226 (2023). https://doi.org/10.1038/s42003-023-04591-x.

Beheshti-Maal, Alireza, Shabnam Shahrokh, Saham Ansari, Elnaz Sadat Mirsamadi, Abbas Yadegar, Hamed Mirjalali, et al. "Gut Mycobiome: The Probable Determinative Role of Fungi in IBD Patients." *Mycoses* 64, no. 5 (2021): 468–476. https://doi.org/10.1111/myc.13238.

Berlow, Mae, Haruka Wada, and Elizabeth P. Derryberry. "Experimental Exposure to Noise Alters Gut Microbiota in a Captive Songbird." *Microbial Ecology* 84, no. 4 (2022): 1264–1277. https://doi.org/10.1007/s00248-021-01924-3.

Buret, Andre G., Thibault Allain, Jean-Paul Motta, and John L. Wallace. "Effects of Hydrogen Sulfide on the Microbiome: From Toxicity to Therapy. Antioxidants & Redox Signaling." *Antioxidants & Redox Signaling* 36, no. 4–6 (2022): 211–219. https://doi.org/10.1089/ars.2021.0004.

Capuron, Lucille, and Andrew H. Miller. "Immune System to Brain Signaling: Neuropsychopharmacological Implications." *Pharmacology & Therapeutics* 130, no. 2 (2011): 226–238. https://doi.org/10.1016/j.pharmthera.2011.01.014.

Chacón, M. R., J. Lozano-Bartolomé, M. Portero-Otín, M. M. Rodríguez, G. Xifra, J. Puig, et al. "The Gut Mycobiome Composition is Linked to Carotid Atherosclerosis." *Beneficial Microbes* 9, no. 2 (2018): 185–198. https://doi.org/10.3920/BM2017.0029.

Chen, Haiwei, Phu-Khat Nwe, Yi Yang, Connor E. Rosen, Agata A. Bielecka, Manik Kuchroo, et al. "A Forward Chemical Genetic Screen Reveals Gut Microbiota Metabolites That Modulate Host Physiology." *Cell* 177, no. 5 (2019): 1217–1231. https://doi.org/10.1016/j.cell.2019.03.036.

Chen, Hongguang, Xing Mao, Xiaoyin Meng, Yuan Li, Jingcheng Feng, Linlin Zhang, et al. "Hydrogen Alleviates Mitochondrial Dysfunction and Organ Damage via Autophagy Mediated NLRP3 Inflammasome Inactivation in Sepsis." *International Journal of Molecular Medicine* 44, no. 4 (2019): 1309–1324. https://doi.org/10.3892/ijmm.2019.4311.

Chen, Yijing, Jinying Xu, and Yu Chen. "Regulation of Neurotransmitters by the Gut Microbiota and Effects on Cognition in Neurological Disorders." *Nutrient* 13, no. 6 (2021): 2099. https://doi.org/10.3390/nu13062099.

Clark, Allison, and Núria Mach. "The Crosstalk Between the Gut Microbiota and Mitochondria During Exercise." *Frontiers in Physiology* 8 (2017): 319. https://doi.org/10.3389/fphys.2017.00319.

Cui, Bo, Huimin Chi, Wa Cao, Donghong Su, Honglian Yang, Zhe Li, et al. "Noise Exposure-Induced Intestinal Flora Dysbiosis Disrupts Homeostasis of Oxi-Inflamm-Barrier in the Gut–Brain Axis of APP/PS1 Mice: Implications for Early Onset Alzheimer's Disease." *Research Square* (2020). https://doi.org/10.21203/rs.3.rs-19045/v1.

Cui, Bo, Zhihui Gai, Xiaojun She, Rui Wang, and Zhuge Xi. "Effects of Chronic Noise on Glucose Metabolism and Gut Microbiota–Host Inflammatory Homeostasis in Rats." *Scientific Reports* 6, no. 36693 (2016).

Damiola, F., N. Le Minh, N. Preitner, B. Kornmann, F. Fleury-Olela, and U. Schibler. "Restricted Feeding Uncouples Circadian Oscillators in Peripheral Tissues from the Central Pacemaker in the Suprachiasmatic Nucleus." *Genes & Development* 14, (2021): 2950–2961. https://doi.org/10.1101/gad.183500.

Deaver, Jessica A., Sung Y. Eum, and Michal Toborekl. "Circadian Disruption Changes Gut Microbiome Taxa and Functional Gene Composition." *Frontiers in Microbiology* 9, no. 737 (2018). https://doi.org/10.3389/fmicb.2018.00737.

Desmet, Louis, Theo Thijs, Anneleen Segers, Kristin Verbeke, and Inge Depoortere. "Chronodisruption by Chronic Jetlag Impacts Metabolic and Gastrointestinal Homeostasis in Male Mice." *Acta Physiologica* 233, no. 4 (2021). https://doi.org/10.1111/apha.13703.

Dong, Yin, and Chun Cui. "The Role of Short-Chain Fatty Acids in Central Nervous System Diseases." *Molecular and Cellular Biochemistry* 477, no. 11 (2022): 2595–2607. https://doi.org/10.1007/s11010-022-04471-8.

Donohoe, Dallas R., Nikhil Garge, Xinxin Zhang, Wei Sun, Thomas M. O'Connell, Maureen K. Bunger, et al. "The Microbiome and Butyrate Regulate Energy Metabolism and Autophagy in the Mammalian Colon." *Cell Metaboolism* 13, no. 5 (2011): 517–526. https://doi.org/10.1016/j.cmet.2011.02.018.

Eda, Nobuhiko, Saki Tsuno, Nobuhiro Nakamura, Ryota Sone, Takao Akama, and Mitsuharu Matsumoto. "Effects of Intestinal Bacterial Hydrogen Gas Production on Muscle Recovery Following Intense Exercise in Adult Men: A Pilot Study." *Nutrients* 14, no. 22 (2022): 4875. https://doi.org/10.3390/nu14224875.

Eshel, Yoni, Uri Peskin, and Nadav Amdursky. "Coherence-Assisted Electron Diffusion Across the Multi-Heme Protein-Based Bacterial Nanowire." *Nanotechnology* 31, no. 31 (2020): 314002.

Flemming, Hans-Curt, Jost Wingender, Ulrich Szewzyk, Peter Steinberg, Scott A. Rice, and Staffan Kjelleberg. "Biofilms: An Emergent Form of Bacterial Life." *Nature Reviews Microbiology* 14 (2016): 563–575. https://doi.org/10.1038/nrmicro.2016.94.

Frank, Alexander, Cleverson C Matiolli, Américo J. C. Viana, Timothy J. Hearn, Jelena Kusakina, Fiona E. Belbin, et al. "Circadian Entrainment in Arabidopsis by the Sugar-Responsive Transcription Factor bZIP63." *Current Biology* 28, no. 16 (2018): 2597–2606. https://doi.org/10.1016/j.cub.2018.05.092.

Franzago, Marica, Elisa Alessandrelli, Stefania Notarangelo, Liborio Stuppia, and Ester Vitacolonna. "Chrono-Nutrition: Circadian Rhythm and Personalized Nutrition." *International Journal of Molecular Sciences* 24, no. 3 (2023): 2571. https://doi.org/10.3390/ijms24032571.

Furusawa, Yukihiro, Yuuki Obata, Shinji Fukuda, Takaho A. Endo, Gaku Nakato, Daisuke Takahashi, et al. "Commensal Microbe-Derived Butyrate Induces the Differentiation of Colonic Regulatory T Cells." *Nature* 504 (2013): 446–450. https://doi.org/10.1038/nature12721.

Gamal, Ahmed, Mohammed Elshaer, Mayyadah Alabdely, Ahmed Kadry, Thomas S. McCormick, and Mahmoud Ghannoum. "The Mycobiome: Cancer Pathogenesis, Diagnosis, and Therapy." *Cancers* 14, no. 12 (2022): 2875. https://doi.org/10.3390/cancers14122875.

Gao, Haichun, Soumitra Barua, Yili Liang, Lin Wu, Yangyang Dong, Samantha Reed, et al. "Impacts of Shewanella Oneidensis C-Type Cytochromes on Aerobic and Anaerobic Respiration." *Microbial Biotechnology* 3, no. 4 (2010): 455–466. https://doi.org/10.1111/j.1751-7915.2010.00181.x.

Gasaly, Naschla, Paul de Vos, Marcela A. Hermoso. "Impact of Bacterial Metabolites on Gut Barrier Function and Host Immunity: A Focus on Bacterial Metabolism and Its Relevance for Intestinal Inflammation." *Frontiers in Immunology* 12 (2021): 658354. https://doi.org/10.3389/fimmu.2021.658354.

Ge, Yanshan, Xinhui Wang, Yali Guo, Junting Yan, Aliya Abuduwaili, Kasimujiang Aximujiang, et al. "Gut Microbiota Influence Tumor Development and Alter Interactions with the Human Immune System." *Journal of Experimental & Clinical Cancer Research* 40, no. 42 (2021). https://doi.org/10.1186/s13046-021-01845-6.

Geesink, Patricia, and Thijs J. G. Ettema. "The Human Archaeome in Focus." *Nature Microbiology* 7 (2022): 10–11. https://doi.org/10.1038/s41564-021-01031-6.

Haase, Stefanie, Nicola Wilck, Aiden Haghikia, Ralf Gold, Dominik N. Mueller, and Ralf A. Linker. "The Role of the Gut Microbiota and Microbial Metabolites in Neuroinflammation." *European Journal of Immunology* 50, no. 12 (2020): 1863–1870. https://doi.org/10.1002/eji.201847807.

Hao, Fengqi, Miaomiao Tian, Xinbo Zhang, Xin Jin, Ying Jiang, Xue Sun, et al. "Butyrate Enhances CPT1A Activity to Promote Fatty Acid Oxidation and iTreg Differentiation." *Proceedings of the National Academy of Sciences of the United States of America* 118, no. 22 (2021): e2014681118. https://doi.org/10.1073/pnas.2014681118.

Haydon, Michael J., Olga Mielczarek, Fiona C. Robertson, Katharine E. Hubbard, and Alex A. R. Webb. "Photosynthetic Entrainment of the Arabidopsis Thaliana Circadian Clock." *Nature* 502 (2013): 689–692. https://doi.org/10.1038/nature12603.

Higgins, Jacob S., Lawson T. Lloyd, Sara H. Sohail, Marco A. Allodi, John P. Otto, Rafael G. Saer, et al. "Photosynthesis Tunes Quantum-Mechanical Mixing of Electronic and Vibrational States to Steer Exciton Energy Transfer." *Proceedings of the National Academy of Sciences* 118, no. 11 (2021). https://doi.org/10.1073/pnas.2018240118.

Hoare, Joseph I., Ann M. Rajnicek, Colin D. McCaig, Robert N. Barker, and Heather M. Wilson. "Electric Fields are Novel Determinants of Human Macrophage Functions." *Journal of Leukocyte Biology* 99, no. 6 (2016): 1141–1151. https://doi.org/10.1189/jlb.3A0815-390R.

Hu, Yongjia, Zhouzhou Chen, Chengchen Xu, Shidong Kan, and Daijie Chen. "Disturbances of the Gut Microbiota and Microbiota-Derived Metabolites in Inflammatory Bowel Disease." *Nutrients* 14, no. 23 (2022): 5140. https://doi.org/10.3390/nu14235140.

Jackson, Dakota N., and Arianne L. Theiss. "Gut Bacteria Signaling to Mitochondria in Intestinal Inflammation and Cancer." *Gut Microbes* 11, no. 3 (2020): 285–304. https://doi.org/10.1080/19490976.2019.1592421.

Jiang, Junxia, Yu He, Honghong Kou, Zongqi Ju, Xuebin Gao, and Hongfeng Zhao. "The Effects of Artificial Light at Night on Eurasian Tree Sparrow (Passer Montanus): Behavioral Rhythm Disruption, Melatonin Suppression and Intestinal Microbiota Alterations." *Ecological Indicators* 108 (2020): 105702. https://doi.org/10.1016/j.ecolind.2019.105702.

Kar, Rajiv K., Anne-Frances Miller, and Maria-Andrea Mroginski. "Understanding Flavin Electronic Structure and Spectra." *WIREs Computational Molecular Science* 12 (2022): e1541. https://doi.org/10.1002/wcms.1541.

Kar, Rajiv K., Sam Chasen, Maria-Andrea Mroginski, and Anne-Frances Miller. "Tuning the Quantum Chemical Properties of Flavins via Modification at C8." *The Journal of Physical Chemistry B* 125, no. 46 (2021): 12654–12669. https://doi.org/10.1021/acs.jpcb.1c07306.

Kim, Chang H. "Control of Lymphocyte Functions by Gut Microbiota-Derived Short-Chain Fatty Acids." *Cellular & Molecular Immunology* 18 (2021): 1161–1171. https://doi.org/10.1038/s41423-020-00625-0.

Kobayashi, Mamiko, Daisuke Mikami, Hideki Kimura, Kazuko Kamiyama, Yukie Morikawa, Seiji Yokoi, et al. "Short-Chain Fatty Acids, GPR41 and GPR43 Ligands, Inhibit TNF-α-Induced MCP-1 Expression by Modulating p38 and JNK Signaling Pathways in Human Renal Cortical Epithelial Cells." *Biochemical and Biophysical Research Communications* 486, no. 2 (2017): 499–505. https://doi.org/10.1016/j.bbrc.2017.03.071.

Kothari, Vijay, Pooja Patel, Chinmayi Joshi, Brijesh Mishra, Shashikant Dubey, and Milan Mehta. "Quorum Sensing Modulatory Effect of Sound Stimulation on Serratia Marcescens and Pseudomonas Aeruginosa." *bioRxiv* (2016): 072850. https://doi.org/https://doi.org/10.1101/072850.

Kothari, Vija, Pooja Patel, Chinmayi Joshi, Brijesh Mishra, Shashikant Dubey, and Milan Mehta. "Sonic Stimulation can affect Production of Quorum Sensing Regulated Pigment in Serratia Marcescens and Pseudomonas Aeruginosa." *Current Trends in Biotechnology and Pharmacy* 11, no. 2 (2017): 122–129.

Kowacz, Magdalena, and Gerald H. Pollack. "Propolis-Induced Exclusion of Colloids: Possible New Mechanism of Biological Action." *Colloid and Interface Science Communications* 38 (2020): 100307. https://doi.org/10.1016/j.colcom.2020.100307.

Kowalski, Karol, and Agata Mulak. "Small Intestinal Bacterial Overgrowth in Alzheimer's Disease." *Journal of Neural Transmission* 129, no. 1 (2022): 75–83. https://doi.org/10.1007/s00702-021-02440-x.

Li, Zhen, Huijing Xia, Thomas E. Sharp III, Kyle B. LaPenna, John W. Elrod, Kevin M. Casin, et al. "Mitochondrial H2S Regulates BCAA Catabolism in Heart Failure." *Circulation Research* 131, no. 3 (2022): 222–235. https://doi.org/10.1161/CIRCRESAHA.121.319817.

Light, Samuel H., Lin Su, Rafael Rivera-Lugo, Jose A. Cornejo, Alexander Louie, Anthony T. Iavarone, et al. "A Flavin-Based Extracellular Electron Transfer Mechanism in Diverse Gram-positive Bacteria." *Nature* 562, no. 140 (2018). https://doi.org/10.1038/s41586-018-0498-z.

Lin, Lan, and Jianqiong Zhang. "Role of Intestinal Microbiota and Metabolites on Gut Homeostasis and Human Diseases." *BMC Immunology* 18, no. 1 (2017): 2. https://doi.org/10.1186/s12865-016-0187-3.

Liu, Jian, Wei Zhao, Zi-Wei Gao, Ning Liu, Wei-Hua Zhang, and Hong. "Effects of Exogenous Hydrogen Sulfide on Diabetic Metabolic Disorders in db/db Mice Are Associated With Gut Bacterial and Fungal Microbiota." *Frontiers in Cellular and Infection Microbiology* 12 (2022): 801331. https://doi.org/10.3389/fcimb.2022.801331.

Livernois, William, and M. P. Anantram, "Quantum Transport in Conductive Bacterial Nanowires." Presented at 2021 IEEE 16th Nanotechnology Materials and Devices Conference (NMDC), Vancouver, BC, Canada, (2021), 1–5. https://doi.org/10.1109/NMDC50713.2021.9677490.

Logan, Bruce E., Ruggero Rossi, Ala'a Ragab, and Pascal E. Saikaly. "Electroactive Microorganisms in Bioelectrochemical Systems." *Nature Reviews Microbiology* 17 (2019): 307–319. https://doi.org/10.1038/s41579-019-0173-x.

Lu, Xurui, Weiliang Hu, Xuejian Wang, Zhifeng Wang, Pingyu Yang, and Wenjie Wang. "Protective Role of Methane in Traumatic Nervous System Diseases." *Medical Gas Research* 14, no. 3 (2024): 159–162. 2024. https://doi.org/10.4103/mgr.mgr_23_23.

Lundberg, Jon. O., Eddie Weitzberg, and Mark T. Gladwin. "The Nitrate-Nitrite-Nitric Oxide Pathway in Physiology and Therapeutics." *Nature Reviews Drug Discovery* 7 (2008): 156–167. https://doi.org/10.1038/nrd2466.

Luu, Mark, Sabine Pautz, Vanessa Kohl, Rajeev Singh, Rossana Romero, Sébastien Lucas, et al. "The Short-Chain Fatty Acid Pentanoate Suppresses Autoimmunity by Modulating the Metabolic-Epigenetic Crosstalk in Lymphocytes." *Nature Communications* 10, no. 760 (2019). https://doi.org/10.1038/s41467-019-08711-2.

Ma, Yuanhang, Chao Xu, Wensheng Wang, Ligang Sun, Songwei Yang, Dingsong Lu, et al. "Role of SIRT1 in the Protection of Intestinal Epithelial Barrier Under Hypoxia and Its Mechanism." *Zhonghua Wei Chang Wai Ke Za Zhi* 17, no. 6 (2014): 602–606. https://doi.org.10.1371/journal.pone.0138307.

Malvankar, Nikhil S., Madeline Vargas, Kelly P. Nevin, Ashley E. Franks, Ching Leang, Byoung-Chan Kim, et al. "Tunable Metallic-Like Conductivity in Microbial Nanowire Networks." *Nature Nanotechnology* 6, (2011): 573–579. https://doi.org/10.1038/nnano.2011.119.

Matsuhashi, Michio, Alla N. L. Pankrushina, Satoshi Takeuchi, Hideyuki Ohshima, Housaku Miyoi, Katsura Endoh, et al. "Production of Sound Waves by Bacterial Cells and the Response of Bacterial Cells to Sound." *Journal of General and Applied Microbiology* 44, no. 1 (1998): 49–55. https://doi.org/10.2323/jgam.44.49.

Mishra, Suryakant, Sahand Pirbadian, Amit Kumar Mondal, Mohamed Y. El-Naggar, and Ron Naaman. "Spin-Dependent Electron Transport through Bacterial Cell Surface Multiheme Electron Conduits." *Journal of the American Chemical Society* 141, no. 49 (2019): 19198–19202. https://doi.org/10.1021/jacs.9b09262.

Nelson, James W., Sharon C. Phillips, Bhanu P. Ganesh, Joseph F. Petrosino, David J. Durgan, and Robert M. Bryan. "The Gut Microbiome Contributes to Blood-Brain Barrier Disruption in Spontaneously Hypertensive Stroke Prone Rats." *FASEB Journal* 35, no. 2 (2021): e21201. https://doi.org/10.1096/fj.202001117R.

Neu, Jens, Catharine C. Shipps, Matthew J. Guberman-Pfeffer, Cong Shen, Vishok Srikanth, Jacob A. Spies, et al. "Microbial Biofilms as Living Photoconductors Due to Ultrafast Electron Transfer in Cytochrome OmcS Nanowires." *Nature Communications* 13, no. 5150 (2022). https://doi.org/10.1038/s41467-022-32659-5.

Page, Amanada J. "Jetlagged Microbiota: A Problem for Gut and Metabolic Function." *Acta Physiologica* 233, no. 4 (2021). https://doi.org/10.1111/apha.13722.

Park, Jeongho, and Chang H. Kim. "Regulation of Common Neurological Disorders by Gut Microbial Metabolites." *Experimental & Molecular Medicine* 53 (2021): 1821–1833. https://doi.org/10.1038/s12276-021-00703-x

Parker, Aimée, Sonia Fonseca, and Simon R. Carding. "Gut Microbes and Metabolites as Modulators of Blood-Brain Barrier Integrity and Brain Health." *Gut Microbes* 11, no. 2 (2020): 135–157. https://doi.org/10.1080/19490976.2019.1638722.

Paterson, Marissa J., Seeun Oh, and David M. Underhill. "Host–Microbe Interactions: Commensal Fungi in the Gut." *Current Opinion in Microbiology* 40 (2017): 131–137. https://doi.org/10.1016/j.mib.2017.11.012.

Paulose, Jiffin K., John M. Wright, Akruti G. Patel, and Vincent M. Cassone. "Human Gut Bacteria Are Sensitive to Melatonin and Express En-Dogenous Circadian Rhythmicity." *PLOS One* 11, no. 1 (2016): e0146643. https://doi.org/10.1371/journal.pone.0146643.

Paulose, Jiffin K., Charles V. Cassone, Kinga B. Graniczkowska, and Vincent M. Cassone. "Entrainment of the Circadian Clock of the Enteric Bacterium Klebsiella Eerogenes by Temperature Cycles." *iScience* 19 (2019): 1202–1213. https://doi.com/10.1016/j.isci.2019.09.007.

Peng, Luying, Zhong-Rong Li, Robert S. Green, Ian R. Holzman, and Jing Lin. "Butyrate Enhances the Intestinal Barrier by Facilitating Tight Junction Assembly Via Activation of AMP-Activated Protein Kinase in Caco-2 Cell Monolayers." *Journal of Nutrition* 139, no. 9 (2009): 1619–1625. https://doi.org/10.3945/jn.109.104638.

Peng, Song-Yang, Xin Wu, Ting Lu, Gang Cui, and Gang Chen. "Research Progress of Hydrogen Sulfide in Alzheimer's Disease from Laboratory to Hospital: A Narrative Review." *Medical Gas Research* 10, no. 3 (2020): 125–129. https://doi.org/10.4103/2045-9912.296043.

Puneet, Seth, Paishiun N. Hsieh, Suhib Jamal, Liwen Wang, Steven P. Gygi, Mukesh K. Jain, et al. "Regulation of MicroRNA Machinery and Development by Interspecies S-Nitrosylation." *Cell* 176, no. 5 (2019). https://doi.org/10.1016/j.cell.2019.01.03.7.

Radjabzadeh, Djawad, Jos A. Bosch, André G. Uitterlinden, Aeilko H. Zwinderman, M. Arfan Ikram, Joyce B. J. van Meurs, et al. "Gut Microbiome-Wide Association Study of Depressive Symptoms." *Nature Communications* 13, no. 7128 (2022). https://doi.org/10.1038/s41467-022-34502-3.

Ridlon, Jason M., Dae Joong Kang, Phillip B. Hylemon, and Jasmohan S. Bajaj. "Bile Acids and the Gut Microbiome." *Current Opinion in Gastroenterology* 30, no. 3 (2014): 332–338. https://doi.org/10.1097/MOG.0000000000000057.

Robinson, Jake M., Ross Cameron, and Brenda Parker. "The Effects of Anthropogenic Sound and Artificial Light Exposure on Microbiomes: Ecological and Public Health Implications." *Frontiers in Ecology and Evolution* 9 (2021). https://doi.org/10.3389/fevo.2021.662588.

Rowe, Annette R., Farshid Salimijazi, Leah Trutschel, Joshua Sackett, Oluwakemi Adesina, Isao Anzai, et al. "Identification of a Pathway for Electron Uptake in Shewanella Oneidensis." *Communications in Biology* 4, no. 1 (2021): 957. Htps://doi.org/10.1038/s42003-021-02454-x.

Sarvaiya, Niral, and Vijay Kothari. "Effect of Audible Sound in Form of Music on Microbial Growth and Production of Certain Important Metabolites." *Microbiology* 84 (2015): 227–235. https://doi.org/10.1134/S0026261715020125.

Sato, Miho, Mariko Murakami, Koichi Node, Ritsuko Matsumura, and Makoto Akashi. "The Role of the Endocrine System in Feeding-Induced Tissue-Specific Circadian Entrainment." *Cell Reports* 8, no. 2 (2014): 393–401. https://10.1016/j.celrep.2014.06.015.

Scott, Samantha A., Jingjing Fu, and Pamela V. Chang. "Microbial Tryptophan Metabolites Regulate Gut Barrier Function via the Aryl Hydrocarbon Receptor." *Proceedings of the National Academy of Sciences of the United States of America* 117, no. 32 (2020): 19376–19387. https://doi.org/10.1073/pnas.2000047117.

Shah, Abheelasha, Akanksha Raval, and Vijay Kothari. "Sound Stimulation Can Influence Microbial Growth and Production of Certain Key Metabolites." *The Journal of Microbiology, Biotechnology and Food Sciences* 5, no. 4 (2016): 330–334. https://doi.org/10.15414/jmbfs.2016.5.4.330-334.

Silva, Ygor Parladore, Andressa Bernardi, and Rudimar Luiz Frozza. "The Role of Short-Chain Fatty Acids from Gut Microbiota in Gut-Brain Communication." *Frontiers in Endocrinology* 11 (2020): 25. https://doi.org/10.3389/fendo.2020.00025.

Simpson, Carra A., Carmela Diaz-Arteche, Djamila Eliby, Orli S. Schwartz, Julian G. Simmons, and Caitlin S. M. Cowan. "The Gut Microbiota in Anxiety and Depression—A Systematic Review." *Clinical Psychology Review* 83 (2021): 101943. https://doi.org/10.1016/j.cpr.2020.101943.

Stokkan, K., A. S. Yamazaki, H. Tei, Y. Sakaki, and M. Menaker. "Entrainment of the Circadian Clock in the Liver by Feeding." *Science* 291, no. 5503 (200): 490–493. https://doi.org/10.1126/science.291.5503.490.

Sun, Yaohui, Brian Reid, Fernando Ferreira, Guillaume Luxardi, Li Ma, Kristen L. Lokken, et al. "Infection-Generated Eelectric Field in Gut Epithelium Drives Bidirectional Migration of Macrophages." *PLOS Biology* 17, no. 4 (2019): e3000044. https://doi.org/10.1371/journal.pbio.3000044.

Yardeni, Tal, Ceylan E. Tanes, Kyle Bittinger, Lisa M. Mattei, Patrick M. Schaefer, Larry N. Singh, et al. "Host Mitochondria Influence Gut Microbiome Diversity: A Role for ROS." *Science Signaling* 12, no. 588 (2019): eaaw3159. https://doi.org/10.1126/scisignal.aaw3159.

Tessaro, Lucas W. E., Blake T. Dotta, and Michael A. Persinger. "Bacterial Biophotons as Non-Local Information Carriers: Species-Specific Spectral Characteristics of a Stress Response." *MicrobiologyOpen* 8, no. 6 (2019): 8:e761. https://doi.org/10.1002/mbo3.761.

Thaiss, Christoph A., David Zeevi, Maayan Levy, Gili Zilberman-Schapira, Jotham Suez, Anouk C. Tengeler, et al. "Transkingdom Control of Microbiota Diurnal Oscillations Promotes Metabolic Homeostasis." *Cell* 159, no. 3 (2014): 514–529. https://doi.org/10.1016/j.cell.2014.09.048.

Thaiss, Christoph A., Maayan Levy, Tal Korem, Lenka Dohnalová, Hagit Shapiro, Diego A. Jaitin, et al. "Microbiota Diurnal Rhythmicity Programs Host Transcriptome Oscillations." *Cell* 167 (2016): 1495–1510. https://doi.org/10.1016/j.cell.2016.11.003.

Thursby, Elizabeth, and Nathalie Juge. "Introduction to the Human Gut Microbiota." *Biochemical Journal* 474, no. 11 (2017): 1823–1836. https://doi.org/10.1042/BCJ20160510.

Waclawiková, Barbora, and Sahar El Aidy. "Role of Microbiota and Tryptophan Metabolites in the Remote Effect of Intestinal Inflammation on Brain and Depression." *Pharmaceuticals* 11, no. 3 (2018): 63. https://doi.org/10.3390/ph11030063.

Walker, David J. F., Ramesh Y. Adhikari, Dawn E. Holmes, Joy E. Ward, Trevor L. Woodard, Kelly P. Nevin, et al. "Electrically Conductive Pili from Pilin Genes of Phylogenetically Diverse Microorganisms." *ISME Journal* 12 (2018): 48–58. https://doi.org/10.1038/ismej.2017.141.

Wang, Wei, Yahui Du, Shuai Yang, Xiaochen Du, Min Li, Bingqian Lin, et al. "Bacterial Extracellular Electron Transfer Occurs in Mammalian Gut." *Analytical Chemistry* 91, no. 19 (2019): 12138–12141. https://doi.org/10.1021/acs.analchem.9b03176.

Wei, Hai-Jun, Xiang Li, and Xiao-Qing Tang. "Therapeutic Benefits of H_2S in Alzheimer's Disease." *Journal of Clinical Neuroscience* 21, no. 10 (2014): 1665–1669. https://doi.org/10.1016/j.jocn.2014.01.006.

Wei, Lin, Fangzhi Yue, Lin Xin, Shanyu Wu, Ying Shi, Jinchen Li, et al. "Constant Light Exposure Alters Gut Microbiota and Promotes the Progression of Steatohepatitis in High Fat Diet Rats." *Frontiers in Microbiology* 11 (2020): 1975. https://doi.org/10.3389/fmicb.2020.01975.

Yadav, Meeta, Soham Ali, Rachel L. Shrode, Shailesh K. Shahi, Samantha N. Jensen, Jemmie Hoang, et al. "Multiple Sclerosis Patients Have an Altered Gut Mycobiome and Increased Fungal to Bacterial Richness." *PLOS One* 17, no. 4 (2022): e0264556. https://doi.org/10.1371/journal.pone.0264556.

Yalcin, Sibel Ebru, J. Patrick O'Brien, Yangqi Gu, Krystle Reiss, Sophia M. Yi, Ruchi Jain, et al. "Electric Field Stimulates Production of Highly Conductive Microbial OmcZ Nanowires." *Nature Chemical Biology* 16 (2020): 1136–1142. https://doi.org/10.1038/s41589-020-0623-9.

Yano, Jessica M., Kristie Yu, Gregory P. Donaldson, Gauri G. Shastri, Phoebe Ann, Liang Ma, et al. "Indigenous Bacteria from the Gut Microbiota Regulate Host Serotonin Biosynthesis." *Cell* 161 (2015): 264–276. https://doi.org/10.1016/j.cell.2015.02.047.

Yao, Yao, Xiaoyu Cai, Weidong Fei, Yiqing Ye, Mengdan Zhao, and Caihong Zheng. "The Role of Short-Chain Fatty Acids in Immunity, Inflammation and Metabolism." *Critical Reviews in Food Science and Nutrition* 62, no. 1 (2022): 1–12. 2020. https://doi.org/10.1080/10408398.2020.1854675.

Ye, Zhou-Heng, Ke Ning, Bradley P. Ander, and Xue-Jun Sun. "Therapeutic Effect of Methane and Its Mechanism in Disease Treatment." *Journal of Zhejiang University: Science B* 21, no. 8 (2020): 593–602. https://doi.org/10.1631/jzus.B1900629.

Ye, Zhou-Heng, Dan-Feng Fan, and Tian-Yi Zhang. "A Narrative Review of Methane in Treating Neurological Diseases." *Medical Gas Research* 13, no. 4 (2023): 161–164. https://doi.org/10.4103/2045-9912.372663.

Yousif, Aziz, Jingyi Zhang, Francis Mulcahy, and Om. V. Singh. "Bio-Economics of Melanin Biosynthesis Using Electromagnetic Field Resistant Streptomyces Sp.-EF1 Isolated from Cave Soil." *Annals of Microbiology* 65 (2015): 1573–1582. https://doi.org/10.1007/s13213-014-0996-7.

Yu, Xiaolan, Abdel-Malek Shahir, Jingfeng Sha, Zhimin Feng, Betty Eapen, Stanley Nithianantham, et al. "Short-Chain Fatty Acids from Periodontal Pathogens Suppress Histone Deacetylases, EZH2, and SUV39H1 to Promote Kaposi's Sarcoma-Associated Herpesvirus Replication." *Journal of Virology* 88, no. 8 (2014): 4466–4479. https://doi.org/10.1128/JVI.03326-13.

Zarrinpar, Amir, Amandine Chaix, Shibu Yooseph, and Satchidananda Panda. "Diet and Feeding Pattern Affect the Diurnal Dynamics of the Gut Microbiome." *Cell Metabolism* 20 (2014): 1006–1017. https://doi.org/10.1016/j.cmet.2014.11.008.

Zhang, Yiming, Zhang Jindong, and Duan Liping, "The Role of Microbiota-Mitochondria Crosstalk in Pathogenesis and Therapy of Intestinal Diseases." *Pharmacological Research* 186 (2022): 106530. https://doi.org/10.1016/j.phrs.2022.106530.

Zhang, Yi-Qiong, Yi-Ming Hua, Chen-Xing Li, Bei-Di Lan Xiao-Ke Wang, Qi Wang, et al. "Gut Microbiota, Metabolites, and Cardiovascular Diseases." *Cardiology Plus* 6, no. 1 (2021): 41–47. https://doi.org/10.4103/2470-7511.312593.

Zhu, Yao, Ying Li, Qiang Zhang, Yuanjian Song, Liang Wang, and Zuobin Zhu. "Interactions Between Intestinal Microbiota and Neural Mitochondria: A New Perspective on Communicating Pathway From Gut to Brain." *Frontiers in Microbiology* 13 (2022). https://doi.org/10.3389/fmicb.2022.798917.

Zou, Yeqing, Anxing Ge, Brako Lydia, Chen Huang, Qianying Wang, and Yanbo Yu. "Gut Mycobiome Dysbiosis Contributes to the Development of Hypertension and Its Response to Immunoglobulin Light Chains." *Frontiers in Immunology* 13 (2022): 1089295. https://doi.org/10.3389/fimmu.2022.1089295.

Borbolis, Fivos, Eirini Mytilinaiou, and Konstantinos Palikaras. "The Crosstalk between Microbiome and Mitochondrial Homeostasis in Neurodegeneration." *Cells* 12, no. 429 (2023). https://doi.org/10.3390/cells12030429.

CHAPTER NINE

Bryan, Cyril P. *The Papyrus Ebers: Ancient Egyptian Medicine*. Martino Fine Books, 2021. ISBN: 978-0890050040.

Cajete, Gregory. *Native Science: Natural Laws of Interdependence*. 1st edition. Clear Light Publishers, 2016. ISBN: 978-1574160413.

Cusack, Carole. "Scotland's Sacred Waters: Holy Wells and Healing Springs." *Sydney Society for Scottish History Journal* 16 (2016): 67–83.

Declercq, Nico, Joris Degrieck, Rudy Briers, and Oswald Leroy. "A Theoretical Study of Special Acoustic Effects Caused by the Staircase of the EI Castillo Pyramid at the Maya Ruins of Chichen-Itza in Mexico." *The Journal of the Acoustical Society of America* 116 (2005): 3328–3335. https://doi.org/10.1121/1.1764833.

Fatangare, Mrunal, and Sukhada Bhingarkar. "A Comprehensive Review on Technological Advancements for Sensor-Based Nadi Pariksha: An Ancient Indian Science for Human Health Diagnosis." *Journal of Ayurveda and Integrative Medicine* 15, no. 3 (2024): 100958. https://doi.org/10.1016/j.jaim.2024.100958.

García, Hernán, Antonio Sierra, and Gilberto Balam. *Wind in the Blood: Mayan Healing & Chinese Medicine*. North Atlantic Books, 1999. ISBN: 978-1556433047.

Hajar, Rachel. "Medicine from Galen to the Present: A Short History." *Heart Views* 22, no. 4 (2021): 307–308. https://doi.org/10.4103/heartviews.heartviews_125_21.

Jacques Jouanna, and Neil Allies. "The Legacy of the Hippocratic Treatise The Nature of Man: The Theory of the Four Humours." In *Greek Medicine from Hippocrates to Galen: Selected Papers* Brill, 2012, 335–60. http://www.jstor.org/stable/10.1163/j.ctt1w76vxr.21.

Kahn-John Diné, Michelle, and Mary Koithan. "Living in Health, Harmony, and Beauty: the Diné (Navajo) Hózhó Wellness Philosophy." *Global Advances in Integrative Medicine and Health* 4, no. 3 (2015): 24–30. https://doi.org/10.7453/gahmj.2015.044.

Kumar, P. Venkata Giri, Sudheer Deshpande, and H. R. Nagendra. "Traditional Practices and Recent Advances in Nadi Pariksha: A Comprehensive Review." *Journal of Ayurveda and Integrative Medicine* 10, no. 4 (2019): 308–315. https://doi.org/10.1016/j.jaim.2017.10.007.

Maoshing, Ni. *The Yellow Emperor's Classic of Medicine: A New Translation of the Neijing Suwen with Commentary.* Revised ed. Shambhala, 1995.

McVeigh, Mary Jo. "The Light within the Light: An Exploration of the Role of Anam Ċara in Irish Celtic Spiritualty and its Application to 21st-Century Therapy." *Australian and New Zealand Journal of Family Therapy* 38, no. 1 (2017): 61–71. https://doi.org/10.1002/anzf.1204.

Meymandi, Assad. "Music, Medicine, Healing, and the Genome Project." *Psychiatry (Edgmont)* 6, no. 9 (2009): 43–5. PMID: 19855860.

Nerlich, Andreas G., Eduard Egarter Vigl, Angelika Fleckinger, Martina Tauber, and Oliver Peschel. "Ötzi" [The Iceman: Life Scenarios and Pathological Findings from 30 Years of Research on the Glacier Mummy "Ötzi"]." *Journal of Pathology* 42, no. 5 (2021): 530–539. https://doi.org/10.1007/s00292-021-00961-6.

Nunn, John F. *Ancient Egyptian Medicine*. University of Oklahoma Press, 2002.

Pandey, Anjali, Bhumika Bhardwaj, and Divyashree Shirvadkar. "Critical Review and Analysis of Nadi Vigyan: A Boon to Ayurvedic Methodology." *Journal of Ayurveda and Integrated Medical Sciences* 8, no. 2 (2023): 68–73. https://www.jaims.in/jaims/article/view/2281.

Ritner, Robert K. "The Cardiovascular System in Ancient Egyptian Thought." *Journal of Near Eastern Studies* 65, no. 2 (2006): 99–109. https://doi.org/10.1086/504985.

Schelberg, Dirk. *Didgeridoo: Ritual Origins and Playing Techniques*. Binkey Kok, 1995.

Shah, Chandana, Ravi Warkhedar, Chandrakishor Ladekar, and Sachin Gandhi. "Fundamentals of Nadi Pariksha: A Review of Ancient Ayurvedic Holistic Diagnostic Tool." *AIP Conference Proceedings* 3013 (2024): 020004. https://doi.org/10.1063/5.0203386.

Wagner, Charles, Jillian De Gezelle, and Slavko Komarnytsky. "Celtic Provenance in Traditional Herbal Medicine of Medieval Wales and Classical Antiquity." *Frontiers in Pharmacology* 11 (2020): 105. https://doi.org/10.3389/fphar.2020.00105.

Young, Philip H. "Fighting in the Shade: What the Ancient Greeks Knew About Humor." *Soundings: An Interdisciplinary Journal* 74, no. 1/2 (1991): 289–307. http://www.jstor.org/stable/41178600.

Zampieri, Fabio, Gaetano Thiene, and Alberto Zanatta. "Cardiocentrism in Ancient Medicines." *IJC Heart & Vasculature* 48 (2023): 101261. https://doi.org/10.1016/j.ijcha.2023.101261.

ACKNOWLEDGMENTS

I want to express my gratitude to Professor Gerald Pollack for reviewing part of this book and offering valuable feedback. I want to thank Gina Bria, founder of the Hydration Foundation, for her helpful feedback on early editions of the book.

I offer my respect and appreciation to the scientists and researchers in this field, furthering our understanding of the body and its ability to heal.

ABOUT THE AUTHOR

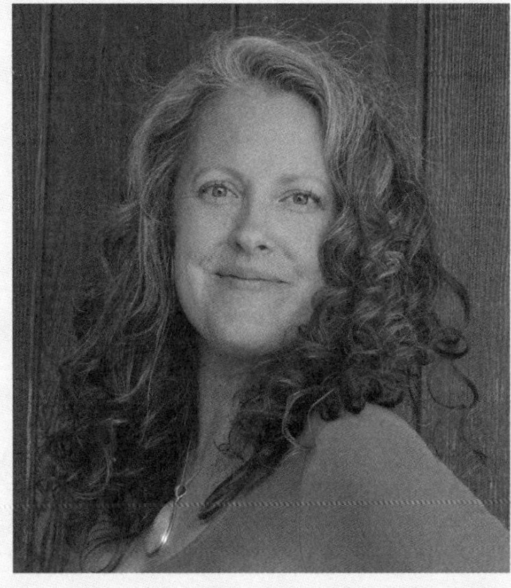

DR. CATHERINE CLINTON, a licensed naturopathic physician, has spent over eighteen years helping people overcome their health issues. She completed her Doctor of Naturopathic Medicine degree from the National University of Natural Medicine. Diagnosed with two autoimmune conditions and Lyme disease while in medical school, Dr. Catherine began the long and difficult journey of healing, a path that led to the commitment to help others to not only heal physically but also to return to the relationships we evolved over millennia for a deeper sense of health and belonging.

Dr. Catherine founded the Quantum Biology Health Institute in 2024. The institute focuses on research in the field of quantum biology and offers training in the application of quantum biology to health. She has published multiple articles in peer-reviewed research journals and maintains a small practice in Eugene, Oregon.

Dr. Catherine teaches doctors, health care practitioners, and health enthusiasts from around the world how to apply the principles of quantum biology for health and is a sought-after speaker with engagements across the globe. Her mission is to empower as many people as she can with knowledge of quantum biology for health and to help them explore a new perspective on healing.

INDEX